CHEMOTHERAPY

Volume 6
Parasites, Fungi, and Viruses

CHEMOTHERAPY

CHEMOTHERAPY

Volume 6
Parasites, Fungi, and Viruses

Edited by
J.D. Williams
The London Hospital Medical College
London, U.K.

and
A.M. Geddes
East Birmingham Hospital
Birmingham, U.K.

Springer Science+Business Media, LLC

Library of Congress Cataloging in Publication Data

International Congress of Chemotherapy, 9th, London, 1975.
    Parasites, fungi, and viruses.

    (Chemotherapy; v. 6)
    Includes index.
    1. Chemotherapy—Congresses. 2. Anti-infective agents—Congresses. I. Williams,
John David, M.D. II. Geddes, Alexander McIntosh. III. Title. IV. Series.
RM260.2.C45   vol. 6   615′.58s   [616.9′6′061]   76-1932

ISBN 978-1-4684-3131-5   ISBN 978-1-4684-3129-2 (eBook)
DOI 10.1007/978-1-4684-3129-2

Proceedings of the Ninth International Congress of Chemotherapy
held in London, July, 1975 will be published in eight volumes,
of which this is volume six.

©1976 Springer Science+Business Media New York
Originally published by Plenum Press, New York in 1976.
Softcover reprint of the hardcover 1st edition 1976

A Division of Plenum Publishing Corporation
227 West 17th Street, New York, N.Y. 10011

United Kingdom edition published by Plenum Press, London
A Division of Plenum Publishing Company, Ltd.
Davis House (4th Floor), 8 Scrubs Lane, Harlesden, London, MW10 6SE, England

CHEMOTHERAPY

Proceedings of the
9th International Congress of Chemotherapy
held in London, July, 1975

Editorial Committee

K. Hellmann, *Chairman* (Anticancer)
Imperial Cancer Research Fund, London.

A. M. Geddes (Antimicrobial)   J. D. Williams (Antimicrobial)
East Birmingham Hospital.   *The London Hospital Medical College.*

Congress Organising Committee

W. Brumfitt	I. Phillips	H.P. Lambert
K. Hellmann	M.R.W. Brown	P. Turner
K.D. Bagshawe	D.G. James	A.M. Geddes
H. Smith	C. Stuart-Harris	D. Armitage
E.J. Stokes	R.G. Jacomb	D. Crowther
F. Wrigley	D.T.D. Hughes	D.S. Reeves
J.D. Williams	T. Connors	R.E.O. Williams

International Society
of Chemotherapy Executive - to July 1975

P. Malek	H.P. Kuemmerle	H. Ericsson
C. Grassi	Z. Modr	G.M. Savage
G.H. Werner	K.H. Spitzy	H. Umezawa
	P. Rentchnick	

Preface

The International Society of Chemotherapy meets every two years to review progress in chemotherapy of infections and of malignant disease. Each meeting gets larger to encompass the extension of chemotherapy into new areas. In some instances, expansion has been rapid, for example in cephalosporins, penicillins and combination chemotherapy of cancer - in others slow, as in the field of parasitology. New problems of resistance and untoward effects arise; reduction of host toxicity without loss of antitumour activity by new substances occupies wide attention. The improved results with cancer chemotherapy, especially in leukaemias, are leading to a greater prevalence of severe infection in patients so treated, pharmacokinetics of drugs in normal and diseased subjects is receiving increasing attention along with related problems of bioavailability and interactions between drugs. Meanwhile the attack on some of the major bacterial infections, such as gonorrhoea and tuberculosis, which were among the first infections to feel the impact of chemotherapy, still continue to be major world problems and are now under attack with new agents and new methods.

From this wide field and the 1,000 papers read at the Congress we have produced Proceedings which reflect the variety and vigour of research in this important field of medicine. It was not possible to include all of the papers presented at the Congress but we have attempted to include most aspects of current progress in chemotherapy.

We thank the authors of these communications for their cooperation in enabling the Proceedings to be available at the earliest possible date. The method of preparation does not allow for uniformity of typefaces and presentation of the material and we hope that the blemishes of language and typographical errors do not detract from the understanding of the reader and the importance of the Proceedings.

K. HELLMANN, Imperial Cancer Research Fund
A. M. GEDDES, East Birmingham Hospital
J. D. WILLIAMS, The London Hospital Medical College

Contents

WHAT ARE THE PROBLEMS IN TROPICAL INFECTIONS?

Anthony Bryceson

Hospital for Tropical Diseases

London, U.K.

Our forefathers had quinine, mercury and tartar emetic; smallpox
and typhoid vaccines and diphtheria antitoxin. The epidemiology of
sleeping sickness, Chagas disease, leishmaniasis, onchocerciasis,
schistosomiasis, plague and yellow fever was unknown. We have
certainly come a long way since then. Vaccine has the upper hand
of yellow fever, smallpox, measles. Vector control has gone a long
way in some areas to combat malaria and sleeping sickness.
Education and sanitation are diminishing the terrors of schistosomiasis, plague, cholera and typhus. Chemotherapy is biting slowly
into the mass of leprosy and tuberculosis - and some of the more
recent successes attributable to chemotherapy will be presented in
the middle section. But one of the scourges has gone and each one
still represents either a continuing pool of misery and debility or a
threat of another decimating epidemic. We have no cause for
complacency.

Indeed we have cause for very great concern, because in some
fields progress has halted and to this we intend to draw your
attention. This is a heavy task because this has to deal with
problems of 7/10ths of the world's population.

Neglact then, is the first problem and ignorance among our own
profession. Take onchocerciasis for example. This year 300,000
adult males, the breadwinners of their families and the backbone of
the socities will be blind of this disease, and next year the same
number and the year after too. What have we to offer? Two weeks'
course of tablets which cause devastating reaction and 6 weeks of
injections which cause nephritis. A clinical and logistic imposs-
ibility. There has been no advance since Suramin was introduced
exactly 50 years ago. Ernst Friedheim, whose solo efforts deserve

more praise than the whole of the pharmaceutic industry, did introduce
a new arsenical, but unfortunately there were a few deaths and it was
dropped. Not one University Department or Pharmaceutical Company is
showing the slightest interest in this devastating disease.

It is very difficult to develop any new chemotherapeutic agent
now. The criteria laid down by W.H.O., Food and Drug Administration
and the Committee of Safety of Medicines for example, are so strict
that they have virtually stopped progress in certain parasitic diseases. What a mercy we had arsenic and antimony before these
Committees were born, for we still use both. Costs too, inhibit
progress. We have no new drug for sleeping sickness since Melarsopral
was introduced full 30 years ago; and the facts are such now that it
is not worth the while a pharmaceutical company to develop a drug
even if a promising lead were offered. For even if the drug was given
to every patient with the disease in Africa, that company would still
not cover its development costs. These very important, perhaps the
most important and ever lowering problems of cost and development are
aired in the last section, and you will be pleased to hear that there
is at last a chink in the clounds.

Even the best drug is no good if you cannot deliver it to the
patient, and in Africa, Asia and South America, the problems of space
and time and their practical expression - communications - pose
problesm which we paleo- and neo-artic citizens constantly fail to
appreciate.

There is a prevalent myth that tropical infections are all due
to "parasites" (i.e. big parasites - the protozoa and helminths). They
are not. It is, however, under the steady burden of these big
parasites that the battle against the little parasites is fought, and
it is becoming increasingly clear that the one drastically lowers
resistance to the other. The annual mortality of meningococcal
meningitis in Northern Nigeria makes this point.

EPIDEMIC DISEASES

D.A. Warrell, P.L. Perine and D.W. Krause

Radcliffe Infirmary, Oxford OX2 6HE, U.K. and U.S.
Naval Medical Research Unit No 5, P.O. Box 1014
Addis Ababa, Ethiopia

The chemotherapy of epidemic diseases in tropical countries poses important practical problems which tend to be underestimated in those western countries where patients can be admitted to hospital, precisely diagnosed and given the drug appropriate to the sensitivity of the infecting organisms.

1. Particular social and environmental conditions may give rise to mixed epidemics of clinically-similar diseases spread by the same vector. Since laboratory facilities may be very limited and immediate confirmation of diagnosis impossible, it is important to consider drugs which are active against both infections, even though they may not be the first choice for either infection alone (e.g. chloramphenicol for bacterial meningitis : doxycycline for relapsing fever and typhus).

2. In the rush of an epidemic it may be impossible to admit patients for prolonged, supervised, courses of chemotherapy. The use of single dose long acting preparations has great advantages in this situation, provided that relapses can be prevented (e.g. doxycycline for relapsing fever and typhus).

3. Drugs effective in killing organisms may endanger the patient's life by causing complications such as Jarisch-Herxheimer type reactions (J-HR) (e.g. relapsing fever and plague).

4. Chemoprophylaxis and the treatment of carriers are important in those infections in which immunisation is not an entirely adequate method of protecting the population. Mass therapy creates problems which include encouragement of the emergence of resistant strains and significant incidence of unpleasant side effects (e.g. meningococcal meningitis).

These problems are illustrated by considering recent progress in the chemotherapy of four important epidemic diseases : louse-borne

3

relapsing fever (LBRF), louse-borne typhus (LBT), meningococcal
meningitis and plague.

LOUSE-BORNE RELAPSING FEVER

The main endemic focus of LBRF is in the Ethiopian highlands
where there may be 100,000 cases per year (Bryceson et al. 1970) and
there have been recent reports of epidemics in adjacent Sudan
(Abdalla 1969; Perine and Reynolds 1974). Various antibiotics are
highly effective in eliminating Borrelia recurrentis spirochaetes
from the blood, but, unfortunately, a severe J-HR usually results
(Parry, Bryceson and Leithead 1967) and may kill the patient as a
result of hyperthermia or hypotension (Warrell et al. 1970). Tetracycline eliminates spirochaetes within 2-3 hours but invariably
causes a J-HR which is not prevented by cortico-steroid. Slow
release penicillins seem less likely to cause a reaction, but
eliminate spirochaetes more slowly and may allow relapses. (Rijkels
1970; Knaack et al. 1972)

In Addis Ababa, Ethiopia, a group of 12 male patients (ages 18-
38 years) with proven LBRF were randomly allocated for treatment
with either pyrrolidino-methyl-tetracycline (Reverin, Hoechst, 275mg
intravenously) or procaine penicillin with aluminium monostearate
(PAM) (Specia-Paris 600,000 units intramuscularly). This dose of PAM
was found to be very effective against syphilis and yaws and to
produce therapeutic blood levels of penicillin for at least four days
(Ovčinnikov and Korbut 1965; Hume and Facio 1956).

Physiological measurements were made before treatment, near the
peak of the febrile response and 24 hours after treatment. Temperature, electrocardiogram and intravascular blood pressures were
monitored continuously and the patients closely observed throughout.

The two groups were comparable before treatment. Spirochaetes
were eliminated much more rapidly by tetracycline (Fig. 1). After
PAM, spirochaetaemia and fever persisted for up to 48 hours, whereas
spontaneous crisis with disappearance of spirochaetes was observed
in five out of 19 patients who were admitted overnight for treatment
the next day. In the tetracycline-treated group peak temperature was
higher, occurred sooner and was always associated with rigors,
whereas only one of the PAM-treated patients had rigors. At the
peak of the febrile response and 24 hours after treatment there was
no significant difference between the groups in cardiac or respiratory rates, pulmonary venous admixture, cardiac output, mean brachial
artery pressure, systemic vascular resistance and arterial pH. There
were significant differences ($P < 0.05$) at the peak of the reaction in
total expired ventilation, oxygen consumption, arterial PO_2 and PCO_2
and dead space : tidal volume ratio. (Fig. 2) These were consistent
with a greater respiratory stimulus in the tetracycline treated
group, perhaps related to higher body temperature and the added

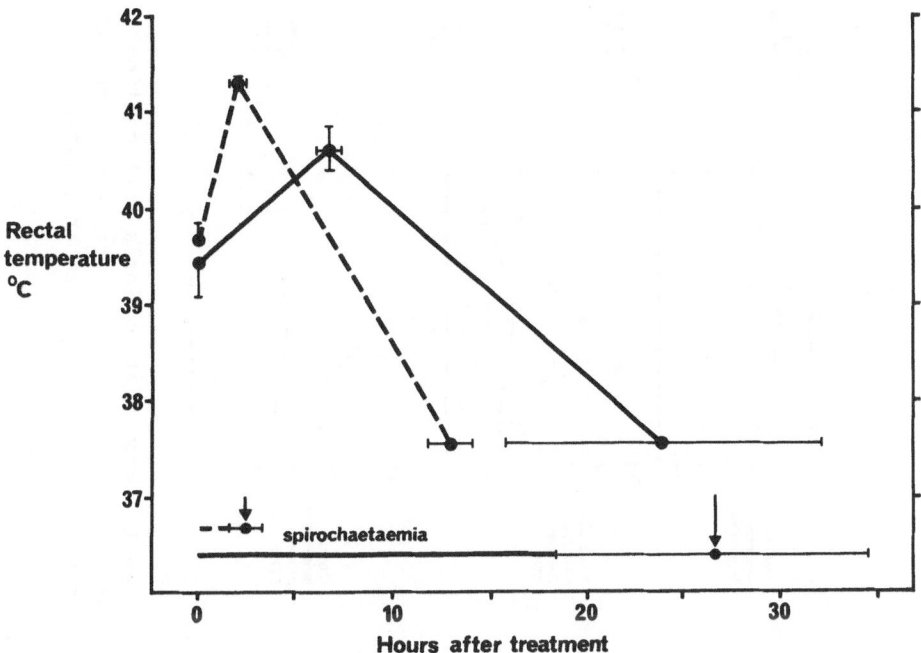

Fig. 1 Course of fever and persistence of spirochaetaemia in
six patients treated with tetracycline (dashed line) and six
treated with PAM (solid line). (Mean ± 1 standard error).

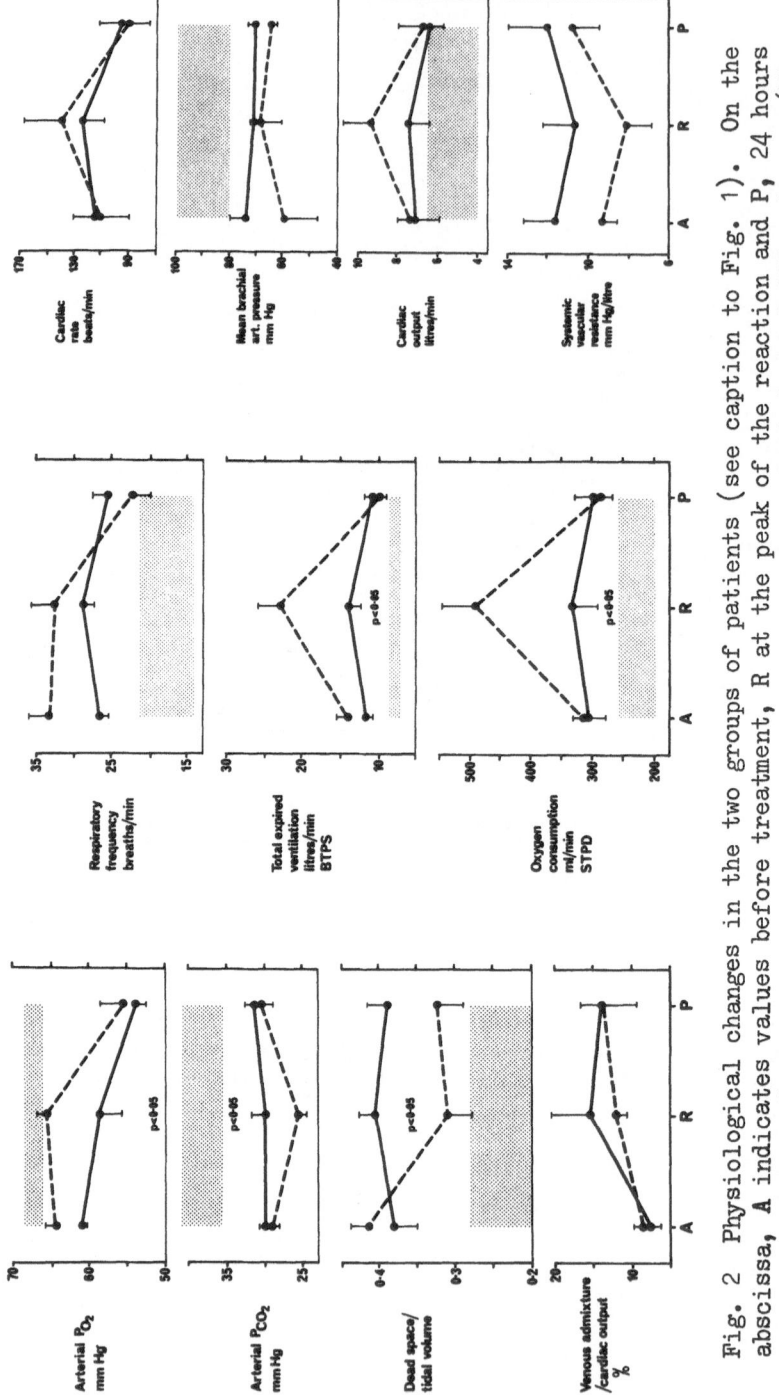

Fig. 2 Physiological changes in the two groups of patients (see caption to Fig. 1). On the abscissa, A indicates values before treatment, R at the peak of the reaction and P, 24 hours after treatment. Shaded areas represent normal values at an altitude of 2,250 metres. (Mean ± 1 tandard deviation).

muscular exercise of rigors. Platelet counts, fibrin degradation
products and complement C3 levels were similar in the two groups.
Thus, although PAM causes a milder respiratory reaction, it is slow
to eliminate spirochaetes. Provided patients can be kept lying for
the first 24 hours after treatment and well hydrated, the risk of
fatal J-HR is small, and we recommend the use of tetracycline as a
rapid cure. Another important advantage of tetracycline is that it
is also effective in typhus.

The problem of J-HR has been encountered in bacterial infections other than syphilis and LBRF: leptospirosis, rat bite fever,
Vincent's angina, brucellosis melitensis, tularaemia, glanders and
plague. There is good evidence that the reactions in syphilis
(Graciansky and Grupper 1961; Gudjonsson and Skogg 1963) and
brucellosis melitensis (Abernathy and Spink 1959) can be prevented
or ameliorated by corticosteroid, but in LBRF, infusions of 20mg
hydrocortisone/kg/hour did not alter the reaction but depressed the
pre-reaction fever (Warrell et al. 1970).

LOUSE-BORNE TYPHUS

Epidemic typhus remains an important problem in Rwanda, Burundi
and Ethiopia (Weekly Epidemiological Record 1973; Brezina et al.
1973), and like LBRF could cause another major pandemic. LBRF and
LBT may be indistinguishable clinically, and during large mixed
epidemics laboratory differentiation may be impracticable. Huys
et al.(1973) found that a single 200mg oral dose of doxycycline
("Vibramycin") was effective in 63 patients in Rwanda: there was
only one relapse. Perine et al. (1974) used a single 100mg oral
dose of doxycycline in 26 patients with LBRF and 10 with LBT in
Ethiopia. All were cured without relapses. Unfortunately, typhoid
may be confused with LBT and can be associated with LBRF (Anderson
and Zimmerman 1955). Diagnosis of LBT is confirmed by an absolutely
high Weil-Felix titre or rise in titre which are unlikely to be
demonstrable early in the disease. Tetracycline is also the drug
of choice for scrub typhus and murine typhus (Sheehy et al. 1973;
Miller et al. 1974). Sulphonamides are ineffective or even deleterious in LBT (Snyder 1948; Huys et al. 1973).

MENINGOCOCCAL MENINGITIS

In the meningitis belt of the northern savanna of Africa there
are annual dry season epidemics of meningococcal meningitis with at
least 25,000 reported cases. Long acting sulphonamides had reduced
mortality to 10-15% (Lapeyssonnie 1963), but their extensive use for
treatment and prophylaxis has resulted in the emergence of sulphonamide resistance in 30-90% strains of the group A meningococcus
responsible for these epidemics. Consequently penicillin has become
the treatment of choice, but large doses need to be given frequently

for at least five days. Chloramphenicol which proved to be as
effective as penicillin in a controlled trial involving 123 patients
in Zaria, Nigeria, had the advantages that it was much cheaper and
could be given by mouth after the first two or three days (Whittle
et al. 1973).

Unexpected variation in the group and sensitivity of the epidemic strain can create difficulties in planning the protection of
a population by immunisation with sero group specific meningococcal
polysaccharide (Gotschlich et al. 1969) or with anti microbial
agents. Thus, the 1975 epidemic in Zaria in the north of Nigeria
was caused mainly by group C strains rather than the usual Group A
(Greenwood, B.M., personal communication). Sulphonamide-resistant
group C organisms were responsible for the recent epidemic in São
Paulo, Brazil involving more than 13,000 cases. In the U.S.A.
sulphonamide resistant strains constituted 68% of the isolates in
1974, whereas in Europe the proportion was 13-20% (Morbidity and
Mortality 1975; British Medical Journal 1975).

The value of selective chemoprophylaxis of high risk contacts
has been suggested by the results of a study of an outbreak of group
C, sulphonamide-resistant meningococcal meningitis in Dade County,
Florida (Kaiser et al. 1974). Amongst close household contacts a
pharyngeal carrier rate of 35% was discovered, compared to 1% in
controls : 6% developed the disease. Rifampicin eradicated carriage
in 92% of contacts. During the São Paulo epidemic Munford et al.
(1974) treated oropharyngeal carriers discovered in the families of
meningitis patients. Minocycline and rifampicin were equally
effective in eradicating the carrier state in 9-17% of contacts
(compared to 49% with sulphadiazine), but 10% of rifampicin-treated
subjects yielded rifampicin-resistant meningococci after two weeks.
Apart from this disadvantage it is unwise to consider wide scale use
of this anti mycobacterial agent for chemoprophylaxis, even in combination with minocycline. At present, minocycline is the most
promising chemoprophylactic drug for sulphonamide resistant organisms
(Guttler and Beaty 1972). Its drawbacks include the dental effects
common to other tetracyclines when used in pregnant women and children, and other side effects, particularly a reversible vestibular
defect.

PLAGUE

In bubonic plague the untreated mortality of around 60% can be
reduced to less than 1% using streptomycin, chloramphenicol or tetracycline. Primary pneumonic plage and septicaemic bubonic plague
pose added problems including circulatory failure, disseminated
intravascular coagulation and J-HR (Butler et al. 1974; Conrad et
al. 1968; Poland 1972). Development of heat killed Yersina pestis
vaccines and vector control offer the best hope of controlling

epidemics, but chemoprophylaxis with sulphonamides or tetracycline is important to protect close contacts. Preliminary results of treatment with trimethoprin and sulphamethoxazole (co-trimoxazole) have been encouraging (Nguyen-Van-Ai et al. 1973; Butler et al. 1974).

REFERENCES

Abdalla, R.E. (1969), Journal of Tropical Medicine and Hygiene, 72, 125.

Abernathy, R.S. and Spink, W.W. (1958), Journal of Clinical Investigation, 37, 219.

Anderson, T.R. and Zimmerman, L.E. (1955), American Journal of Pathology, 31, 1083.

Brezina, R., Murray, E.S., Tarizzo, M.L. and Bögel, K. (1973), Bulletin of the World Health Organization, 49, 433.

British Medical Journal (1975), 2, 625.

Bryceson, A.D.M., Parry, E.H.O., Perine, P.L., Warrell, D.A., Vukotich, D. and Leithead, C.S. (1970), Quarterly Journal of Medicine, 39, 129.

Butler, T., Bell, W.R., Linh, N.N., Tiep, N.D. and Arnold, K. (1974), Journal of Infectious Diseases, 129, S 78.

Conrad, F.G., Lecocq, F.R. and Krain, R. (1968), Archives of Internal Medicine, 122, 193.

Gotschlich, E.C., Goldschneider, I. and Artenstein, M.S. (1969), Journal of Experimental Medicine, 129, 1385 and 1367.

Graciansky, P.De. and Grupper, C. (1961), British Journal of Venereal Diseases, 37, 247.

Gudjonsson, H. and Skog, E. (1968), Acta dermato-venereologica, 48, 15.

Guttler, R.B. and Beaty, H.N. (1972), Antimicrobial Agents and Chemotherapy, 1, 397.

Hume, J.C. and Facio, G. (1956), Bulletin of the World Health Organization, 15, 1057.

Huys, J., Freyens, P., Kayihigi, J. and Van Den Berghe, G. (1973), Transactions of the Royal Society of Tropical Medicine and Hygiene, 67, 718.

Kaiser, A.B., Hennekens, C.H., Saslaw, M.S., Hayes, P.S. and Bennet, J.V. (1974), Journal of Infectious Diseases, 130, 217.

Knaack, R.H., Wright, L.J., Leithead, C.S., Kidan, T.G. and Plorde, J.J. (1972), Ethiopian Medical Journal, 10, 13.

Lapeyssonnie, L. (1963), Bulletin of the World Health Organization, 28, supplement.

Miller, M.B., Bratton, J.L., Hunt, J., Blankenship, R., Lohr, D.C. and Reynolds, R.D. (1974), Military Medicine, 139, 184.

Morbidity and Mortality Weekly Report (1975), 24, 227.

Munford, R.S., De Vasconceles, Z.S.S., Phillips, C.J., Gelli, D.S., Gorman, G.W., Risi, J.B. and Feldman, R.A. (1974), Journal of Infectious Diseases, 129, 644.

Nguyen–Van–Ai, et al. (1973), British Medical Journal, 4, 108.
Ovčinnikov, N.M., and Korbut, S.E. (1965), Bulletin of the World
    Health Organization, 32, 861.
Parry, E.H.O., Bryceson, A.D.M. and Leithead, C.S. (1967), Lancet,
    1, 81.
Perine, P.L., Krause, D.W., Awoke, S. and McDade, J.E. (1974),
    Lancet, 2, 742.
Perine, P.L. and Reynolds, D.F. (1974), Lancet, 2, 1324.
Poland, J.D., (1972) in Infectious Diseases, ed. P.D. Hoeprich,
    Harper and Row, Hagerstown, p. 1141.
Rijkels, D.F. (1971), Tropical and Geographical Medicine, 23, 335.
Sheehy, T.W., Hazlett, D. and Turk, R.E. (1973), Archives of
    Internal Medicine, 132, 77.
Snyder, J.C. (1948) in Rickettsial Diseases of Man, ed. F.R. Moulton,
    American Association for the Advancement of Science, Washing-
    ton, p. 169.
Warrell, D.A., Pope, H.M., Parry, E.H.O., Perine, P.L. and Bryceson,
    A.D.M. (1970), Clinical Science, 39, 123.
Weekly Epidemiological Record (1973), 48, 221.
Whittle, H.C., Dadvidson, N.McD., Greenwood, B.M., Warrell, D.A.,
    Tomkins, A., Tugwell, P., Zalin, A., Bryceson, A.D.M., Parry,
    E.H.O., Brueton, M., Duggan, M. and Rajković, A.D. (1973),
    British Medical Journal, 3, 379.

PROGRESS ACHIEVED IN THE CHEMOTHERAPY OF SOIL-TRANSMITTED HELMINTHS

F. Arfaa and I. Farahmandian

School of Public Health and Institute of Public

Health Research, University of Teheran

Human infection with various helminth parasites still remains as one of the most important public health problems in many developing countries. Among various types of helminthiasis, soil-transmitted helminths (geohelminths), because of their wide distribution and high prevalence among a large proportion of the world's population and their damaging effects, constitute one of the most important infections and diseases.

From the standpoint of overall prevalence and severity of diseases caused, the most important soil-transmitted helminths are: _Ascaris lumbricoides_, _Trichuris trichiura_, _Necator americanus_, _Ancylostoma duodenale_ and _Strongyloides stercoralis_. In addition, in a few areas of the world the prevalence of infection with other soil-transmitted helminths is very high, such as the high prevalence of trichostrongyliasis found in Iran (Ghadirian & Arfaa, 1975).

In spite of the very wide distribution and high prevalence, and sometimes high incidence, of helminthic infections in many parts of the world, successful control of helminthiasis has been achieved in only a few countries. Among the various control methods used, mass-chemotherapy has been and still is the most effective approach. Fortunately, in recent years, access to newly introduced and very effective anthelminthics has created considerable hope for individual management and mass-control of these prevalent infections.

In this paper the results of studies on the effect of new drugs on soil-transmitted helminths as well as the results

TABLE 1

Results of drug trials on various soil-transmitted helminths conducted in Khuzestan, southwest Iran (1970-1975)

Author and Date	Drug(s) Used	Number Treated	Percent Cure Rate and Reduction in Egg Count*		
			Ascaris	Trichos-trongylus	Ancy-lostoma
Farahmandian et al. 1970	Bephenium hydroxy-naphthoate	39	56.3	43.7	79.5
	Thiabendazole	38	55.3	94.8	26.4
Farahmandian et al. 1971	Bephenium hydroxy.	50	52.9 (61.7)	56 (10.8)	92 (76.5)
	Pyrantel Pamoate	75	90.2 (78)	45.4 (0)	96 (92.4)
Arfaa et al., 1973	Bitoscanate	71	6.6	38.6	39.3
Farahmandian et al. 1974	Levamisole	83	98.8 (99.9)	93.9 (88.7)	95.2 (98.1)
Farahmandian et al. 1975	Pyrantel Pamoate		50 (7)	50 (7)	90 (69)
	Levamisole		96 (83)	98 (25)	100 (100)
	Thiabendazole		47 (12.6)	92 (8)	51 (33.7)
	Mebendazole		54 (91)	82 (5.7)	35 (40.8)
	Bephenium hydroxy.		53 (15)	34 (0)	85 (78)
Farahmandian et al. 1975	Pyrantel Oxantel	42	91.4	50	86.3

* Figures in parentheses indicate the percent reduction in egg count.

of mass-chemotherapy in the control of these infections in Iran will be presented. A summary of the results obtained from large-scale mass-chemotherapy in a few other countries will also be discussed.

MATERIAL AND METHOD

Because of the very high prevalence of soil-transmitted helminths in Iran, infecting a majority of the rural population and the inhabitants of some large cities (Arfaa, 1972), and because of long-term plans for their control, the evaluation of new drugs has been underway for the past 10 years.

The inhabitants of several villages in infested areas in the vicinity of 3 field stations of the Institute of Public Health Research in the north, central and southern parts of the country, having different ecologies and fauna of soil-transmitted helminths, were stool examined. Two or more methods, such as the sulphate zinc flotation method (WHO, 1967) combined with direct smear or Kato thick smear, formaline ether, and Stoll egg count methods, were used. Persons found infected with one or more species of parasite were then treated with anthelminthic drugs with the dosage recommended by the manufacturer. Treated persons were examined 2-4 weeks after therapy and the reduction in prevalence and intensity of various intestinal helminthiasis with different drugs was determined and compared. In some studies, persons treated were re-examined at different intervals and the trend of re-infection was established. In other studies, other methods of control alone or in combination with mass-treatment were also evaluated. The anthelminthic drugs used during these studies were Piperazine derivatives, Bitoscanate, Tetrachloroethylene, Bephenium hydroxynaphtoate, Pyrantel Pamoate, Thiabendazole, Levamisole, Mebendazole, Diphetarsone (for Trichuris only) and Oxantel-Pyrantel.

RESULTS

The cure rate and percent reduction in egg count for various intestinal helminths by using a variety of anthelminthic drugs in different areas are shown in Tables 1-3.

As indicated in Table 1, the most prevalent soil-transmitted helminths in Khuzestan, southwestern Iran, are Ascaris, Trichostrongylus and Ancylostoma duodenale. Of the various drugs used for Ascaris, the highest reduction in prevalence and intensity of infection (percent reduction in eggs) were found when Levamisole was administered. Other drugs, in order

TABLE 2

Results of drug trials on various soil-transmitted helminths conducted in the Caspian Littoral, north Iran

Author and Date	Drug(s) Used	Number Treated	Percent Cure Rate and Reduction in Egg Count*		
			Ascaris	Necator	Trichuris
Barzegar et al., 1974	Piperazine & Tetrachloroethyl		62 (88)	56 (79)	
Ghadirian & Sanati, 1972	Pyrantel Pamoate 10 mg/kg	40	100	75	
	20 mg/kg	80	100	92.5	
Amini et al., 1974	Tetrachloroethylene		--	67.8 (89.9)	
	Pyrantel Pamoate		90 (94.6)	35.5 (87)	22 (48)
	Bephenium hydroxy.			27.7 (64.8)	76 (93.6)
	Mebendazole		98.6 (99)	14.5 (70.5)	
	Bitoscanate 300 mg			17.7 (75.8)	
	150 mg			2.7 (54.5)	

TABLE 3

Results of drug trials on various soil-transmitted helminths conducted in Isfahan, central Iran

Author and Date	Drug(s) Used	Number Treated	Percent Cure Rate and Reduction in Egg Count*		
			Ascaris	Trichuris	Trichos-trongylus
Ghadirian et al., 1972	Pyrantel Pamoate	205	100 (100)	–	–
Ghadirian & Arfaa, 1975	Pyrantel Pamoate	648	94.5 (93.8)	4	30
Arfaa et al., 1975	Levamisole	834	90.4	136*	91.4
Farahmandian et al. 1975	Pyrantel-Oxantel	30	93	83	50

* The percent positive with Trichuris has increased after treatment.

of their effectivity, were Pyrantel Pamoate, Oxantel-Pyrantel, Mebendazole, Bephenium hydroxynaphtoate, Thiabendazole and Bitoscanate.

For Trichostrongylus the most effective drug was found to be Levamisole, followed by Thiabendazole, Mebendazole, Bephenium hydroxynaphtoate, Pyrantel Pamoate and Bitoscanate. For hookworm (Ancylostoma duodenale) the highest cure rate was achieved with Levamisole; other drugs, in order of their effectivity, were Pyrantel Pamoate, Oxantel-Pyrantel, Bephenium hydroxynaphtoate, Thiabendazole and Bitoscanate.

Table 2 indicates the results of evaluation of anthelminthic drugs in the Caspian Littoral in the north of Iran, where the most prevalent species of soil-transmitted helminths are Necator americanus, Trichuris, Ascaris and Trichostrongylus. The anthelminthics used in this area were Tetrachloroethylene, Pyrantel Pamoate, Mebendazole, Bephenium hydroxynaphtoate and Bitoscanate (300 mg in 3 doses at 12-hour intervals and 150 mg in a single dose).

For Necator americanus, the highest cure rate and reduction in number of eggs were achieved with Tetrachloroethylene, which resulted in a 67.8% cure rate and 89.9% reduction in the number of eggs of Necator. The cure rates observed by using other drugs were less than 36%.

For Ascaris the highest cure rate was achieved with Pyrantel Pamoate and Mebendazole. For Trichuris, the only satisfactory drug was Mebendazole, which achieved a cure rate of 76% and a 93.6% reduction in the number of eggs.

In Isfahan villages, where Ascaris, Trichuris and Trichostrongylus spp. are infecting more than 90% of the population with a very heavy worm load, the highest cure rate observed for Ascaris was 90-100% achieved by the administration of Pyrantel Pamoate or Levamisole, and Oxantel-Pyrantel. Levamisole gave better results in the treatment of trichostrongyliasis, but the effect of Pyrantel Pamoate and Levamisole on trichuriasis was very low. The only satisfactory results in the treatment of trichuriasis were achieved by administration of Oxantel-Pyrantel in a trial in which an 83% cure rate was achieved among 42 people treated with a combination of 10 mg/kg Oxantel and 10 mg/kg Pyrantel.

Side-effects observed when using the above-mentioned drugs were usually low for most of the compounds. However, mild nausea, vomiting and abdominal pain were reported among patients taking Bephenium hydroxynaphtoate, Bitoscanate, Thiabendazole and large doses of Levamisole. The severity of

TABLE 4

Reduction in positivity rate of various soil-
transmitted helminths achieved by using
different control measures,
Khuzestan, South West Iran

Type of Operation	Reduction in Positivity Rate:		
	Ascaris	Ancy-lostoma	Trichostron-gylus spp.
Sanitation + mass-chemotherapy	86.2	68.5	38.5
Mass-chemotherapy alone	81.6	71.6	22.9
Sanitation alone	31.9	13.3	35.0
Control	21.5	26.2	14.2

side-effects differed among the various drugs and was very low for some of the drugs such as Pyrantel Pamoate, Levamisole and Mebendazole.

In other trials, the effect of mass-treatment in the control of helminthiasis was compared with other methods in various parts of the country. In a trial in the rural area of Dezful, southwestern Iran, where the majority of inhabitants are infected with Ascaris, Ancylostoma and Trichostrongylus, the effect of different methods such as mass-treatment alone or together with sanitation, and sanitation alone, were compared in 16 villages (Arfaa et al., 1973). The drugs used for mass-treatment were Piperazine salts for Ascaris and Bephenium hydroxynaphtoate for Ancylostoma, given alternately every 4 months. Sanitation measures consisted of the construction of one latrine for every family and the provision of a sanitary water supply in each village. Reduction in the positivity rates of Ascaris, Ancylostoma and Trichostrongylus spp. with the 3 above-mentioned methods, indicated 3-4 years later, was respectively as follows: sanitation, 31.9, 13.3 and 35%; mass-treatment, 81.6, 71.6 and 22.9%; sanitation plus mass-treatment, 86.2, 68.3 and 38.5%. In the control villages this reduction was 21.3, 13.1 and 14.2% respectively (Table 4). The results obtained from the above studies indicate the effectiveness of mass-chemotherapy in the control of helminthiasis in this region.

In another study undertaken for the control of Ascaris in Isfahan villages by mass-chemotherapy (Ghadirian & Arfaa, 1974), using a more effective drug, i.e. Pyrantel Pamoate, the mean prevalence of infection, which was 91% before mass-treatment, dropped to 5% 3 weeks after treatment. However, it started increasing again in such a way that it reached 25% two months, 62% 4 months, 77% 6 months and 87% one year after treatment. A sudden and significant reduction in the mean number of eggs also occurred after treatment; it started building up again after treatment but did not reach its original number up to one year after therapy. This observation confirms once again the need for repeating mass-chemotherapy at least once every 3 months for a long period of time.

Based on this finding, in another trial already underway in Isfahan villages, the inhabitants of several villages are treated once every 3 months with a Levamisole compound.

Mass-chemotherapy for the control of hookworm infection (Necator americanus) has also been started 2 years ago in the Caspian Sea area in the north of Iran, where about 70% of the people are infected with this parasite with an intensity of more than 3000 eggs/g of faeces. The drug being used for the

mass-treatment of about 500,000 inhabitants of 1788 villages
in the age group 8-45 is Tetrachloroethylene (a single dose of
0.1 mg/kg b.w.), given after the administration of a single
dose of Piperazine to reduce the side-effects (Samsar-Yazdi
et al., 1975).

DISCUSSION AND CONCLUSION

Human infection with various intestinal helminthiasis,
especially soil-transmitted helminths, is not only very prevalent in most developing countries but is also important in
some of the highly developed countries of the world. For example, according to an estimation recently made by Warren
(1974), there are 54.2 million worm infestations, giving a
26.7% infection rate, in North America.

Fortunately, great efforts made in a few developed countries such as Japan and the U.S.S.R. have resulted in the
dramatic reduction and even eradication of some helminthiasis
in these countries. In Japan, as the result of a large-scale
campaign begun after World War II, the overall prevalences of
Ascaris and hookworm have been reduced from 61.3% and 23.3% in
1922-1926 to 1.1% and 0.3% in 1971 respectively (Morishita,
1973). These successful results have been achieved mainly by
mass-chemotherapy combined with other control methods such as
night-soil disposal and sanitation measures. The anthelminthics used were Santonin and Kainic acid, Santonin and Piperazine compounds for Ascaris and Tetrachloroethylene, 1 Bromo-
naphtoal 2; Iod-thymol and Bephenium hydroxynaphtoate.

Similar progress has also been achieved in the control of
helminthiasis in various parts of the Soviet Union by using
mass-treatment, sanitation and health education. The first
All-Union Helminthiasis Control Plan was drawn up in 1937, and
from 1960-1966 more than 50 million people were examined each
year throughout the U.S.S.R. (WHO, 1966). Some helminthiasis
have even been eradicated from some areas (Arfaa, 1974).

In Korea, organized efforts of the Korean Association for
Parasite Eradication and the Korean Society for Parasitology
have resulted in a reduction of the prevalence of Ascaris,
Trichuris, hookworm and Trichostrongylus from 80%, 80%, 45%
and 27% respectively in 1949 to 55%, 0.5%, 11% and 7% respectively in 1971. The control methods used were mass-chemotherapy twice annually, using a Piperazine compound for Ascaris
and other appropriate drugs for other helminths, combined with
health education and the construction of latrines.

The above-mentioned examples indicate the effectiveness

TABLE 5

The Effects of Various Anthelminthics
on Trichuris trichiura in Iran

Author and Date	Drug(s) Used	No. Treated	Cure Rate and Reduction in the Egg-Count*
Farahmandian et al., 1975	Diphetarsone	32	93.7
Semsar-Yazdi et al.	Pyrantel pamoate	97	22 (48)
	Mebendazole	97	76 (93.6)
Farahmandian et al.	Oxantel-Pyrantel	72	83

*Figures in parantheses indicate percent reduction
in the number of eggs.

of mass-chemotherapy in the control of soil-transmitted helminths. In selecting an anthelminthic compound as the drug of
choice for the mass-treatment of helminthiasis in a given area,
other criteria such as the effect of the drug as a broad-
spectrum anthelminthic, low toxicity and side-effects, the
number of doses required, the price of the drug and its acceptance by the people should be considered.

For example, in Iran, in regions where the prevalent soil-
transmitted helminths consist of Ascaris, Trichostrongylus and
hookworm, such as is the case in most parts of Khuzestan,
southwest Iran, Levamisole has been selected as the drug of
choice because of its high effect on all of these helminths,
producing more than 90% cure rates for existing soil-transmitted helminths and possessing the other criteria mentioned
above. In areas where, in addition to other soil-transmitted
helminths, Trichuris is also prevalent, Mebendazole can also
be considered as the drug of choice because of its high effect
on Trichuris, with the disadvantage that this drug should be
given in 2 doses daily for 3 consecutive days. It is clear
that in any mass-chemotherapy campaign, drugs which are administered in a single dose significantly reduce the cost of
operation.

It should be noted that most of the anthelminthics, except Mebendazole, Diphetarsone and Oxantel-Pyrantel, have a
poor effect on trichuriasis. The results of investigations on
these 3 drugs in Iran are shown in Table 5. Of these drugs,
Diphetarsone, although very effective, cannot be considered
for mass-chemotherapy because of the long duration required
for treatment. Mebendazole, on the other hand, is highly
effective with low side-effects but should be given in 6 doses.
Oxantel-Pyrantel, a new compound, has given encouraging results
on Trichuris and some other helminths.

One interesting observation made during the mass-chemotherapy of soil-transmitted helminths using some newly introduced drugs, was the increase of the prevalence of trichuriasis
after treatment. This might be due to the fact that, because
of the high cure rate induced for Ascaris, Trichostrongylus and
hookworm, the ova of Trichuris can be more easily detected
after treatment.

In conclusion, access to the highly effective anthelminthic drugs introduced recently may be a solution to the problem
of very high infection of man with soil-transmitted helminths
in many parts of the world.

REFERENCES

Amini, F. and Barzegar, M.A. (1972) Evaluation of the effect of Tetrachloroethylene for the mass-treatment of hookworm in the Caspian Sea area, north of Iran. Iran.J.Pub.Hlth.

Amini, F. et al (1974) The effect of anthelminthic compounds on hookworm and other intestinal helminths in the north of Iran. Presented at the 1st National Seminar on Parasitic Diseases, Teheran, 1-3 July 1974.

Arfaa, F. (1972) Present status of human helminthiasis in Iran. Trop.Geog.Med., 24, 353-362.

Arfaa, F., Sahba, G.H., Jamshidi, Ch. and Jalali, H. (1973) Trial of Phenylen di-isothiocyanata (Jonit) in the mass-treatment of intestinal helminthiasis. Bull.Soc.Path.Exot., 66, 191-195.

Arfaa, F., Sahba, G.H., Farahmandian, I., Mansoori, A. and Jalali, H. (1974) Evaluation of different methods of control of soil-transmitted helminths in Khuzestan, South West Iran. Presented at the 1st National Seminar on Parasitic Diseases, Teheran, 1-3 July 1974.

Arfaa, F. (1974) Report on a visit to the U.S.S.R. under a WHO Exchange of Research Workers Grant. Unpublished document.

Chin-Thack Soh (1973) Control of soil-transmitted helminths in Korea, a progress report. Presented at the 9th International Congress of Tropical Medicine and Malaria, Athens.

Farahmandian, I., Sahba, G.H. and Sadeghi, A. (1970) Prevalence of intestinal helminthiasis in a village in Dezful and comparative trial on the effect of Alcopar and Mintezole. J.Gen.Med., 9, 305-307 (in Persian)

Farahmandian, I., Arfaa, F., Sahba, G.H. and Jalali, H. (1972) A comparative evaluation of the therapeutic effect of Pyrantel Pamoate and Bephenium Hydroxynaphtoate on Ancylostoma duodenale and other intestinal helminths. J.Trop.Med.Hyg., 75, 205-207.

Farahmandian, I., Arfaa, F., Jalali, H. and Reza, M. (1974) Comparison of the effects of new anthelminthic drugs on various intestinal helminthiasis in Iran. Presented at the 1st National Seminar on Parasitic Diseases, Teheran, 1-3 July 1974.

Farahmandian, I., Arfaa, F., Sahba, G.H. and Jalali, H. (1974) Preliminary trial on the effect of Leavo-tetramisole on various intestinal helminthiasis in Iran. Iran J.Pub.Hlth, 3, 92-96.

Farahmandian, I., Arfaa, F., Jalali, H. and Hedaiati, M.A. (1975) The effect of Oxantel-Pyrantel on Trichuris and other intestinal helminths (in preparation).

Ghadirian, E., Sanati, A., Missaghian, G. and Yossefi, A. (1972)
    Treatment of ascariasis with Pyrantel Pamoate in Iran.
    J.Trop.Med.Hyg., 75, 195-197.

Ghadirian, E. and Arfaa, F. (1975) Present status of tricho-
    strongyliasis in Iran (in press).

Ghadirian, E. and Arfaa, F. (1975) Evaluation of the effect of
    Pyrantel Pamoate on various intestinal helminthiasis in
    Isfahan, Central Iran (in preparation)

Morishita, K. (1973) Report of "The Japan Association of Parasite
    Control" and its activities

Semsar-Yazdi, M.M., Amini, F. and Barzegar, M.A. (1975) Mass-
    chemotherapy in the control of hookworm infection in the rural
    areas of the Caspian Sea region, North Iran. Presented at the
    2nd Asian Congress of Agricultural Medicine and Rural Health,
    Teheran, 21-24 April 1975.

Warren, K.S. (1974) Helminthic diseases endemic in the United
    States. Amer.J.Trop.Med.Hyg., 23, 723-730.

World Health Organisation (1966) Report of the WHO Inter-Regional
    Travelling Seminar on Helminthic Diseases, U.S.S.R., 12 May -
    2 June 1966, unpublished document, WHO/Helminth/66.72.

World Health Organisation (1967) Control of ascariasis. Report
    of a WHO Expert Committee. Tech.Rep.Ser. 372, Geneva,
    Switzerland.

THE TREATMENT OF CHLOROQUINE-RESISTANT FALCIPARUM MALARIA

A.P. Hall

SEATO Medical Reseach Laboratory

Bangkok, Thailand

INTRODUCTION

The severity of the falciparum infection is a much more important factor than its response to chloroquine.

The two major mistakes in the management of malaria are a delay in diagnosis and therapy which is excessive (especially quinine) or inappropriate (e.g., heparin).

DIAGNOSIS

A thick blood film should be performed on any person who is sick and who has been in a malarious area. A thin film rapidly fixed in methanol should also be prepared. The slide should be dried in cold air and then stained for 30 minutes with 1:50 Giemsa or another suitable stain. The films should be dried in cold air and then examined under an oil-immersion lens. If plasmodia are note readily apparent, then 400 high power fields should be examined on the thick film. The thin film may help in differentiating between P. falciparum and P. vivax, etc.

If malaria is suspected but the blood film is negative in a seriously ill person, a therapeutic test with a four hour intravenous infustion of quinine should be made.

OVERALL MANAGEMENT

Severe falciparum malaria is a medical emergency. The following are guidelines for optimum management. The patients are continuously supervized by experienced nurses and physicians examine the patients regularly throughout the 24 hours. The temperature, heart rate, blood pressure and respiratory rate are recorded at least every four hours. The body weight is recorded daily. A fluid intake and output chart is maintained. The urinary bladder is catheterized if the patient cannot urinate spontaneously. Venous blood is obtained a least once daily for biochemistry (for example, serum bilirubin, creatinine and quinine) and hematology (parasite count and packed cell volume). Parasite counts are determined at regular intervals, for example every eight hours. The value of drugs other than antimalarials has not been prove. No controlled studies have been performed with respect to corticosteriods, anticoagulants, dextran and mannitol.

QUININE THERAPY

Quinine by intermittent intravenous infusions (IVQ) is the only regimen currently available that is effective in patients seriously ill with chloroquine-resistant falciparum malaria. There is evidence that quinine is more effective than chloroquine in patients with falciparum malaria acquired in Africa (an area considered chloroquine sensitive). The half-life of quinine is about 10 hours in health but is usally prolonged in falciparum malaria, presumably because of hepatic impairment. Therefore, the required dosage is inversely related to the severity of the disease. The optimum daily dose of quinine in patients with severe renal or hepatic failure is 10 mg. per Kg. Most seriously ill patients are best treated with 15 to 20 mg per Kg. daily. After the initial response to therapy, 20 mg. per Kg. usually rapidly reduces the parasitemia to zero but 30 mg. to Kg. is occasionally necessary in infections showing resistance to quinine.

A two hours infusion is the most effective method of administering quinine, especially if the blood is free of the drug before therapy. A four hour infusion is safer, especially for subsequent doses.

COMPLICATIONS OF FALCIPARUM MALARIA

The manifestations of cerebral malaria include coma, convulsion, stupor, confusion, aphasia, delusional states and psychosis.

Deep coma is often irreversible whereas the other forms of
cerebral malaria usally respond to therapy. However, convulsions
in children are an ominous sign. In many patients falciparum
coma is light and ephermeral and responds to a small dose of
intravenous quinine. In more severe cases, intermittent infusions
of quinine are needed, the optimum dose is usally 10 mg. per Kg.
every 12-14 hours. Most patients in coma respond satisfactorily
to quinine. Intravenous dexamethazone may heasten recovery in the
occasional case but a controller study has not been performed.

Clinically obvious jaundice commonly occurs in patients
with falciparum malaria and is usually associated with a high
parasite density. Both hemolysis and liver damage contribute
to falciparum jaundice. Apart from jaundice, abnormality of
hepatic function in falciparum malaria is common as is hepatomegaly.
A thick film should be examined for malaria on all patients
presenting with jaundice in an area endemic for the disease.
Jaundice in falciparum malaria does not require any specific
treatment.

Anemia is common in falciparum malaria is mainly due to
hemolysis. The degree og anemia is usally related to the severity
of the infection. The anemia improves steadily once the infection
has been brought under control and blood transfusion is rarely
required.

Blackwater fever refers to the passage of hemoglobin in the
urine secondary to rapid or severe lysis of erythrocytes and is
not always associated with any impairment of renal function.
Blackwater fever is usally caused by the disease, less commonly
by quinine therapy. It commonly dollows blood transfusion given
for the disease. There is no specific proof for the claim that
adrenocorticosteroids are useful in the management of blackwater
fever.

Acute renal insufficiency is a rare complication of falciparum
malaria. This probelm is usually associated with anemia or
oliguria (urine output less than 400 mg. daily). Prompt but
limited intravenous infusion of fluids on admission probably
presents A.R.I. in many patients. Peritoneal dialysis has been
effective in many patients. Hemodialysis has also been used.
Nephrotic syndrome due to Plasmodium malariae is common in Africa
and is associated with the deposition of soluble immune complexes
in the glomerular basement membrane. The nephrotic syndrome is
rare in falciparum malaria but immune complexes have been detected
in the glomerular basement membrane of patients with varying degrees
of urinary abnormality.

Pulmonary edema rarely occurs in falciparum malaria if fluid
input is controller but may occur if large volumes of intravenous
fluids are infused. Dehydration is not a common feature in the
disease Indeed there is evidence of an increased plasma volume
and an increase in tissue catabolism and fluid production in the
disease. Hyponatremia is also common. Thus, samll volumes of
intravenous saline are a logical vehicle for quining therapy.
There is a rapidly fatal pulmonary complication which occurs
rarely. The patients develops acute dyspnoea but evidence of
gross fluid overload is not present.

Abnormal bleeding is an occasional complication in severe
falciparum malaria but is rarely clinically significant. The
excessive bleeding is either due to decreased production of
clotting factors by a damaged liver or to disseminated intravascular coagulation (D.I.C). However, the complete syndrome of
D.I.C. is rare. The use of heparin for D.I.C. is controversial
and there is a report in which heparin appeared to cause D.I.C.
Fatal hemorrhages have occurred in several falciparum patients
treated with heparin. Heparin or any other anticoagulant should
not be used in malaria.

Rupture of the spleen is a frequently missed diagnosis in
malaria. The treatment is splenectomy.

Myocardial involvement in falciparum malaria does occur but
has never been delineated. Tachycardia, low cardiac output and
dealth are the manifestations. Serial electrocardiograms should
be performed in seriously ill patients.

CHLOROQUINE-RESISTANT FALCIPARUM MALARIA

The most effective regiments are now briefly discussed.

Quinine (at least four doses given at an interval of eight
to twelve hours) (followed by a single dose of pyrimethamine
with sulfadoxine (Fansidar[R]) (is the most effective treatment for
chloroquine-resistant falciparum malaria. In about 80 per cent
of patients admitted to hospital, at least the first does of
quinine should be administered as a two or four hours infusion.
Fansidar is very effective as a secondary drug but is often slow
acting when used alone. No adequate substitute for intravenous
quinine has yet been tested but mefloquine is a worthy substitute
for Fansidar[R].

Mefloquine (WR142490) is a quinoline methanol, developed by
the U.S. Army Malaria Research Program. In Thailand, mefloquine
cleared parasitemia and fever more rapidly than did pyrimethamine
with sulfadoxine in a controlled study of each drug given alone as
a single dose. However, mefloquine like Fansidar was slow acting

in several patients especially those seriously ill. The cure rates with each regimen were 88 per cent (14/16) for mefloquine and 80 per cent (12/15) for Fansidar. Mefloquine will probably prove to be especially useful as single-dose therapy in patients treated on an outpatient basis and for chemoprophylaxis.

THE ROLE OF UNIVERSITY RESEARCH DEPARTMENTS IN THE

DEVELOPMENT OF ANTIPARASITIC CHEMOTHERAPY

Professor W. Peters

Department of Parasitology, Liverpool School of Tropical

Medicine, Pembroke Place, Liverpool L3 5QA

1   THE INITIATION OF A CHEMICAL SYNTHESIS PROGRAMME

An extensive programme of chemical synthesis designed to seek new antiparasitic drugs is a costly undertaking that can seldom be accepted within a university department. If such research is performed it is usually either because the work itself is of genuine academic interest, or because the acceptance of a contract from an outside organisation may, incidentally, provide funds that can then be used for other items of research of primary interest to that particular department.

Money for research is a major problem, and university government funds at least in this country are limited. The head of the department must often seek financial support for research from other sources. Non-governmental funds may be obtainable from international organisations such as WHO, or trusts such as the Rockefeller Foundation or Wellcome Trust. Alternatively, the department may succeed in winning a research and development (R and D) contract from a different governmental body, for example the Ministry of Overseas Development in UK, or a branch of some military establishment, such as the US Army. Generally speaking the type of support that a university department receives for fundamental research is of a temporary nature ("soft money"), but occasionally permanent benefits are derived, for example new laboratory equipment or even new buildings. However, this is exceptional and normally something that is only achieved when a long term and unusually large R and D contract is granted. Chemical synthetic programmes have been undertaken in some university departments, for example those of Professors Urbanski and Serafin of Warsaw, and Professor Dann of Erlangen who have produced several series of potential antimalarial compounds with substantial support from WHO and, in the latter case, also from the West German government. In the last decade several research departments, particularly in North American universities have received R and D contracts for the synthesis of antimalarials in the course of the current US Army antimalarial programme. On the whole however, it is unusual for university departments to act as the initiators of programmes to synthesise antiparasitic drugs.

2 DEVELOPMENT LEADING FROM AN ESTABLISHED CHEMICAL LEAD

On the contrary, in the further development of chemical leads discovered elsewhere chemical research departments of universities can play a significant role. Here the example of the US Army antimalarial programme again comes to the fore. To date nearly one quarter million chemical structures have been provided for the primary screen of the US Army programme. The majority of these have been developed on contract by various research organisations including, besides pharmaceutical and other chemical concerns, a number of university departments.

Academic workers can contribute to such a programme in several areas. Among them are, for example, the production of analogues leading from the initial discovery. Another is the development of improved synthetic approaches for the production of specified target compounds. A third is the development of new procedures to produce increased quantities of a particular target compound. Examples of such collaboration between universities and the pharmaceutical industry are too common to need further emphasis here.

3   BIOLOGICAL SCREENING

The next most important place for university departments lies in the field of biological screening. The problem today is that the pharmaceutical industry has, for essentially commercial reasons, largely lost interest in the development of new antiparasitic drugs. It is at present difficult to persuade pharmaceutical companies to include, for example, a biological screening system for activity against trypanosomiasis, leishmaniasis or filariasis in their general screening procedures. This is true even if good screening techniques are already available, but certainly in the case of leishmaniasis and filariasis ideal laboratory models have yet to be developed. Here academic workers can make a significant contribution by attempting to develop new screening models that can eventually be passed on to pharmaceutical laboratories. Large scale drug screening is not the function of a university research department, although there are a number of exceptions. For example, the late Dr. Louis Rane and his wife developed the primary rodent malaria screen through which have passed these $\frac{1}{4}$ million compounds in a simple test

of blood schizontocidal activity. Those of you who have had the good fortune
to visit the Rane laboratories in the University of Miami will appreciate the
smooth production line process that was developed there, in a special building
funded on a US Army R and D contract. In Belo Horizonte, Brazil a highly
efficient screen was developed by Professor Pellegrino for the evaluation of
potential schistosomicides. While undoubtedly both these programmes have
benefited their respective universities, they have demanded a considerable
proportion of the time and energy of the principal investigators, and it is
questionable whether this is justified for individuals who have, after all,
major academic responsibilities.

Fund giving bodies such as the Wellcome Trust are understandably
cautious about providing grants that they feel are going to be used for drug
screening. It is however an entirely different matter when a university
worker engages in the investigation of a new screening technique, where
such a technique is lacking and where industry will not provide the effort and
manpower needed for its development. Once a new technique has been
produced it is up to the academic to persuade the pharmaceutical industry to
take up this screen and put it to practical use.

4   PHARMACOLOGY AND TOXICOLOGY

Once promising new target compounds have been developed there
remains the complete gamut of basic pharmacological and toxicological testing,
and eventually pre-clinical and clinical pharmacology. These are essentially
development types of activity that can sometimes be farmed out to university
departments on R and D contracts. There are numerous examples where this
has been done. Professor Aviado of Pennsylvania University for example, has
contributed considerably to the pharmacological testing of potential antimalarials for the current US Army programme. Again this demands an academic
interest as well as expertise on the part of the research worker since it is not
the function of a university department, generally speaking, to undertake
such work purely on a commercial basis. In many cases it is possible to give
a particular problem to a research student working for a higher degree. In
this way not only is the investigation carried out, but the salary and expenses
of the student are provided.

Studies designed to elucidate the mode of action of a new compound
are also suitable research areas for university workers. While many pharmaceutical concerns maintain sophisticated departments for this type of research,
generally speaking they are less inclined to devote time to drug mode of
action studies than to the discovery of new drugs. The old argument says
that, if we knew more about how drugs work we would be able to produce
more new drugs on a rational basis, rather than the empirical basis of large
scale synthesis and screening. In general the hard-headed leaders of the

pharmaceutical industry are not very impressed by this argument. They know too well from experience that the empirical approach usually has paid off the best and it is difficult to persuade them otherwise. This means in effect that investigations on the mode of drug action frequently are left to the academic world. It is however remarkably difficult to obtain research grants for this purpose, particularly from the pharmaceutical industry itself. Even the Research Councils in UK, like the research trusts are reluctant to provide money for what they feel is the type of investigation that should be funded by the pharmaceutical industry.

5   CHANCE AND DESIGN IN DRUG DEVELOPMENT

In a recent review of the current US Army antimalarial programme Kinnamon and Rothe (1975) showed that for each 3,000 compounds examined in the primary screen only one was finally tested against a human malaria parasite, and that only in a simian model. In fact this is not a bad average compared with drug screening programmes in the pharmaceutical industry. The US Army programme began in December 1961. Out of the $\frac{1}{4}$ million compounds examined probably one completely new drug, mefloquine, a quinoline-methanol, will appear before too long on the market. It has already been tested in patients infected with multiple drug resistant Plasmodium falciparum, and has proved to be remarkably effective. At the peak of the US Army programme something in the order of $6 million per year were being spent, mainly on drug screening. This gives some indication of the scale of money required to produce one new compound for one specific indication.

The current large scale programme to eliminate onchocerciasis from the Volta River Basin, financed largely by the UNDP and World Bank and organised by WHO, is estimated to cost over $6 million yearly for the next 20 years. The scheme is based primarily on the use of insecticides against the Simulium vectors and relatively little attention has been paid so far to the chemotherapeutic aspects of the disease. We do not possess today any drug safe enough for mass chemotherapy either to kill the microfilaria or the adult worms. Were we to possess such a drug we could undoubtedly cut down, perhaps even by years, the duration of this project and thus improve its chances of success. The necessity of developing new macro and microfilaricides, not only against onchocerciasis, but also against other forms of filariasis in man is paramount. The majority of the pharmaceutical companies are reluctant to explore this field, although indeed a few are still pursuing active filariasis research programmes. In this case we are faced with a lack of really adequate laboratory screening models and undoubtedly university research workers could make a major contribution. However, whereas in the case of the US Army malaria programme money was relatively easily produced for large scale screening and development, this is not yet the case for filariasis. It may well

cost between 10 and 20 million US$ to discover and develop the type of drug
we need for the treatment of patients with filariasis. Although the development of new screening techniques and the investigation of new filaricidal
drugs could be carried out in university departments, the major problem of
synthesising large numbers of new compounds would have to depend primarily
on the pharmaceutical industry. Moreover, the eventual clinical testing of
new drugs is best carried out by experienced clinical pharmacologists, most
of whom are employed in industry, although there are still a few specialists
within the academic world who can provide this type of expertise.

6   THE WHO TASK FORCE PROGRAMME, THE INDUSTRY
AND THE UNIVERSITIES

WHO has recently established a programme to explore research
priorities and to initiate research in the areas of chemotherapy and immunisation, aimed at combatting six major tropical diseases, five of them parasitic
i.e. malaria, trypanosomiasis, schistosomiasis, filariasis and leishmaniasis.
The sixth disease is leprosy. It is hoped that experts in the various fields
called together by WHO will pinpoint the main needs, and outline programmes
for their resolution. The actual conduct of the research will depend upon
independent research workers, particularly within the universities. In this
particular situation WHO recognises very clearly the reluctance of the
pharmaceutical industry to engage in this type of research and it would not
be surprising if WHO in time actually offers research contracts to the
pharmaceutical industry to work on specified chemotherapeutic problems.
This is an interesting twist since, in the past, it has always been the academic
world that has depended on the pharmaceutical industry for grants of this type.

7   FUTURE CONSIDERATIONS

It is clear that there is an immense need for close collaboration
between the pharmaceutical industry, international organisations, other
research initiating bodies (such as the US Army) and the academic world, in
the development of new antiparasitic drugs. This collaboration could be
strengthened by several simple measures. First of all there should be more
cooperation between academics, the industry and other organisations at the
very first stage, namely the pinpointing of research needs. Secondly, there
should be more exchange visits of personnel between the various organisations
so that the progress of research can be freely discussed. Thirdly, there is
surely a place for more experienced academic research workers as consultants
within industrial research groups. Fourthly, the pharmaceutical industry
could second some of its own personnel to assist in university research departments, for example in the development of new screening techniques. Finally,
the universities badly need additional money to carry out their research.

This problem is not unique to Britain, and throughout the Western world the universities are seriously feeling the economic pinch. Ultimately most of the new antiparasitic drugs that are being sought are for the benefit of the peoples of the developing world and not those of the developed world. This would surely be the moment to create an internationally controlled fund for research into the chemotherapy of parasitic diseases. The major oil-producing countries are among those that suffer most from parasitic diseases, and any benefits derived from the development of new antiparasitic drugs would be of primary interest to their inhabitants. Could not the OPEC countries provide a substantial fund for this purpose to be distributed, for example, through the WHO Task Forces to university departments, or even to the pharmaceutical industry itself? This would breathe new life into the universities, giving them at the same time increased opportunities to train young research workers from the developing nations. As to the pharmaceutical industry, it could thus make a major contribution to world health. While the industry would not obtain large profits, it would certainly gain a handsome return in terms of goodwill.

Kinnamon, K. E. and Rothe, W. E. (1975). Am. J. trop. Med. Hyg., 24, 174-178.

CURRENT PROBLEMS IN THE CHEMOTHERAPY OF PARASITIC DISEASES - THE

ROLE OF THE PHARMACEUTICAL INDUSTRY

O.D. Standen

The Wellcome Research Laboratories

Langley Court, Beckenham, Kent, U.K.

Summary: The last decade has seen the progressive withdrawal
of industrial Research and Development from the field of tropical
parasitic disease. If the downward trend persists at the same rate,
the already acute situation of absence of suitable drugs for control
programmes in high prevalence diseases such as filariasis, schistosomiasis, malaria and trypanosomiasis could become irreversible. The
reason for this withdrawal is essentially one of economics.
Industry is concentrating its effort in disease areas offering
reasonable chance of return on investment. The problem is how to
equate the humanitarian needs of the increasing population of
developing countries with the need for profitability adequate to
maintain viability in industry. A possible answer lies in current
WHO policy for establishing collaboration with industry and the
recruitment of external expertise and funding supportive to
industrial effort.

The last thrity years has been a period of intense activity in
the search for therapeutic and prophylactic agents for a very wide
range of diseases of man and animals. This has resulted in considerable advances in many fields, notably in antibacterials and drugs
for diseases of the Western World. However, there has been markedly
less success in the field of tropical diseases.

Exceptions to this are drugs for the treatment of infection with
intestinal nematodes and amoebiasis, among which excellent specifics
are now available. Far less well served are the great vector-borne
diseases such as filariasis, schistosomiasis, malaria and trypanosomiasis. In filariasis, drug research has been at a very low level
and no new drug has been produced since diethylcarbamazine was
introduced as a microfilaricide in 1948. In schistosomiasis, the

35

trivalent antimonials have been largely replaced by niridazole,
hycanthone and, latterly, oxamniquine. However, all have their
shortcomings and are unlikely to be suitable for mass treatment for
all three types of schistosome infection.

      In malaria, chloroquine, pyrimethamine, proguanil and primaquine
were thought to meet most likely requirements for treatment and
prophylaxis but the emergence of drug resistant strains has materially
altered the picture. New antimalarials, effective against drug
resistant strains are now needed. In African trypanosomiasis, the
drugs availabel are toxic and by no means satisfactory whereas in
Chagas disease only one drug, 'Lampit', has emerged and has yet to
demonstrate widespread utility.

      Future development of better drugs for these four diseases of
high and increasing prevalence is now much at risk. A highly
disturbing feature has been the progressive pull-out of the pharmaceutical industry from this field over the last 10 years. Major
effort in drug research has been based in the Western World and
many large firms in Europe and Ajerican made considerable investment
in tropical medicine during the 15 to 20 post-war years. However, the
progressive decline in this endeavour offers a current situation
where no major company is now operative in the United States and
probably no more than six remain active in Europe. In the present
investment climate, European programmes may also be at risk for
precisely the same reasons of withdrawal in U.S.A. The significance
of this situation is best seen against the background of global
population trends. At present, the world population of about 3.8
billion is distributed in the ratio of 30% in the developed world and
70% in the developing countries. By 1990, with world population
estimated at 5.5 billion the change in distribution pattern will be
20% and 80%. With the exception of malaria, there is little to
indicate that the prevalence rate of these diseases has decreased
over the past 30 years or that this situation is likely to change
for the better in the foreseeable future.

      Thus, it is not difficult to anticipate a situation of increased
incidence of diseases of already astronomical prevalence coupled with
diminishing prospect of development of the means for treatment or
contribution from chemotherapy to control or prophylaxis.

      It is of importance to reach an understanding of how this
dangerous circumstance has come about. Essentially, it is related
to the economics of drug development within the pharmaceutical
industry.

      Unfortunately, the same economic pressures are operating
against investment in research to find better agents for vector
control where, for instance, resistance to established insecticides
presents an increasing problem. This downward trend of support to

development of better agents for servicing two essential arms of disease control presents a bleak future in the face of likely increased incidence and prevalence of disease in tropical countries.

Two salient facts relating to drug development are apparent. The first is that discovery of new and better drugs is almost entirely confined to industry while development of such discoveries is wholly dependent upon industrial resource and expertise. The second is that within this responsibility, deployment of resorces is inevitably linked largely, if not entirely, to the profit motive.

The costs involved in industrial R&D have been escalating steeply over recent years. The failure rate along this road establishes such work as being highly speculative. Continuity in investment in drug development is therefore dependent upon likelihood of a reasonable profit margin to provide a return to investors and to make provision to finance further work. Many factors have conspired to increase the difficulties in expanding investment to embrace R&D involvement in all fields of potential interest to a given company. Among these are the steep increase in inflation and greater expenditure to meet regulatory requirements for drug registration and for manufacturing standards. Whatever the causes of increased cost, the effect has been for companies to concentrate their resources on fewer programmes and to select those with the greatest likelihood of return on investment. This refinement of policy is reflected by the figure (Table 1) for new single chemical entities marketed in the U.S.A. since 1959 (de Haen, 1973).

Similarly, the figures for annual increase in R&D investment in the U.S.A. pharmaceutical industry (Table 11) show a decline from +12.5% in 1970 to +4.5% in 1973 against a rising inflationary situation, meaning that the resource availability in real terms has been falling.

TABLE 1 : Number of new chemical entities arising from pharmaceutical research, U.S.A. for the years 1959 - 1972.

1959	63	1966	13
1960	45	1967	27
1961	41	1968	14
1962	28	1969	11
1963	18	1970	16
1964	17	1971	14
1965	23	1972	11

TABLE II : Rate of annual increase in Research and Development
Budgets in the Pharmaceutical Industry, U.S.A., for
the years 1970 - 1973. (With acknowledgement to
the Stanford Research Institute).

	Increase over previous year
1970	+ 12.6%
1971	+ 10.6%
1972	+ 6.5%
1973	+ 4.5%

The priority given to any one subject for research in industry
must be seen in the context of the cost of the total R&D programme.
Whereas R&D budgets will vary in size as between companies, the
relationship of expenditure to return will be of much the same order.
Davey (1974) offers an example where R&D costs of about £10m per year
operating in a facility of £30m investment value might, with luck,
discover one significant new drug within the total operation every 2
to 3 years. Because of the time scale of R&D, no return could be
expected on this investment for at least 7 years, with annual investment on-going during this period. On this basis he arrives at a
figure of overall investment of £90m before any return can be expected
from the original discovery.

Against this background it is not surprising that industry has
tended to reject programmes with potentially low return on investment
in favour of programmes relevant to those diseases of countries of the
Western World with high gross national product. Casualties in this
category include those areas of tropical medicine now seen as at risk.
The completed fact of withdrawal in the U.S.A. is in part matched by
the downward trend in Europe. The danger is that if this trend should
continue to its logical conclusion the process could be reversed with
only the greatest difficulty or not al all. The question now arises
as to how to solve this dilemma. It is inconceivably that by 1990,
industry will be meeting the drug development requirements of only
20% of the world population. On the other hand, if industry is to
remain viable it may not be able to afford adequate investment in
fields of research and development which are unlikely to provide
reasonable return.

Before considering possible answeres to these problems of drug
development it must be asked whether it is essential. Certainly,
treatment of individuals infected with these diseases is as essential
for the same moral reasons as treatment of any other disease but this
alone is unlikely to make any significant impression on prevalence or

incidence rates. Only control programmes on a national scale are
likely to achieve this end. Again, whereas chemotherapy is unlikely to achieve control on its own it could be an important con-
tributory factor in association with other measures such as vector
control, artificial modification of local environments, provision of
sanitary facilities and health education.

Success in the bacterial and viral fields suggests that the ideal
answer lies with antiparasitic vaccines. So far, there is no vaccine
available for prevention of any human parasitic disease. In terms of
practical availability of vaccines we are rather in the position of
seeing a cloud no bigger than a man's hand. This may presage things
to come, perhaps more quickly with some diseases than with others,
but realization may be a long way off. Again, the economic factor
intrudes. That is to say, where will the onus lie for long-term
investment in antiparasitic vaccine research? Assuming therefore
that, in the short to medium term, chemotherapeutic support to control
programmes is deemed to be of considerable significance, ways have to
be found to reverse the decline in Research and Development towards
evaluation of new and better drugs suitable for mass application under
conditions of minimal medical monitoring.

It is of value to indicate briefly the approaches which can be
made towards discovery of new or better chemotherapeutic agents for
use against parasitic diseases. Essentially, these approaches may be
classified as Basic and Direct. The Basic appraoches may include
the study of comparative physiology and biochemistry of host and
parasite in search of a better understanding or even characterization
of the coexistent life-support systems. In ultimate chemotherapeutic
terms, the objective here is exposure of similarities and differences,
thus offering guidelines to selective inhibition of essential enzyme
activity. Even more fundamental and long term would be the detailed
characterization of such enzyme systems and rational design of
specific inhibitors of their activity. Additionally, is an approach
to greater understanding of the biochemical basis for the mode of
action of existing drugs and, with supportive chemistry, the design
of substances with enhanced specificity and hence higher therapeutic
index. Again, basic contribution can be made through study of host-
parasite relationships, response to exisitng drugs and the design of
improved laboratory models as tools for research.

The Direct approach is that commonly referred to as screening,
where in vivo or in vitro model systems are challenged by the
introduction of chemical substances. This procedure may be selective
where chemical thought has progressed from the point of known active
molecular configuration or selectively empirical where the structure
of compounds tested relates to configurations of known biological
activity or purely empirical where activity potential is not known
to exist. Essentially, both Basic and Direct approaches are in
search of a chemical lead which may be subsequently extended by

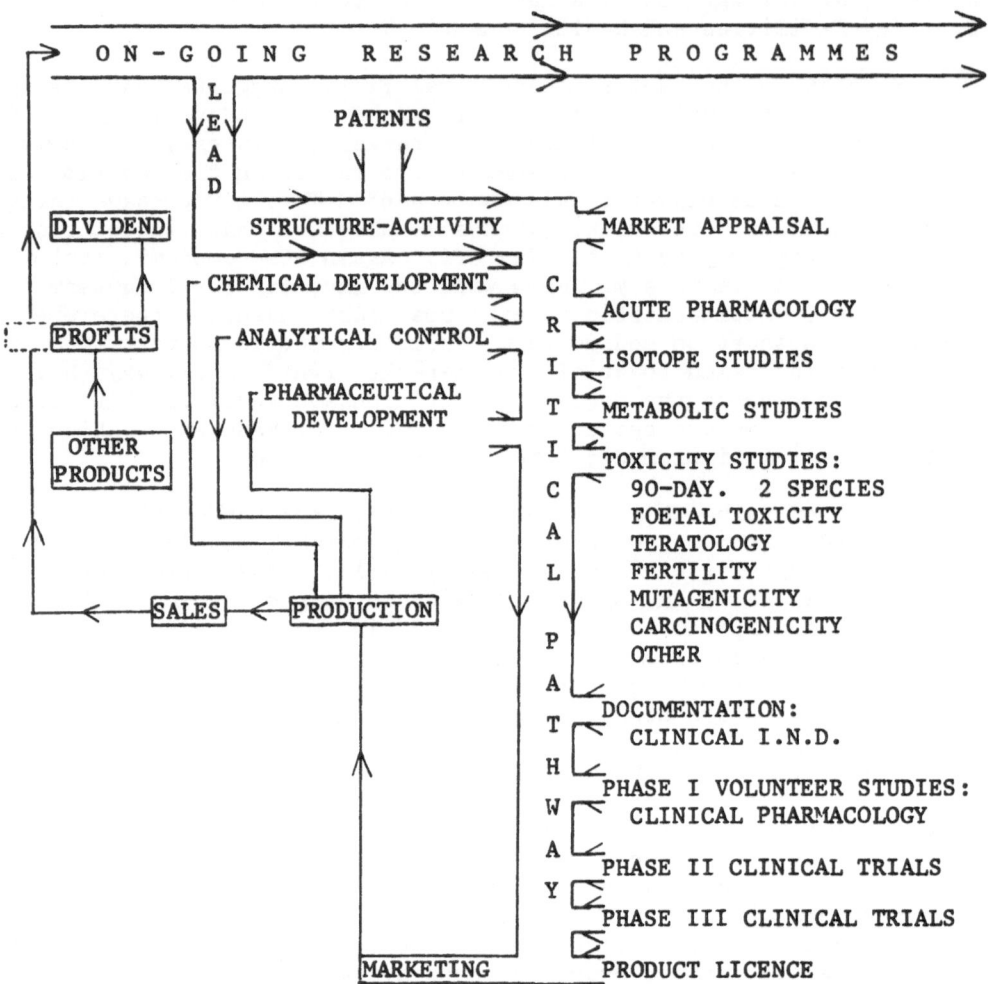

Fig. 1.   Diagramatic representation of a typical flow
           chart of Drug Evolution in the Pharmaceutical
           Industry covering the main features of Research,
           Development, Production and Sales.

application of intensive chemical and biological research to reach a structure of optimal therapeutic index.

The screening approach is almost completely confined to industry because of its need for extensive chemical support. Depth of involvement in basic approaches varies with individual industrial research policy but related research of this kind is to be found in academic institutions although by no means necessarily related to chemotherapeutic objectives. In terms of drug development, establishment of the chemical lead is but the tip of the iceberg. Diagramatic representation of a flow chart in drug development (Fig. 1) indicates the range of studies required to be completed for drug registration and sale. The time scale from the point of lead to sale of a product is highly unlikely to be less than 5 years and can be as long as 7 or 10 years. Moreover, the Critical Path presents a formidable array of resource utilization of high cost and failure rate which may be as high as 9 out of 10 candidate drugs entering this system. Thus, even when arrived at the lead discovery stage, future investment cost in development is high and the chance of success is low. Furthermore, with candidate drugs for development arising from a whole range of other and unrelated programmes, there can be severe competition for these development resources and consequent priority allocation to projects with greatest likelihood of lucrative return. Unfortunately, drugs for human parasitic disease have not proved highly competitive in this respect.

The reasons, therefore, are clear for the progressive withdrawal of industry from the tropical research field. If the incentive to justify high risk development costs is absent, then the economic justification for maintaining the originating research programme is hard to find. Thus, the dilemma arises as how to equate humanitarian needs with the need to provide return reasonable enough to retain investment in industry.

Only in very recent years has international concern been apparent for a likely shortfall in drug development for diseases of importance to developing countries. Now, ways and means are being sought to halt and reverse this trend. The World Health Organization with interest in principle from other international and national agencies, has set up a Special Programme for Research and Training embracing a positive policy aimed at collaboration with the pharmaceutical industry. One interesting possibility envisaged is much closer integration of objectives through collaboration of industry with academic institutions and another is recruitment of external resources for funding development of discoveries of potential value. Clearly, the very international nature of the problem requires interest and support at international level. It is much too early to report progress but the hazard has been defined and understood in anticipation of finding a sensible solution to the problem of

drug development as required to meet some of the future needs of
developing countries in the tropics.

REFERENCES

1.   Davey, D.G. (1974) A.B.P.I. News (53), November 1974.

2.   de Haen, P. (1973) "Pharmaceutical Specialities Marketed
      Nationally". FDC Reports (Pink Sheet) 5th February 1973.

3.   Stanford Research Institute. Report. The United States Health
      Product Market to 1980. June 1973.

NEW NITROIMIDAZOLES WITH A CHEMOTHERAPEUTIC ACTIVITY

E. Winkelmann

W. Raether

Hoechst AG., Frankfurt(M)-Höchst, W.-Germany

The nitroimidazole preparation >Tinidazole< (Pfizer),
compound I, used for combating trichomoniasis is substituted at the imidazole ring in the 1-position by
an ethylsulfonylethyl group. If this is replaced by
an ethylthioethyl group, compound II, an intermediate
of >Tinidazole< , a practically ineffective compound
is obtained. Our studies have shown, this structure-
activity relation is almost reversed when changing
from the corresponding alkyl to aryl sulfur compounds,
especially with electronegative radicals. For example,
the 1-(4-nitrophenylsulfonylethyl) compound III is
practically ineffective, the 1-(4-nitrophenylthio-
ethyl) compound IV exhibits a pronounced action
against trichomonads. This effect is increased when
heterocyclic radicals are introduced. Thus the 1-(4-
pyridylsulfonylethyl) compound V also has a weak
effect, whilst the 1-(4-pyridylthioethyl) compound VI
has a comparable effect to >Metronidazole< . These
results promted us to extend the studies also to the
2-position of the 5-nitroimidazoles.
However, these structure-activity studies produced a
result that was different again. The 2-ethylsulfonyl-
methyl compound VII and the 2-ethylthiomethyl compound VIII, prepared by Merck, Rahway, have only a
weak but equal activity against trichomonads. Studies
of our own demonstrated that analogous aryl sulfur
compounds substituted by an electronegative radical,
for example the 2-(4-nitrophenylsulfonylmethyl) compound IX and the 2-(4-nitrophenylthiomethyl) compound
X, have an effect that is almost comparable to that

of the analogous compound III and IV in the series
substituted in the 1-position. It was possible, as in
the series substituted in the 1-position, to increase
the effect markedly by the introduction of heterocyclic radicals. Thus the 2-(2-pyridylsulfonylmethyl)
compound XI and the 2-(2-pyridylthiomethyl) compound
XII have an optimum effect in this series. If the
pyridyl radical is replaced by other heterocyclic
radicals, preparations are nearly always obtained
which are highly effective in vivo against trichomonads and other protozoas.
After extensive research in this field the following
basic structure can be given. As is generally known,
the nitro group must be in the 5-position. Analogous
4-nitro compounds or compounds without a nitro group
are ineffective. Compounds in which the 5-nitro group
is replaced by an amino or acetamino group are ineffective. The most favourable radical R 1 is a
methyl group. A hydrogen atom or a hydroxyethyl group
in the 1-position result in a loss of activity in this
series, whilst an ethyl group reduces the activity
considerably. However, a hydrogen atom or a methyl
group in the radical R 2 produces compounds of equal
high efficacy. The bridgeforming sulfur atom can be
replaced by the sulfoxide or sulfone group. The compounds thus obtained have an equally good effect.
Corresponding compounds with an analogous oxygen link
exhibit a reduced effect. The heterocyclic radical
can be varied within wide limits, with the good activity maintained. An electropositive substituent R 3
at the heterocycle, for example a methyl, hydroxy,
methoxy, amino or dimethylamino group reduced the
effectiveness considerably, and so does the carboxyl
or the carboxamide group. An electronegative substituent R 3, for example a halogen atom, a nitro or cyano
group, also results in highly effective preparations
without a further increase being attained. A very
goog effect is also exhibited by the nitrogenoxide
derivatives of various heterocycles.
Of the numerous 5-nitroimidazoles of this series prepared and tested, preparation HOE 088, >Pirinidazole<,
1-methyl-2-(2-pyridylthiomethyl)-5-nitroimidazole has
been selected for further investigations.
The following paper will report on the results of the
chemotherapeutic tests.

NEW 5-NITROIMIDAZOLES WITH ANTIPROTOZOAL ACTIVITY:

EFFECT OF HOE 088 (PIRINIDAZOLE)

W. Raether, E. Winkelmann

Hoechst AG, 6 Frankfurt, F.R.G.

Preparation Hoe 088, a 1-Methyl-2-(pyridyl-2-thio-methyl)-5-nitro-imidazole, was found to be the compound from a series of new 5-nitro-imidazoles with the broadest action against protozoans. Its effect against trichomonads is the most pronounced. The comparison of the effective doses of different 5-nitroimidazoles against Trichomonas fetus demonstrates that the compound (Hoe 088) is slightly superior to Tinidazole, distinctly superior to Metronidazole, and very much superior to Nitrimidazine. As a supplementary basic model the subcutaneous abscess in the mouse caused by Trichomonas vaginalis was used for further assessing the trichomonacidal effect. None of the compounds tested could prevent the formation of abscesses in all animals at the dose of 4 times 100 mg/kg. After administration of Hoe 088 the smallest number of abscesses was counted. The next in order were the Tinidazol- and finally the Metronidazole-treated animals. Up to a dosage of 12,5 mg/kg the abscesses were found to be sterile with Hoe 088, followed by Metronidazole and Tinidazole at 25 mg/kg. It is evident that it is more difficult to influence the subcutaneous abscess by an active drug than the trichomonadal peritonitis. This is connected with the higher drug concentration in the peritoneum than in the subcutis. The amoebicidal effect of the compound against liver abscess caused by Entamoeba histolytica in the golden hamster is distinctly weaker than that of several standard preparations. This fact is clearly demonstrated by

the effective dose of Metronidazole, Tinidazole and
Hoe 316, a 1,4-bis-(methyl-5-nitroimidazolyl-methylene-
imino)-piperazine, in comparison with that of Hoe 088.
For this reason the compound is to be further
developed initially only as a drug against trichomonads. Like other 5-nitroimidazoles the compound
has a good effect against Histomonas meleagridis
the causative organism of Blackhead disease in
turkeys and other fowls. Compared with currently
most active preparation Ipronidazole the efficacy
of Hoe 088 is slightly inferior, whereas it is
slightly superior to Dimetrinidazole. The marked
effect of the compound against Trypanosoma cruzi
must be described as some what surprising. After
repeated oral administration of Hoe 088 a favourable
influence on the course of the infection was detected
in mice following an interval treatment. The results
show that after 50 oral applications 11 of 12 mice
were cured and elimination of amastigote forms was
attained. These results are comparable with those
obtained with Nifurtimox, a nitrofurane, or Hoe 036,
a thioisonicotinic acid amide, compounds which were
specially developed for use against chagas' disease .
African trypanosomes are also killed by Hoe 088
however, only after rather high doses (2 x 200 mg/kg).
But the effect against Trypanosoma congolense is
even less pronounced than against T.brucei, so that
particularly in comparison with the highly active
diamidines the trypanocidal effect of Hoe 088 will
only attain academic interest.

The half-life of 15 hours indicates that the
substance is eliminated relatively slow in the
Wistar-rat after a single oral dose of 75 mg/kg;
the maximum serum level (9 mcg/ml) was attained after
7 hours, but relatively high concentrations were
also measured within 2 and 16 hours of application.
The respective sulfoxide is detectable in the urine
of rats as one of the primary metabolites of Hoe 088,
essential within 24 hours after application. It is
found to be highly active against trichomonads and
other protozoans.

Some toxicological data of Hoe 088 show that the
compound is well tolerated. No side-effects were
observed in the mouse after a single oral dose
of 4000 mg/kg. Wistar rats tolerated ten times the
therapeutic dose, applied daily over a period of
30 days, without showing any side-reactions. Up to
30 times 1000 mg/kg the animals suffered a slight

weight loss, very probably due to the large amount
of the substance administered daily, which caused
disturbed absorption of food. Dogs tolerate the
substance equally well. Vomiting which occurred in
isolated cases after administration of 30 times
250 mg/kg was possibly caused by local irritation of
the well known sensitive dog's stomach.

In Summary it can be said that preparation Hoe 088
has a very good effect against pathogenic trichomonads and marked effect against Histomonas meleagridis and Trypanosoma cruzi, with good tolerance
characteristics. The efficacy of the compound against
other protozoans, as Entamoeba histolytica and
African trypanosomes, is notable but meaningless
compared with corresponding standard preparations.

PHARMACOKINETIC AND METABOLIC STUDIES WITH ORNIDAZOLE IN MAN.

COMPARISON WITH METRONIDAZOLE

D.E. Schwartz, F. Jeunet

Departments of Experimental Medicine/Clinical Research
F. Hoffmann-La Roche & Co. Ltd.
CH-4002 B a s l e

Ornidazole[*](1) is a new compound belonging to the group of the 5-nitro-imidazoles (Fig. 1). It showed marked antiprotozoal activity in vitro and in laboratory animals (2, 3). This activity was further confirmed by clinical studies in patients with intestinal and liver amoebiasis (4, 5, 6), lambliasis (7) and vaginal trichomoniasis (8,9). The compound has no basic nor acidic properties, however, due to its secondary alcohol group it is fairly soluble in water. Remarkable also is its high solubility in ether and chloroform which in turn allows us to anticipate a good solubility in lipids. Our aim was to compare the pharmacokinetics and the metabolism of ornidazole to that of metronidazole (FLAGYL) in man (10). For this purpose both drugs were labelled with ^{14}C in position 2 of the imidazole ring. They were administered orally at a dose of 750 mg and at an interval of 2 to 4 weeks to the same 4 adult volunteers. Additional pharmacokinetic studies of ornidazole with single high doses of the drug were carried out with cold material.

Pharmacokinetics

The bioavailability of ornidazole was studied in two dogs, each dog receiving successively the same dose orally and intravenously. Comparison of the areas under the concentration in plasma versus time-curves indicated for ornidazole, when given orally in gelatine cap-sules, a bioavailability of 94 and 99 %.

---

[*] Trade name = TIBERAL Ⓡ Roche

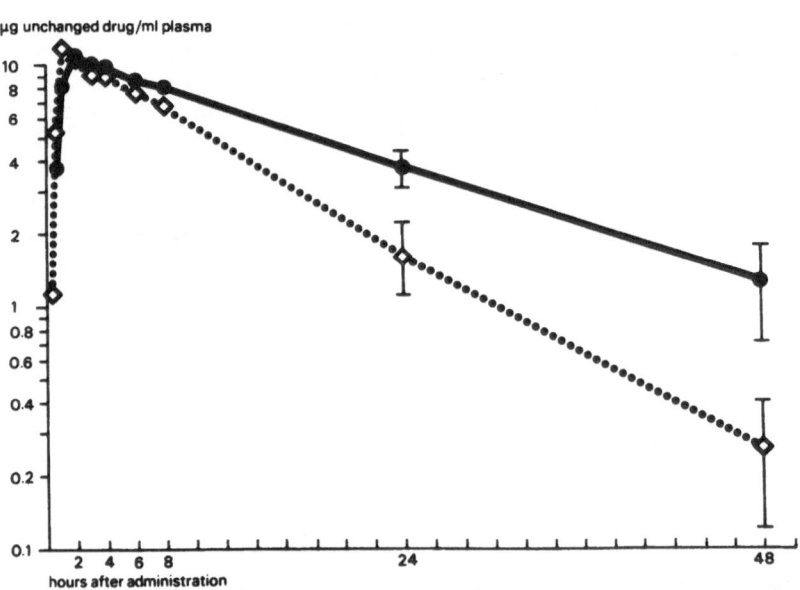

Fig. 1.   Ornidazole

Fig. 2.   Plasma levels of unchanged drug measured in the plasma
of volunteers given 750 mg doses of ornidazole (●————●) or
metronidazole (◇···········◇) orally. Mean values and standards
deviation from the same 4 subjects. (from Chemotherapy 1976 (10)).

Table 1: Half life of elimination from plasma, $t_{1/2}(h)$, of ornidazole and metronidazole in the same subjects.

Subjects	Ornidazole	Metronidazole
1	17.3	10.3
2	13.8	6.6
3	15.5	8.6
4	11.2	8.1
Average	14.4 (∓2.6)	8.4 (∓1.5)

Table 2: Ornidazole: Half life of elimination from plasma $(t_{1/2})$

Dose (mg) Administration	Nr. of Subjects	Sex	Av. Age (y)	Av. weight (kg)	$t_{1/2}$ (h)
750 3 gel. caps. orally	4	m	25	73	14.4 (∓2.6)
2000 4 tablets orally	5	f	36	63	12.6 (∓1.0)
3000 4 tablets orally (2000) 1 tablet vaginally (1000)	4	f	22	54	13.1 (∓1.1)
Average of 13 subjects					13.3 (∓1.7)

Following a single oral dose of 750 mg to man, unaltered ornidazole was found to reach peak plasma concentrations of 8.8 to 14.8 µg/ml within 2 and 3 hours, unaltered metronidazole of 10.1 to 13.9 µg/ml within $\frac{1}{2}$ and 1 hour (Fig. 2). The apparent volume of distribution of the two drugs was found to be practically the same.

The contribution of the unchanged drug to the total radioactivity of plasma progressively decreased with time dropping from the first to the 48th hour, for ornidazole from 80 % to 50 %, for metronidazole from 80 % to 17 %. The remaining part of radioactivity in the plasma represented primarily free extractable metabolites. In the 4 subjects of our study ornidazole was eliminated from plasma with an average half-life of 14.4 hours, metronidazole with one of 8.4 hours (Table 1)

For ornidazole there was further good agreement between half-life values determined in subjects of both sexes given different doses of the drug (Table 2). Figures obtained from 13 individuals amounted on the average to 13.3 $\pm$ 1.7 hours with extreme values of 11.2 and 17.3 hours.

Since the drug is almost entirely metabolized, its rate of elimination from plasma will essentially not be affected by a reduction in renal clearance.

Total radioactivity recovered from urine and faeces during the first 4 days amounted on average for ornidazole and metronidazole to 85 % and 90 % of the dose respectively, 63 % and 77 % being excreted with the urine, 22 % and 14 % with the faeces (Fig. 3).

Metabolism

The urines collected during the first 2 days from 2 subjects were further examined for their content in various metabolites. The unchanged drug together with the free metabolites and those liberated by enzymatic scission of the conjugates were successively extracted with nitromethane.

Unaltered ornidazole found in the urine represented approximately 4 %, its free metabolites 7.9 %, its conjugates (glucuronides and sulfates) 3.7 % of the dose administered, while 44.5 % remained in the aqueous phase (Table 3).

Metronidazole, given to the same subjects, was excreted in somewhat higher percentage unaltered or in the form of free and conjugated metabolites. However, as in the case of ornidazole, the largest part of the radioactivity remained in the aqueous phase.

Extracts of the free metabolites and of the deconjugates were submitted to TL-chromatography. In the case of ornidazole, in addition to the unaltered drug, 6 radioactive compounds could be detected in free form as well as conjugated in the urine (Fig. 4).

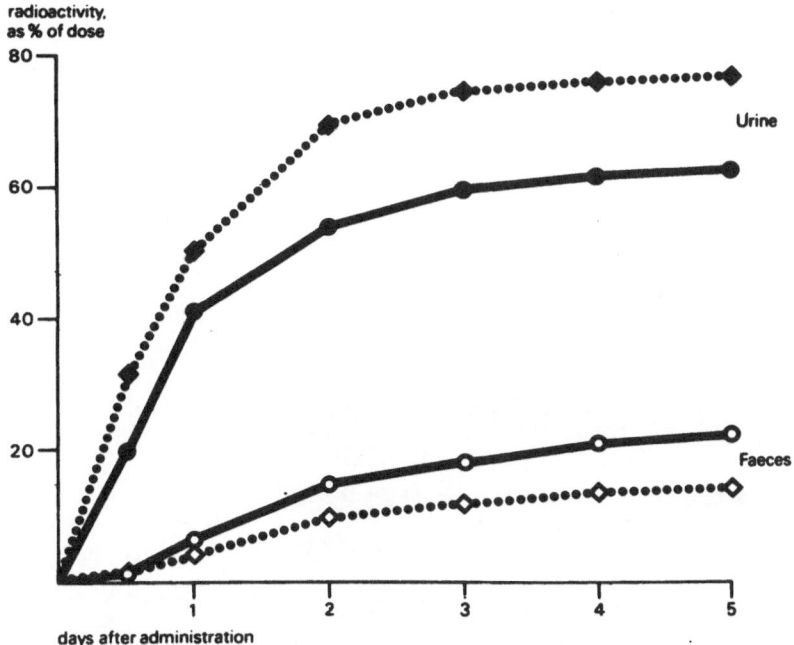

Figure 3. Cumulative values of drug-related readioactivity, expressed as % of dose, recovered in the urine and the faeces from
subjects given 750 mg ^{14}C-labelled ornidazole (● & o) or metronidazole (◆ & ◇) orally. Mean figures from the same 4 subjects.

Table 3: Excretion in the urine – valuesin percent of dose (750mg,
oral).

Drug		Ornidazole		Metronidazole	
Subject		1	2	1	2
Extract A: (direct)	Unchanged drug	3.9	4.0	8.7	6.7
	Free metabolites	9.2	6.7	20.1	14.8
Extract B: (after incubation with glusulase)	Conjugated metabolites (glucu-ronides + sulfates)	3.1	4.3	8.7	12.5
Metabolites remaining in the water phase		47.0	42.0	40.3	38.2

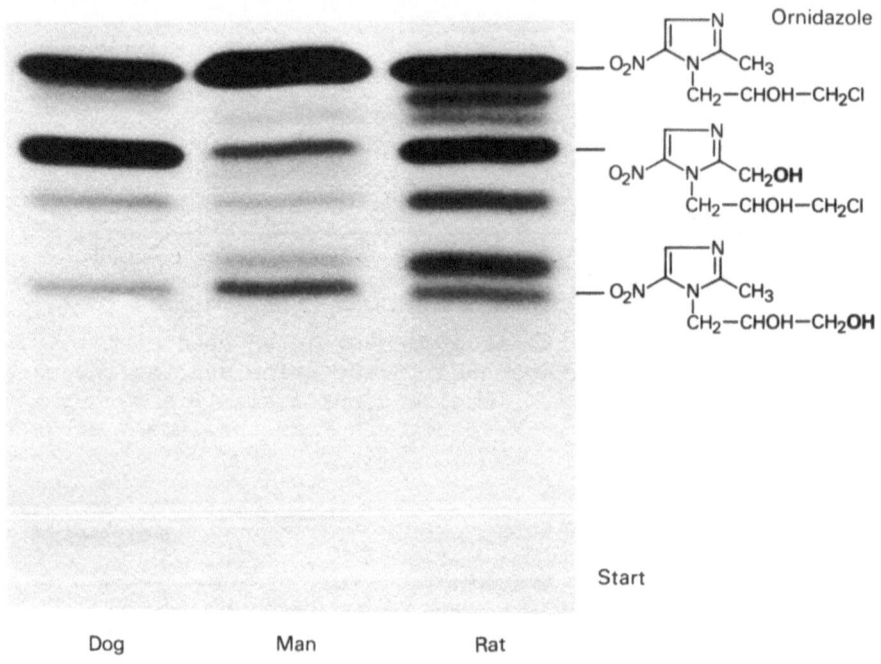

Figure 4. TL-Chromatogram of ornidazole and its free metabolites as present in the urine in three species (Chloroform extract).

In man two of these were present in somewhat larger proportion. After separation by TL-chromatography, their trimethylsilyl derivatives were formed. They were further purified by gas-chromatography and their structure established by mass-spectrometry. One metabolite corresponded to the 2-oxymethyl-derivative, the other to the α-oxymethyl-derivative.

Both metabolites were found to be less active than the parent compound against trichomonas vaginalis.

Until now nothing is known about the structure of the polar, water-soluble metabolites of ornidazole.

The unchanged drug could be detected in the faeces of man. However, its quantitative estimation was not possible due to poor extraction yield.

Single High-dose Therapy in the Treatment of vaginal Trichomoniasis

Single dose therapy with ornidazole, which can easily be controlled by the physician, led to excellent results in the treatment of patients with vaginal trichomoniasis. For such treatment a 2 g oral dose has generally been recommended. For female patients, however, some physicians favor the concomitant topical application of the drug.

For single dose therapy the time during which the drug in the plasma will remain above the minimum inhibitory concentration (MIC) depends primarily upon its initial maximum plasma concentration and its half-life of elimination. On the other hand, maximum plasma levels, if they exceed a certain value, may cause side effects. Thus to develop the full potentialities of a drug it may be necessary to maintain its plasma concentration above the MIC but below toxic levels for as long a period of time as possible. The vaginal application of ornidazole, acting as a slow release form, may prove useful to achieve this goal.

The purpose of our study was to determine to what extent and at what rate the drug was being absorbed from the vagina and how this would influence its plasma levels.

^{14}C-labelled ornidazole, when administered topically in the form of vaginal tablets was slowly absorbed. Total radioactivity measured in the plasma reached maximum values only after approximately 12 hours, as compared to 2 to 3 hours after oral administration (Fig.5). In spite of this slow absorption from the vagina, ornidazole was almost as well absorbed by this route as by the oral one. This is substantiated by the comparison of the areas of total radioactivity of plasma versus time-curves. The total absorption quota of ornidazole, when given vaginally, amounted to 80 % of that obtained after oral administration

Plasma levels of total radioactivity in subjects given a single dose of ^{14}C-ornidazole by different routes
⊙·············⊙ : 750 mg (3 gelatine capsules) orally – Mean and single values of 4 male volunteers –
●————● : 500 mg (1 vaginal tablet) vaginally – Mean and single values of 3 female patients –

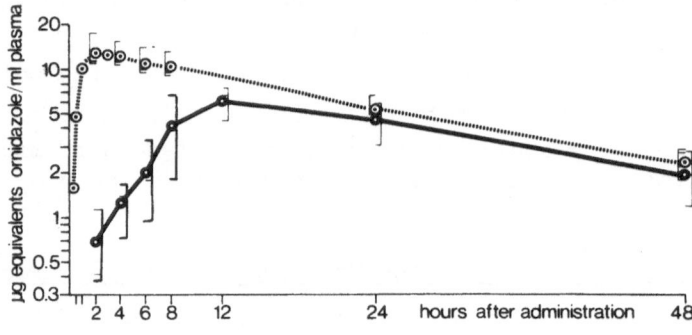

Figure 5

Average plasma levels of ornidazole in female volunteers following administration of:
⊙·············⊙ : 2 g ornidazole orally – 5 subjects –
●————● : 2 g ornidazole orally + 1 g ornidazole vaginally – 4 subjects –

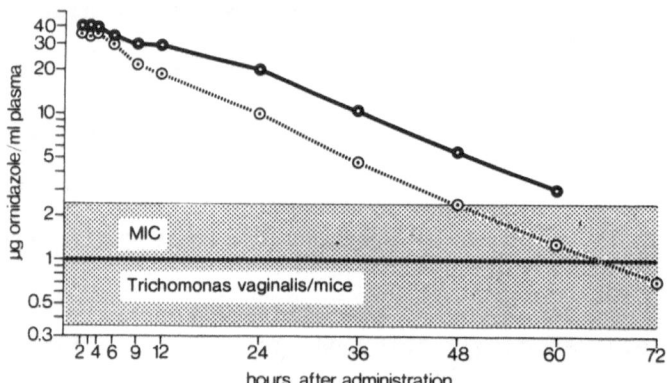

Figure 6

The simultaneous administration of 1 g ornidazole vaginally in addition to 2 g orally did not increase the maximum peak levels but allowed to maintain the MIC in the plasma for an additional 8 hours (Fig. 6).

Confirming this data the cure rate registered in a group of 175 patients given a single 2 g oral dose of ornidazole was 89 % whereas that observed in a group of 102 patients given one dose of 2 g orally + 1 g vaginally amounted to 98 %.

The advantage of the vaginal form may further reside in the fact that, due to its slow absorption, the drug will be present initially in high concentration in this organ. Subsequently, as it gradually reaches the circulatory system, it will sustain the plasma levels and consequently also prolong the time during which it will flow back into the vagina.

Summary

The pharmacokinetics and the metabolism of $2\text{-}^{14}C$-labelled ornidazole and metronidazole have been compared in 4 human subjects.

In spite of great similarities, the two drugs differed essentially by the following:
Ornidazole reached peak concentration in the plasma 2 to 3 hours after administration (metronidazole $\frac{1}{2}$ to 1 hour).
Ornidazole was eliminated from plasma with a mean half-life of 14.4 hours (metronidazole 8.4 hours).
Ornidazole excreted unaltered in the urine amounted to 4 % of the dose (metronidazole 7.7 %).
Of possible further interest were the following observations:
The bioavailability of ornidazole tested in two dogs amounted to 94 and 99 % respectively. In man, unaltered ornidazole and 6 radioactive metabolites were detected in free form as well as conjugated in the urine. Two of these could be identified to the 2-oxymethyl- and α-oxymethyl-derivatives. They were found to be less active against trichomonas vaginalis than the parent compound. Small amounts of ornidazole could be detected in the faeces of man.
Vaginal administration of ornidazole will ensure high initial concentration of the drug in this organ. Subsequently, as it gradually reaches the circulatory system, it will sustain the plasma levels and consequently also prolong the time during which it will flow back into the vagina.

Acknowledgements

We are indebted to Dr. L. Humair, Dept. of Internal Medicine,
Hospital of La Chaux-de-Fonds, Switzerland, to Dr. K. Hernborg-
Johanessen, Dept. of Gynaecology, Haukeland Hospital, Bergen,
Norway,and to Dr. M. Sköld from the Dept. of Dermatology and
Venereal Diseases, and Dr. H. Gnarpe, from the Dept. of Bacteriology,
Gävle Hospital, Sweden, for performing the clinical part of these
investigations.
We also acknowledge the skilful assistance of Miss G.Eckert.

The labelled compounds were synthetized by N. Moser, Dr. R. Barner
and Dr. J. Würsch and mass spectra of metabolites taken and interpreted by M. Oesterhelt and Dr. W. Vetter from the Physical Research
Dept., F. Hoffmann-La Roche & Co. Ltd., Basle, Switzerland.

Bibliography

(1) Hoffer, M. and Grunberg, E.: Synthesis and antiprotozoal activity of 1-(3-Chloro-2-hydroxypropyl)-substituted nitroimidazoles.
J. Med. Chem. 17: 1019-1020 (1974).

(2) Fernex, M., Jeunet, F. and Richle, R.: Development of a nitroimidazole derivative (Ro 7-0207) for the treatment of amoebiasis,
lambliasis and trichomoniasis. 8th Int. Congr. Chemotherapy,
Athens, September 1973.

(3) Richle, R. and Surbek, B.: Entwicklung neuer Nitroimidazol-Deri-
vate als Protozoenmittel. Kongr. Deutschsprachiger Tropenmed.
Ges., Montreux, Juni 1972.

(4) Kee-Mok Cho, Hai-Young Cha and Chin-Thack Soh: Clinical trials
of Ro 7-0207 against Entamoeba histolytica infections (Double
blind trials versus metronidazole). Yonsei Rep. Trop. Med. 3:
123-133 (1972).

(5) Powell, S.J. and Elsdon-Dew, R.: Some new nitroimidazole derivatives. Clinical trials in amoebic liver abscess. Amer. J. trop.
Med. Hyg. 21: 518-520 (1972).

(6) Ruas, A., Ramalho Correia, M.H., Correia do Valle, J. and
Ataide Ribeiro, J.: Ro 7-0207 in amoebic liver abscess. Compara-
tive study of the effects of Ro 7-0207 and metronidazole. Centr.
Afr. J. Med. 19: 128-132 (1973).

(7) Wolfensberger, H.R.: Results of double-blind comparative trials
in amoebiasis and giardiasis with a new nitroimidazole derivative (Ro 7-0207) versus metronidazole. 9th Int. Congr. Trop.
Med. and Malaria, Athens, October 1973.

(8) Lean, T.H. and Vengadasalam, D.: Treatment of vaginal trichomoni-
    asis with a new anti-protozoal compound, α-(chloromethyl)-2-
    methyl-5-nitro-1-imidazole-ethanol. Brit. J. vener. Dis. <u>49</u>:
    69-71 (1973).

(9) Sandront, M.A. and Lambotte, R.: Conception nouvelle de la
    thérapeutique des vaginites à trichomonas vaginalis. Traitement
    minute. Revue Française de Gynecologie <u>69</u>: 623-625 (1974).

(10) Schwartz, D.E. and Jeunet, F.: Comparative Pharmacokinetic
     Studies of Ornidazole and Metronidazole in Man.
     Submitted for publication. Chemotherapy, in press, 1976.

THE DIAGNOSIS AND TREATMENT OF LAMBLIASIS

Dr. W. Altorfer

Specialist in Internal Medicine

Kloten / Switzerland

1. Introduction

   Giardia lamblia is a parasite of the small intestine, which in man is also found in the duodenum. Its occurrence is no longer, as was previously the case, confined to tropical countries, but nowadays is increasingly commoner in temperate countries. Lamblia cysts are transmitted via water which has not been purified or by the consumption of uncooked contaminated foodstuffs. Flies appear to play a part in the spread of the infection : lamblia cysts pass undamaged through the gut of these insects.

   It is well known that lambliasis is asymptomatic in many individuals. The development of symptoms only occurs with massive infestations with invasion of the mucosal villi of the duodenum and small intestine. The principal complaints are abdominal pain, usually confined to the central abdomen, diarrhoea, anorexia, distension and fatigue.

   Increasing attention must be paid to lambliasis with the extension of international air travel. The incidence of the condition in Central Europe has probably been underestimated.

   The trial reported here involves 35 cases of lambliasis in adults, all of whom lived in the neighbourhood of the International Airport at Kloten, and half of whom were employed at the airport.

The diagnosis was made on the basis of the clinical symptoms mentioned above, and the positive results of stool examination. Treatment consisted of the oral administration of 150 mg tinidazole (Fasigyn ®, Pfizer) twice daily for seven days.

2. Material and Methods

Lambliae were identified in 35 patients in the author's practice as a physician, over a period of 16 months. All these patients were adults: no children were included in the trial. The average age was 36 years, and 19 of the patients were women, and 16 men. 17 patients, or nearly half the series, worked at the airport, and one patient was a sewage attendant, and was thus particularly at risk. Two patients had recently returned from the tropics, and one woman patient was employed as a dietetic assistant.

Two separate stool specimens were examined in each patient, a direct smear being examined without using special stains or fixation. Treatment consisted of the oral administration of 150 mg tinidazole twice daily for seven days. Two further stool specimens were examined 14 days after the end of the course of treatment, and a second course prescribed if necessary.

3. Results

The diagnosis was made for the first time in 33 patients; lambliae had been found in one, a sewage attendant, in 1971, and treated with metronidazole. One housewife had been previously unsuccessfully treated with metronidazole.

Reason for Consultation

Abdominal pain	21 Pat.	60 %
Epigastric pain	11 Pat.	31.4 %
Disturbance of appetite	14 Pat.	40 %
Distension	11 Pat.	31.4 %
Diarrhoea	10 Pat.	28.6 %
Pronounced fatigue	4 Pat.	11.7 %
Asymptomatic	8 Pat.	22.9 %

Main Findings on Examination

Tenderness to pressure around umbilicus	26 Pat.	74.3 %
Epigastric tenderness	5 Pat.	14.3 %
Colonic tenderness	6 Pat.	17.1 %
N.A.D.	8 Pat.	22.9 %

Stool Examination

Before treatment	1 x positive	20 Pat.	57.2 %
	2 x positive	15 Pat.	42.8 %
After treatment	negative	30 Pat.	85.7 %
(one course)	positive	5 Pat.	14.3 %

Thus, the success-rate following seven days' treatment with tinidazole was 85.7 %. Five patients were given a second course of treatment, following which the stools were negative in all patients. The success-rate following two courses of treatment was thus 100 %.

A second intestinal parasite was found in three patients. In two cases this was oxyuris and in the third it was whipworm.

Tolerance

Tinidazole was extremely well tolerated, and none of the 35 patients complained of any side-effects.

4. Discussion

The relatively large number of patients suffering from lambliasis may be associated with the area in which they live and their work: all lived near the airport and nearly half were associated with the airport in the course of their work. The introduction of lambliae by international air traffic and transmission to ground personnel and their relations appears to be on the increase, in spite of hygienic measures.

It was striking that 60 % of all patients complained of abdominal pain: epigastric symptoms were present in only 31 % and were therefore much less. This corresponds with the principal site of lamblia infestation - the small intestine. The parasites are less commonly found in the duodenum. In 40 % the disease resulted in anorexia. Diarrhoea is still quoted in the literature as one of the principal symptoms, but was present in only 28.6 % of cases in this series. 22.9 % of the patients were asymptomatic, and this confirms that lambliasis may run a symptom-free course.

Among the results of clinical examination, tenderness around the umbilicus was far the most prominent. Nearly 3/4 of the patients i.e. 74.3 % complained of pain on pressure over the umbilical region. This is an important diagnostic point.

The success-rate following a single course of tinidazole was 85.7 % which is extraordinarily high. The failure-rate of 14.3 % fell to 0 % after a second course of treatment. Lamblia could not be found in the stools of any patients subsequently.

The product was extremely well tolerated and no side-effects were complained of.

In tinidazole, therefore, we have available a highly effective and well tolerated product for the treatment of lambliasis of the small intestine.

Summary

The incidence of lambliasis in adults in Central Europe is probably underestimated.

Over a period of 16 months the author diagnosed lambliasis in 35 adults in his practice. Half of the patients were associated in their work with airport traffic.

The principal symptoms of the disease were abdominal pain, followed by disturbances of appetite and distension. Diarrhoea was seen less often than is described in the literature.

The principal finding on examination of patients with lambliasis was tenderness to pressure restricted to the para-umbilical region, and was found in nearly 3/4 of the patients.

All 35 patients were given tinidazole orally, 150 mg, twice daily for seven days. 30 patients (85.7 %) were cured as a result of this, and a second course of treatment was administered to five patients.

The tolerance of tinidazole was very good, and no side-effects were observed.

TREATMENT OF GIARDIASIS WITH A SINGLE ORAL DOSE OF TINIDAZOLE

Tor Pettersson

Aurora Hospital

Nordensköldinkatu 20   00250 Helskini 25   Finland

Giardia lamblia (intestinalis) is a ubiquitous parasite but it is widespread particularly in tropical countries and in some temperate areas. As a consequence of increased travelling, infestation with the parasite has become more common. It may cause no symptoms but it may also cause longlasting diarrhoea and bowel troubles (4).

In the treatment of giardiasis and trichomoniasis tinidazole (Fasigyn[R]) (ethyl (2-(2-methyl-5-nitro-1-imidazolyl)ethylsulphone) has proved to be an axcellent drug, with a cure rate higher than 90% (2,6,7). The conventional dosage regimen has been 300 mg daily for seven days. However, several investigations have recently shown that treatment of trichomoniasis with a single dose of 2.0 g tinidazole gives excellent results (3,5,8). This "flash therapy" is much more convenient for the patient than the one-week treatment. These reports stimulated me to study the effect of a single-dose treatment of giardiasis with tinidazole.

MATERIAL AND METHODS

Sixty-three adults (24 women and 39 men) whose ages ranged from 18 to 48 years and 14 children between 3 and 10 years who all suffered from symptomatic giardiasis were selected for this study. All the patients had contracted the disease when abroad. The majority had visited East European countries.

The diagnosis of giardiasis was based upon detection of Giardia cysts in two formalin-preserved stool specimens. Salmonella and Shigella infection was excluded by negative culture.

The adults were given 2.0 g of tinidazole in a single dose and the children 1.0 g.

Follow-up examinations were made 1, 4-6 and 12-16 weeks after therapy. On every occasion two stool specimens were examined by the formalin-ether concentration method described by Allen and Ridley (1). The patients were questioned about disappearance of symptoms and whether side effects of the drug had occured.

RESULTS

Table I shows the result of the treatment of the adults. All 63 patients came to the first follow-up, made one week after the drug had been given. In 2 cases cysts of Giardia were demonstrated in stool specimens. Both patients complained of diarrhoea and periodic stomac pains. 59 of these 63 patients attended the second follow-up, performed 4-6 weeks after treatment. In 4 cases cysts of Giardia were detected in the stools. These patients all complained of bowel dysfunction. One of them had been abroad in Eastern Europe during the time between the first and second follow-up. He had a relapse of symptoms shortly after coming home, and reinfection is very probable. 40 patients attended three follow-ups. They were all negative and symptomfree.

Of the 14 children ten were seen at all three follow-up examinations and they all had negative stool samples and were symptomfree, Table II. 2 of these ten had been given 1.0 g tinidazole twice with an interval of 3 days. 3 children had negative results of stool examinations at two follow-ups but were then lost for further check-up because of travelling abroad. One had Giardia cysts in the first stool specimen after treatment. Generally the bowel symptoms disappeared 1 to 3 days after treatment. In a few cases some bowel discomfort lasted about a week.

A second single-dose treatment was given to the 6 adult failures. 2 of these have been cured; one of them was the patient probably reinfected. Two courses of metronidazole (200 mg three times daily for seven days) were given to the other 4 without result. They were then all given mepacrine hydrochloride loo mg three times daily for seven days and have all been cured with that drug.

The single-dose treatment with tinidazole was generally well tolerated by the patients. Only minor side effects, including slight nausea and increased diarrhoea during the day of treatment, were noted in 15% of the cases.

Table I. Treatment of giardiasis with a single dose of 2.0 g
tinidazole. Adults.

No. of patients	Rate of negativity of stool for Giardia in follow-up		
	1 week	4-6 weeks	12-16 weeks
63	61/63	55/59	40/40

No. of failures 6   Cure rate 90%

Table II. Treatment of giardiasis with a single dose of
1.0 g tinidazole. Children.

No. of patients	Rate of negativity of stool for Giardia in follow-up		
	1 week	4-6 weeks	12-16 weeks
14	13/14	13/14	10/10

No. of failures 1   Cure rate 95%

DISCUSSION

The efficacy of the treatment of giardiasis in adults with a single
dose of 2.0 g tinidazole seems to be as good as when the conventional one-week regimen is used. It is much easier for the patient
and well tolerated. The cure rate in this study was 90%. A second
course seems worth trying for the failures but the cure rate was
not very high. As far as can be concluded from the small number
of children included in this study 1.0 g of the drug was an
adequate dosage.

REFERENCES

1   Allen, A.V.H. and Ridley, D.S. (1970). Journal of Clinical
    Pathology, 23, 545.

2   Andersson, T., Forssell, J. and Sterner, G. (1972). British
    Medical Journal, 2, 449.

3   Bedoya, J.M. (1974). Current Medical Research and Opinion,
    2, 165.

4   Leading article (1974) British Medical Journal, 2, 347.

5   Dellenbach, P. and Muller, P. (1974). Current Medical Research
    and Opinion, 2, 142.

6   Howes Jr., H.L., Lynch, J.E. and Kivlin, J.L. (1969).
    Antimicrobial Agents and Chemotherapy, 261.

7   Pettersson, T.(1973). 8th International Congress of Chemo-
    therapy, Athens, Abstract A-453.

8   Schellen, T.M.C.M. and Meinhardt, G. (1974). Current Medical
    Research and Opinion, 2, 158.

A Rural Study in Tanzania of the Chemosuppressant Activity of
Various Regimes of Co-trimoxazole or Chloroquine in Subjects with
P.falciparum Parasitaemia

Th.J. Goosen*, M.A.L. Goosen*, and A.J. Salter**

*East African Institute of Malaria and Vector-borne
 Diseases, Amani Tanzania
**Department of Clinical Investigation
 Wellcome Foundation Ltd., London

INTRODUCTION

Efficacy of co-trimoxazole against a wide range of bacterial
infections is beyond dispute. Both components of this combination
interfere at two sequential points in the folate biosynthetic pathway
of bacteria and plasmodia.

As trimethoprim (TMP) and sulphamethoxazole (SMX) are used in
combination for their antibacterial properties in endemic malarious
areas we considered whether treatment of a bacterial infection in a
patient also suffering from acute malaria might temporarily suppress
the malaria attack only for it to recur with renewed vigour once the
patient had apparently recovered from his infection. This would
obviously be more important in non-immune persons than in semi-immunes.

Although reports in the literature suggest efficacy, we decided
to carry out a controlled study in a semi-immune population unlikely
to be at risk if co-trimoxazole was not properly effective in
malaria.

Furthermore, as chloroquine is an effective drug in Africa we
decided to use chloroquine as the comparative agent. Since pyrexia
of unknown origin (P.U.O.) in malarious areas is frequently treated
blindly with chloroquine plus an antibiotic when there are no
laboratory facilities to make a proper diagnosis, we were also
interested from that point of view.

We wished to know also the minimum effective duration of
co-trimoxazole if used in malaria. Since compliance of patients in
underdeveloped tribal environments is known to be poor, the shortest

treatment course of any drug is advisable. A single dose of therapy is the optimum when follow-up of patients is difficult.

Finally, it has been suggested[1] that the standard three-day course of chloroquine may be marginally less effective in chloroquine-sensitive malaria than a five-day regime.

METHODS

The study was carried out in the Kicheba area of the Muheza sub-district of Tanzania. Kicheba is a group of several villages administered as a settlement scheme, with a population of two to three thousand inhabitants. The villages lie amongst sisal estates on a plain on the coastal side of the Usambara mountains.

Malaria is highly endemic there, and maximum transmission follows the onset of the heavy rains which usually start in about February, although in 1974 these were several months late. The parasite causing malaria in this region is usually P.falciparum.

A Malaria Field Station was constructed and used as a base. It also acted as a dispensary and the laboratory for slide-reading. Transportation around the area for follow-up was by land Rover.

Relations with the inhabitants had been carefully fostered for some time prior to the trial. The administration of the study was facilitated by approaching schools in the area and using the school-child as an introduction to the extended family unit.

Subjects aged 5 to 60 years were chosen for study, unless they were excluded for reasons such as current antimalarial therapy, pregnancy, known hypersensitivity to the study drugs, severe vomiting, or their inability to take oral medication. Patients severely ill with malaria or other diseases were also excluded.

Those eligible for the trial underwent clinical examination, which included body weight, a search for concurrent illness and measurement of spleen size according to Hackett's classification[2].

Thick and thin blood films were examined for malaria parasites, and the thin film was then fixed and the slide stained with Giemsa's stain in saline buffer. Asexual parasites were counted against 200 WBCs and expressed as parasites/mm^3 on the assumption of 8,000 WBCs/mm^3 blood. Gametocytes were counted against 500 WBCs and similarly expressed. Species identification was also recorded.

A table of random numbers was then used to allocate subjects to one of seven treatment groups (Table 1).

TABLE 1

Septrin

Group	Adults		Duration
I	2 tab. b.d.*	1 tab.† b.d. (aged 5-12 years)	1 day
II	"	"	3 days
III	"	"	5 days
IV	"	"	7 days

Chloroquine (expressed as mg base)

Group	Adults		Duration
V	600 mg	10 mg/kg	Single dose
VI	600 mg/day	10 mg/kg/day	2 days)
then	300 mg/day	5 mg/kg/day	1 day) 3 days
VII	600 mg/day	10 mg/kg/day	2 days)
then	300 mg/day	5 mg/kg/day	3 days) 5 days

* Each Septrin tablet contains 80 mg TMP + 400 mg SMX

† or equivalent in suspension

Random allocation appeared to be successful as shown by the age distribution in Table 2. The mean age of the total samples was 12.4 years, as the majority of the subjects were children.

This is also confirmed by the pretreatment parasite densities of the groups (Table 3). The figures do not include P.malariae or P.ovale counts, even though these parasites were present in 45 out of the total 958 cases.

Following randomisation subjects were treated and usually seen daily for parasite counts until these were negative or until two days after treatment stopped. They were then seen once weekly for about four weeks, but the follow-up period did not exceed 40 days.

TABLE 2

Age distribution

		----SEPTRIN----			Treatment Group	------CHLOROQUINE------			
Age in Years	1 day I	3 days II	5 days III	7 days IV	Single dose V	3 days VI	5 days VII	TOTAL
1-10	54	54	61	50	60	59	57	395
11-20	77	75	64	81	70	70	71	510
21-30	3	4	4	5	3	3	6	28
31-40	1	4	1	2	3	2	2	15
41-50	-	1	1	-	1	1	1	5
51-60	1	-	2	-	-	-	1	4
> 61	-	1	-	1	-	-	-	2
N/R	-	-	-	-	1	-	-	1
TOTAL	136	139	133	139	138	135	138	958
MEAN AGE	12.2	12.9	12.4	12.5	12.2	11.9	12.7	12.4

94% of subjects are aged 20 years or less

TABLE 3

Initial parasite densities

Falciparum densities expressed as number/mm^3 blood.

	Treatment group	Mean	sd	n	Observed range
I	1 day Septrin	4301	8145	136	80 - 54400
II	3 days Septrin	3801	7714	139	80 - 48480
III	5 days Septrin	4769	8639	133	80 - 60640
IV	7 days Septrin	3448	6966	139	80 - 44800
V	Single dose Chloroquine	5544	14539	138	80 -105760
VI	3 days Chloroquine	4352	10238	135	80 - 75200
VII	5 days Chloroquine	4410	9271	138	40 - 59560

There are no significant differences in mean initial densities between the treatment groups.

RESULTS

Parasite clearance rates are shown in Table 4, which indicates numbers of cases showing their first negative count after starting treatment. Not one subject became negative and then positive during the initial period of daily observation. The mean time to negativisation was less than three days in all groups, and there was no difference between them ($p > 0.05$).

TABLE 4

Clearance of asexual forms		Post-treatment day when first zero count observed								
Treatment Group		1	2	3	4	5	6	>6	ND	TOTAL
I	1 day Septrin	27	58	25	16	1	4	4	1	136
II	3 days Septrin	24	50	35	18	7	2	3	-	139
III	5 days Septrin	17	63	25	15	7	4	2	-	133
IV	7 days Septrin	22	58	27	24	6	-	2	-	139
V	Single dose Chloroquine	18	52	33	17	9	3	6	-	138
VI	3 days Chloroquine	19	46	42	16	6	4	2	-	135
VII	5 days Chloroquine	15	52	32	24	4	8	3	-	138

TABLE 5

Falciparum (asexual) recurrence –
all asexual falciparum recurrences,
whether or not gametocytes are present.

Group		No. of subjects recurring	No. of subjects not recurring	Total
I	1 day Septrin	41 (30.4%)	94	135
II	3 days Septrin	25 (18.0%)	114	139
III	5 days Septrin	25 (18.8%)	108	133
IV	7 days Septrin	22 (15.8%)	117	139
V	Single dose Chloroquine	21 (15.2%)	117	138
VI	3 days Chloroquine	8 (5.9%)	127	135
VII	5 days Chloroquine	6 (4.4%)	131	137

Recurrence of parasitaemia during the four-week follow-up period is shown in Table 5. The recurrence rate in the one-day co-trimoxazole group was significantly higher than in the other groups (p < 0.05). There was no difference in the recurrence rates between groups II, III, IV and V (p > 0.05). In the three and five-day chloroquine groups these were significantly lower than in the other groups (p < 0.05).

The time to recurrence was taken as the post-treatment day on which parasitaemia recurred (Table 6), and was similar in all the groups.

There were no differences between the groups with respect to the presence of falciparum gametocytes in the follow-up period (Table 7).

TABLE 6

Recurrence during follow-up

Group		Time to recurrence (days)		
		Mean	sd	N
I	1 day Septrin	23.8	5.5	41
II	3 days Septrin	25.5	6.2	25
III	5 days Septrin	26.5	5.2	25
IV	7 days Septrin	26.6	3.8	22
V	Single dose Chloroquine	26.4	5.7	21
VI	3 days Chloroquine	28.5	6.5	8
VII	5 days Chloroquine	25.7	5.6	6

TABLE 7

Falciparum gametocyte presence –
whether or not asexual falciparum were present.

Group		No. of subjects with gametocytes	No. of subjects without	Total
I	1 day Septrin	8 (5.9%)	127	135
II	3 days Septrin	8 (5.8%)	131	139
III	5 days Septrin	12 (9.0%)	121	133
IV	7 days Septrin	9 (6.5%)	130	139
V	Single dose Chloroquine	3 (2.2%)	135	138
VI	3 days Chloroquine	3 (2.2%)	132	135
VII	5 days Chloroquine	7 (5.1%)	130	137

DISCUSSION

The time available does not allow full discussion of the interesting and possibly controversial points arising from this study.

It is clear, however, that co-trimoxazole is rapidly effective in clearing asexual forms in this particular group of subjects even when used for one day. This is also true of even a single dose of chloroquine. In the light of the difficulties now being encountered in malaria eradication schemes these facts should not be lightly dismissed with respect to a mass chemotherapy approach.

As these subjects were presumably semi-immunes and their pretreatment parasite counts only moderately high, equivalent activity cannot be assumed in non-immunes with heavy parasitaemia without further study.

The one-day co-trimoxazole treatment, at least at the dosage given, is clearly unsatisfactory. The three and five-day chloroquine regimes were the most successful.

One cannot definitely exclude the possibility that reinfection, rather than relapse, was higher by chance in the two chloroquine groups VI and VII, but it is unlikely that such bias occurred. Nevertheless, this concept is favoured by the fact that time to recurrence was similar in all the groups. Only a study of subjects with malaria travelling into a non-malarious region and being treated there would conclusively answer that question.

As a result of this study one can only say that the possibility of malaria relapse after co-trimoxazole treatment can not be excluded.

Active search continues for drugs suitable for the treatment of chloroquine-resistant malaria. We recommend that co-trimoxazole is studied in this situation prior to any recommendation to use this combination in chloroquine-resistant malaria. In addition, efficacy against pyrimethamine-resistant and P.vivax malaria should be examined.

Co-trimoxazole should not be considered as a long-term prophylactic agent against malaria. Several reasons exist for this contention, namely that frequent dosing would probably lead to loss of patient compliance, that folate impairment may be induced in populations with poor nutritional states where malaria is endemic, and finally cost.

Should co-trimoxazole be effective, however, in the conditions outlined earlier, then other problems must be considered, such as the possibility of plasmodial and bacterial resistance induction and the vexed question of use in tropical P.U.O.

Whatever the outcome of these considerations, we believe that co-trimoxazole will continue to generate discussion by those interested in the treatment of bacterial infections and malaria.

References

1. Haworth, J. Personal communication.

2. Hackett, L.W. (1944), J. nat. Malar. Soc., 3, 121.

RESULTS OF THE ANTI-T. CRUZI ACTIVITY OF Ro 07-1051* IN MAN

Jose A. Cerisola, Carlos A. Barclay, Humberto Lugones
and Oscar Ledesma
Instituto Nacional de Diagnostico e Investigacion de la
Enfermedad de Chagas 'Dr.M.F.Chaben', Buenos Aires
Argentina

The anti-Trypanosoma cruzi activity of the compound Ro 07-1051
(N-benzyl-2-nitro-1-imidazoleacetamide) was investigated in 107
acute Chagas' disease cases. The dosage used was 3 up to 10 mg/Kg
per day for a one month period. Sero-parasitological follow up
tests were performed monthly and results of a 12 months follow up
are available for 76 cases. The xenodiagnosis became negative in
45 (83.3%) children and 8 (36.4%) infants and both the complement
fixation test and indirect haemaglutination test decreased the
positivity significantly. Immunofluorescence tests showed negative
reactions or a significant decrease of the titres in successfully
treated patients. Skin reactions were observed in 14% of the
patients.

. . . .

The chemotherapeutic agent Ro 07-1051 (N-Benzyl-2-nitro-1-
imidazoleacetamide) (Fig.1) has shown a systemic activity comparable to that of Nitrofurazone in mice experimental infected with
T.cruzi (Richle, 1973). Results of a 12 months follow up of acute
cases (Barclay et al, 1974) and acute and chronic cases (Lugones
et al, 1974) were reported.

MATERIAL AND METHODS

The anti-T.cruzi activity of the compound was investigated in
107 acute Chagas' disease cases with a mean age of 5 years and an
average weight of 12 Kg. Before treatment, the presence of the
parasite was demonstrated in blood smears and/or zenodiagnosis.

*F. Hoffmann-La Roche et Cie, Basle, Switzerland.

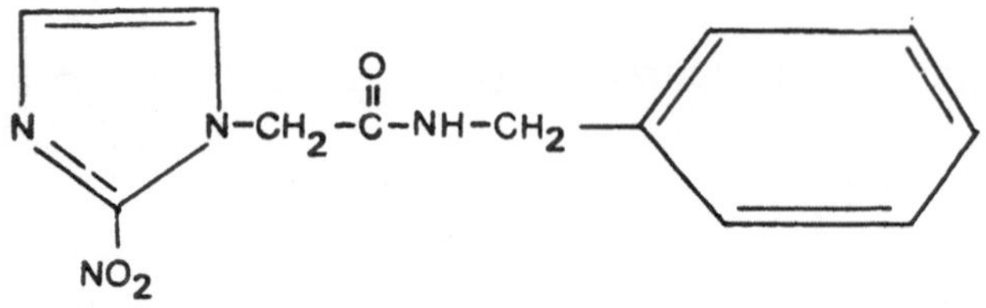

N-Benzyl-2-nitro-1-imidazoleacetamide

Fig. 1. Ro 7-1051.

Table I: Acute Chagas' disease. Serial xenodiagnosis in 76
patients treated with Ro 07-1051.

GROUP	Number of Patients	XENODIAGNOSIS Positive		Negative	
		Total	%	Total	%
Infants	22	14	63.6	8	36.4
Children	54	9	16.7	45	83.3
Total	76	23	30.3	53	69.7

The compound was administered at increasing doses of 3 up to
10 mg/Kg daily for a period of one month. Clinical examinations
and seroparasitological studies were performed in each patient
at regular intervals for a period of 12 months or more, following
the initial diagnosis. Laboratory tests were performed once a
month during the first 5 months and every 3 months thereafter.
It is necessary to point out that re-infection possibility was
carefully avoided.

The demonstration of T.cruzi in peripheral blood was performed by xenodiagnosis, the most sensitive procedure for
recovering the parasite. Essentially it consists in having the
suspect patient bitten by a certain number of nymphs of any of
the varieties of bugs known to develop T.cruzi in the intestinal
tract.

After a predetermined period of time, the intestinal duct or
faeces of the insects are examined for the presence of T.cruzi.
Altogether, this is the equivalent to a blood culture performed
in the natural host.

In the present study, xenodiagnosis was performed with 4 boxes
containing each 10 nymphs of the 3rd. instar of Triatoma infestans.

The antibodies were demonstrated through complement fixation
test (CFT), haemagglutination test (HAT) and fluorescent antibody
test (FAT).

RESULTS

The therapeutic efficacy of a 12 month follow up period is
available for 76 cases (54 children and 22 infants). In this group
a total of 465 xenodiagnosis were applied, which means 1,860 boxes
(18,600 insects) with an average of 6.1 xenodiagnosis for each
patient. Post-treatment xenodiagnosis remained persistently negative in 45 (83.3%) children and 8 (36.4%) infants (Table I). This
discrepancy in the rate of successful treatment between both groups,
perhaps may be related to insufficient or inaccurate administration
of the drug.

The serological findings of the whole group (Fig.2) demonstrated
that in day 0 (when the clinical diagnosis was made and parasites
could be demonstrated in peripheral blood) the positive rate was
57.6% and 20.3% for CFT and HAT respectively. An increase of the
positive rate was observed in both tests at the end of the first
month but, from the second and third months on, however, the
positivity fell clearly and stabilised around 20% up to 12 months.

That means that around 80% of the treated patients became
negatives.

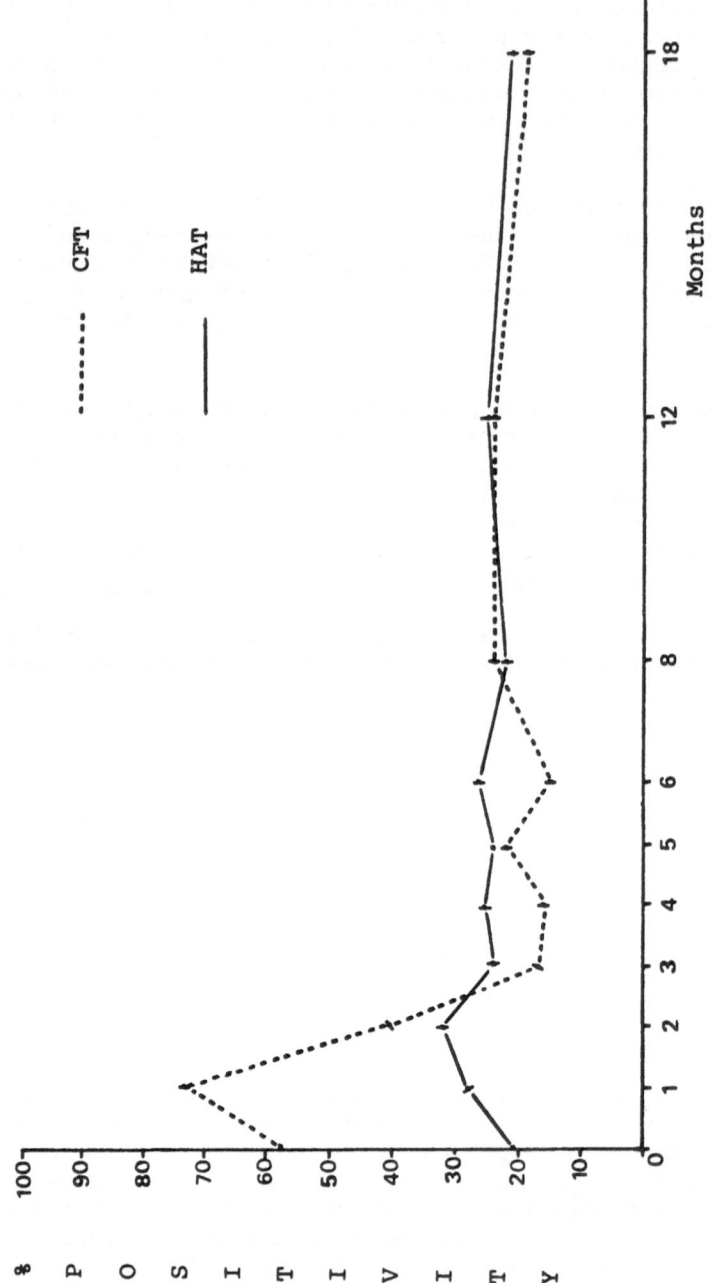

Fig. 2. Acute Chagas' disease. Immunodiagnostic response after
treatmetn with Ro 07-1051 in 76 patients.

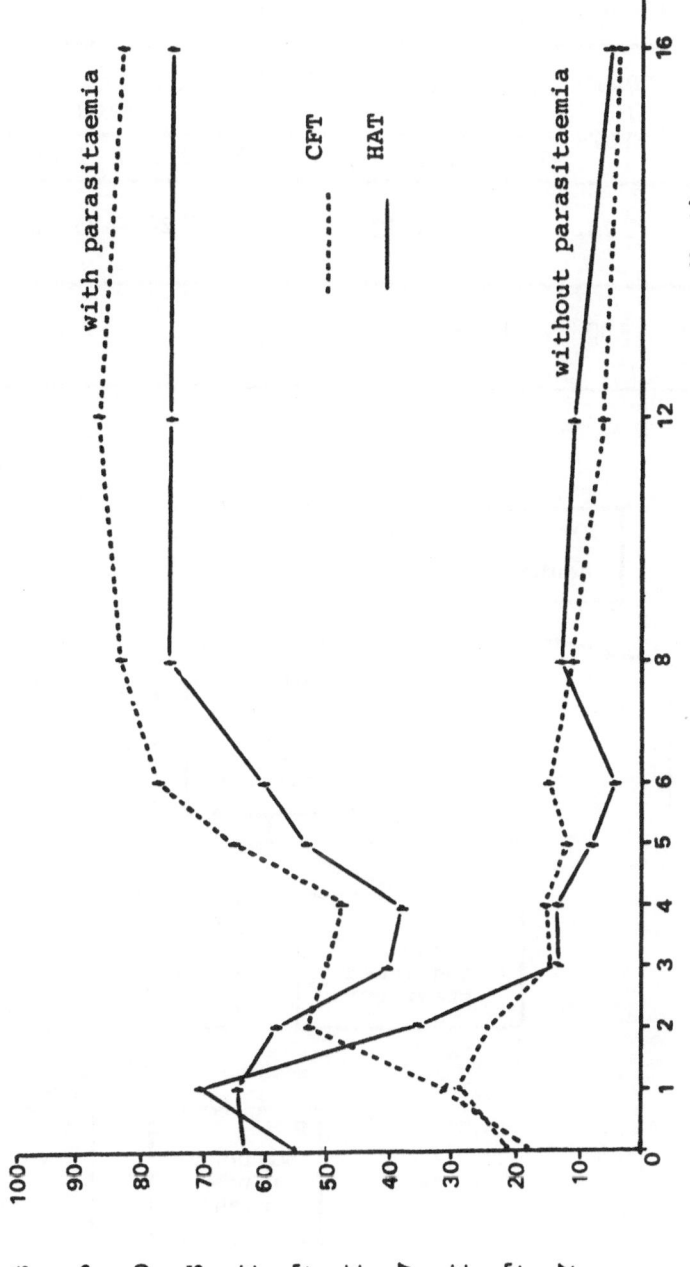

Fig. 3. Acute Chagas' disease. Imunodiagnostic response after treatment with Ro 07-1051 in 76 patients.

Table II. Acute Chagas' disease. Fluorescent antibody test (PAT)
12-18 months follow-up titers after the end of
treatment (128 tests performed).

XENODIAGNOSIS	NUMBER OF TESTS	TITERS						
		LOW				HIGH		
		Neg.	1/30	1/60	1/120	1/240	1/480	1/960
Positive Persistent parasitaemia	28	4 - 14.3%				24 - 85.7%		
Negative Without parasitaemia	100	98 - 98.0%				2 - 2.0%		

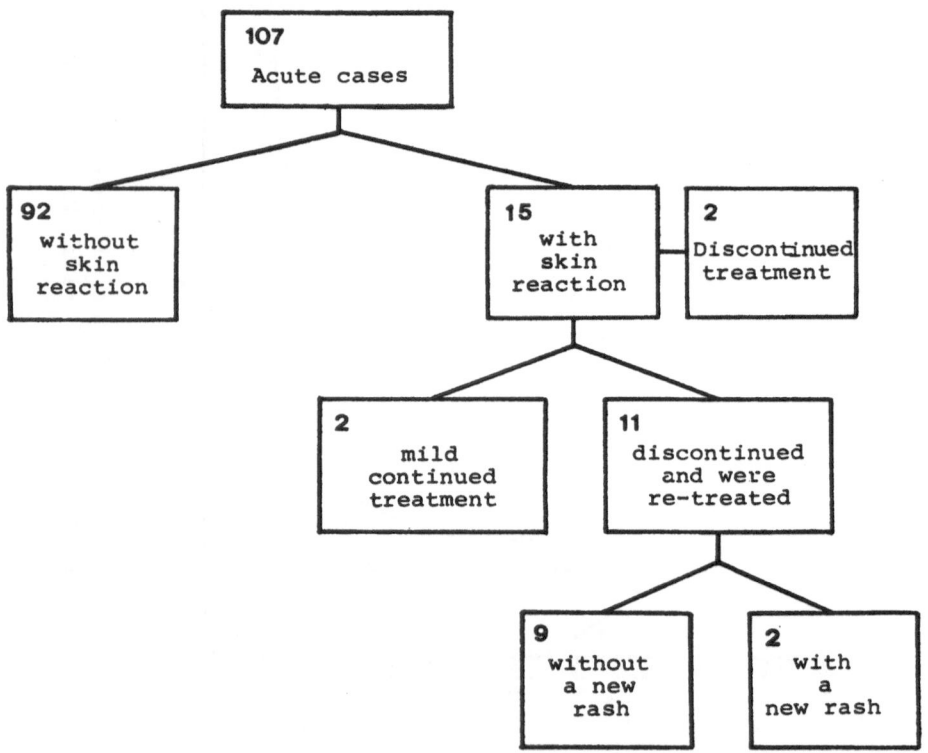

Fig. 4. Acute Chagas' disease. Side effects in 107 patients
treated with Ro 07-1051.

It is of interest to compare the results of the serological reactions in the group of patients parasitologically negatives with those with persistent parasitaemia (Fig. 3).

From the second and third month both groups reach a different percentage of positivity for CFT and HAT. The curve is stable up to 18 months follow up- patients without parasitaemia reach a serological positivity around 4.7% for the CFT and 4.3% for the HAT, whilst in patients with parasitaemia this percentage is 75 and 83.3% respectively. Consequently we verified a correlation between xenodiagnosis and serology.

The fluorescent antibody test (FAT) was performed by means of a semi-quantitative procedure using serum dilutions. The results of the FAT were different when comparing the groups with or without persistent parasitaemia (Table II); negative reactions or smallest titres were observed in 98% of the patients of the second group and in only 14.3% of the first. 87.5% of the patients with positive xenodiagnosis reached high titres and on the contrary only 2% of those with negative xenodiagnosis.

In conclusion, the FAT became negative or had a significantly decreased titre in successfully treated patients.

SIDE EFFECTS

Skin reactions, observed in 14% of the patients (Fig. 4) were the most frequent side effect but in only two the treatment was discontinued.

CONCLUSIONS

The results of our studies to date support the conclusion that at the doses used the compound possesses a marked therapeutic activity in the treatment of the acute stage of Chagas' disease and further trials are necessary both in acute and chronic cases in order to confirm these promising results.

REFERENCES

Barclay, C.A., Cerisola, J.A., Lugones, H., Ledesma, O. and Jozami, L.B. (1974) Proceedings of the XIVth International Congress of Pediatrics, Buenos Aires, 4, 238.

Lugones, H., Rabinovich, B., Cerisola, J.A., Ledesma, O. and Barclay, C.A. (1974) Third International Congress of Parasitology, Munich, 25-31 August.

Richle, R. (1973) Ninth International Congress on Tropical Medicine and Malaria, Athens, 14-21 October.

THE EFFICIENCY OF METRONIDAZOLE 'FLAGYL'* AGAINST <u>TRYPANOSOMA</u> <u>EVANSI</u> IN VIVO

A.M. Mandour and A.M. Abd-El Rahman

Department of Parasitology, Faculty of Medicine

Assiut University, Egypt

INTRODUCTION

<u>Trypanosoma evansi</u> is the cause of an important disease in camels known as Surra. This parasite might also be the cause of an acute and fatal disease in horses and dogs, while the infection results in a chronic disease in donkeys and transient in cattle. (Levine, 1961). According to Chandler and Read (1961) animals were formerly treated, with only fair success, with antimony compounds and antrypol, but recently two new drugs, dimidium bromide (Phenanthridium) and antrycide in the form of methyl sulphate or chloride salts, have greatly brightened the picture. However, antrycide is less effective against <u>Trypanosoma brucei</u>. <u>T.evansi</u> and <u>T.equiperdum</u>. On the other hand, dimidium bromide is ineffective against <u>T.brucei</u>, <u>T.evansi</u> and <u>T.simiae</u>.

The present work has been carried out in attempts to find a potent and safe drug for the treatment of Surra. The senior author in the present work has suggested the possible trypanocidal effects of metronidazole "Flagyl" which already affects some protozoan parasites such as <u>Trichomonas vaginalis</u>, <u>Giardia lamblia</u> and <u>Entamoeba histolytica</u>.

MATERIAL AND METHODS

<u>Trypanosoma evansi</u> has been isolated from naturally infected camels at Bany Ady, Assiut (Upper Egypt). The strain could be transmitted to white rats, white mice and puppies. The rats were inoculated intraperitoneally each with 1 ml, the mice with 0.3 ml and the puppies were inoculated intravenously with 1.5 ml of the virulent citrated blood. The average weight of the white rat was

*A product of Specia Company (France)

about 100 gm, while the average weight of the white mouse was
20 gm. The weight of the puppies was from 6-8 Kgm. The number of
trypanosomes in thin blood films of the infected camel was 3-5 per
high power field. The maximum number of trypanosomes appeared on
the third to fifth day in rats and mice, while in dogs it reached
the maximum on the ninth day after giving the infection.

Attempts to treat rats, mice and dogs with "Flagyl"

1.   Ten infected rats were given the drug (10-25 mg per 100 gm
body weight) through a stomach tube.

2.   Ten mice already infected with the same strain were inoculated intraperitoneally with the drug (1-10 mg per 20 gm body
weight).

3.   Two puppies were inoculated intravenously with two doses
of "Flagyl" with 48 hours interval- the dose being 5'8 mg per Kgm
body weight.

    Blood films were prepared to be examined daily for one
month for the detection of any sign of parasitological cure. Control animals consisted of infected groups of mice and rats, in
addition to two puppies. They were left without being treated.
Their blood was daily examined.

    Parasitological cure was based on the absence of the para-
site in blood films, and when the suspected blood was inoculated
intraperitoneally into mice with negative results.

OBSERVATIONS

    The present experiments have shown that "Flagyl" is curative
when given by intravenous, intraperitoneal, subcutaneous routes
as well as through the stomach tube (per os). The trypanosomes
disappeared from the blood of mice and rats within the first 48
hours of treatment, while the puppies became trypanosome-free
within 72 hours. No side effects were observed on the treated
animals. Follow up of the treated mice, rats and puppies showed
negative results during the course of one month. Control animals
died within 4-9 days for rats and mice, but the puppies died
after 2-6 months. The puppies lost weight, suffered from anaemia
oedema of the dependant parts of the body, conjunctivitis and
before they died they became "bags of skin and bone".

    During the first 24 hours after treatment with "Flagyl"
the trypanosomes were aggregated in groups (Fig. 1). Stumpy
forms and dividing forms were occasionally observed.

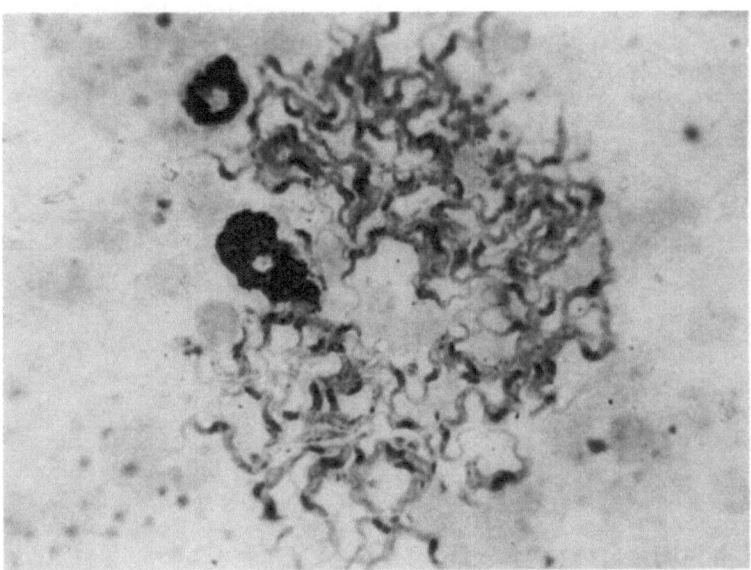

Fig. 1 Photomicrograph showing aggregates of <u>Trypanosoma evansi</u>
24 hours after giving "Flagyl" X6000

DISCUSSION

From the present experiments, it is obvious that "Flagyl"
has a potent effect against <u>Trypanosoma evansi</u> in experimentally
infected mice, rats and puppies. Ormerod (1951) working on
trypanocidal drugs suggested that drugs with heavy molecular
weight and more electric charges could be used as trypanocidal.
According to this suggestion, "Flagyl" has got a heavy molecular
weight with two double bonds, a fact which might support the view
of Ormerod (1951). It has been suggested by the latter author
(Ormerod, 1975) that "Flagyl" may have killed a proposed occult
phase of <u>T.evansi</u>, thus production of blood stages have stopped.
He added (Ormerod, 1975) that "Flagyl" affects the anaerobic
stages considering that the blood stages are aerobic and the proposed occult stages are anaerobic. However, in the present work
it appears that "Flagyl" has affected both. The present drug
might be useful when given to camels and horses which can be
treated with one dose. However, this suggestion needs further
investigation to study the toxicity of this drug in such domestic
animals. If future work shows that "Flagyl" is effective against
<u>T.evansi</u> in our domestic animals, it will be superior to Suramine
(Germanin, Naganol) which may produce toxic effects in treated
animals. Moreover, "Flagyl" is effective when given by mouth,

in addition to other routes, while "Suramine" should be administered intravenously. In addition, it is found by Goodman and Gilman (1963) that "Flagyl" in large doses affects neither the cardio-vascular nor the respiratory systems. The only difficulty in the usage of "Flagyl" is that it is sparingly soluble in water, thus it should be given in a suspension form.

The present work may open the field for research workers to study the efficiency of "Flagyl" against the trypanosomes of sleeping sickness in man in Africa.

SUMMARY

The authors found that metronidazole "Flagyl" produced by Specia Company (France) is efficient against Trypanosoma evansi when it was given by mouth, intravenously and intra-peritoneally. It has no toxic effects to laboratory animals and dogs. The trypanosomes disappeared from the blood within a few days. It has been suggested that its effect in domestic animals should be studied since it is a safe and a potent drug.

REFERENCES

Chandler, C. and Read, C.P. (1961) Introduction to Parasitology with special reference to the parasites of man. Wiley International Edition. Toppan Company, Tokyo, Japan.

Goodman, L.S. and Gilman, A. (1968) The Pharmacological basis of therapeutics. Third edition. The McMillan Co., New York.

Levine, N.D. (1961) Protozoan parasites of domestic animals and of man. First edition. Burgess Pnblishing Co., Minneapolis, Minnesota, U.S.A.

Ormerod, W.E. (1951) A study of basophilic inclusion bodies produced by chemotherapeutic agents in trypanosomes. Brit. J. Pharm., 6, 334-341.

Ormerod, W.E. (1975) Personal communication, London July 1975.

EMERICID (31 559 R.P.) : A NEW ANTICOCCIDIAL

F. BENAZET, J.R. CARTIER, J. FLORENT, C. JOHNSON,
J. LUNEL, D. MANCY
Rhône-Poulenc-Centre Nicolas Grillet, Vitry s/Seine,
France
and Rhodia Inc. Animal Health Division-Ashland-Ohio

During the past 25 years, several different antibiotics
containing an acid group and a cyclic polyether structure have been
discovered, some of which are potent anticoccidial agents.
31,559 R.P. recently isolated in our laboratories belongs to this
family.

PRODUCTION OF 31,559 R.P.

31,559 R.P. is produced from Streptomyces hygroscopicus
DS 24,367 by classical submerged fermentation technics. The active
antibiotic is extracted from the mycelium using an organic solvent
and purified by chromatography and cristallisation.

PHYSICOCHEMICAL PROPERTIES

These are shown in table I. According to its physical characteristics, N.M.R. spectra data and the X ray diffraction studies
it appears that this product is original.

ANTICOCCIDIAL ACTIVITY IN CHICKS

Anticoccidial activity of 31,559 R.P. has been evaluated in a
series of battery trials against single infections of Eimeria
tenella, E. acervulina, E. necatrix, E. maxima, E. brunetti and in
floor pen trials against mixed infections of 5 species. These
studies have involved approximately 8 000 chicks. Only some
representative trials are reported here.

Table 1 - Physicochemical properties of 31,559 R.P., sodium salt

Aspect	white microcrystallized powder	
Melting point	181.5°C	
Molecular formula	$C_{44}H_{75}O_{14}Na$ (851.064)	
Elemental composition	Found %	Calculated %
C	62.3	62.10
H	8.8	8.88
O	27.5	26.32
Na	2.8	2.70
$[\alpha]_D^{20}$ (c = 1 in methanol)	+ 48.6° ± 1°	
Neutral equivalent (perchloric acid)	840	

Controlled Battery Experiments

Customary methods and criteria of efficacy were used. Vantress x Pilch broiler chickens 16 days of age. Sporulated oocysts were inoculated directly into the chicks crop or mixed with the feed. Depending on the species, the inoculum varied from 10^5 to 10^6 oocysts. Broiler starter mash or pellets were used as the basal ration.Concentrations of 31,559 R.P. in the feed were 0.01 % to 0.0045 %. Medication was initiated 72 to 24 hours prior to inoculation for E. tenella and 24 hours prior to inoculation or on the day of exposure for other species and was continued for between 7 to 14 days post exposure. 31,559 R.P. was compared with monensin (0.0121 and 0.01 %), with uninoculated, unmedicated controls and with inoculated, unmedicated controls. Mean weight gain of birds, percentage mortality, gross pathology, fecal droppings and oocyst production were the criteria assessed. The results are summarized in table 2.

E. tenella : At 0.009 %, 31,559 R.P. has a superior effect on weight gain and a comparable effect on mortality, lesion score and pen score to that of monensin at 0.121 %. At 0.0063 % level, 31,559 R.P. is only slightly less active than at the 0.009 %.

E. acervulina : 31,559 R.P. (0.01 to 0.0075 %) is highly effective ; at the lowest level (0.0075 %) it compares favorably with monensin at either of its use levels (0.0121 % and 0.01 %).

E. necatrix : mortality in the nonmedicated infected groups and clinical signs confirm the severity of the infection. The activity demonstrated by 31,559 R.P. at 0.01-0.00875 and 0.0075 % is as good as that of monensin (0.0121 and 0.01 %).31,559 R.P. is capable of permitting normal growth during the critical periods of a severe E. necatrix infection.

Table 2 – Battery evaluation against single infections

Eimeria Treatment	No chicks	awg (g)	mort. %	lesion score	pan score	oocyst %
E. tenella		D + 6		D + 6	D + 6	
umui	79	212.5	0	0	0	0
umi	80	-26	33.7	4	4	100
31,559 R.P. 0.009 %	239	197.7	0	0.21	0.42	3.8
" 0.0063 %	239	174	1.2	0.55	1.33	22
" 0.0045 %	240	171.2	3.7	1.75	2.84	65
monensin 0.0121 %	79	174.1	0	0.16	0.67	10
E. acervulina		D + 5		D + 5	D + 6	
umui	40	174		0	0	0
umi	40	65		4	4	100
31,559 R.P. 0.01 %	40	161		0.4	0	2.2
" 0.00875 %	39	160		0.33	0	5.5
" 0.0075 %	40	161		0.5	0.3	6.5
monensin 0.0121 %	40	128		0	0	10
" 0.01 %	40	159		0	0	7
E. necatrix		D + 7		D + 5	D + 7	
umui	40	243	0	0	0	
umi	40	39	40	3.7	4	
31,559 R.P. 0.01 %	40	231	0	0	0	
" 0.00875 %	40	235	0	0	0	
" 0.0075 %	39	238	0	0	0	
monensin 0.0121 %	40	200	0	0.5	0	
" 0.01 %	40	230	0	0.4	0.25	
E. maxima		D + 7		D + 8	D + 7	
umui	40	227		0	0	0
umi	40	86		100	4	100
31,559 R.P. 0.01 %	40	208		0	0	108
" 0.00875 %	40	208		0	0.5	179
" 0.0075 %	40	207		0	0.75	205
monensin 0.0121 %	37	187		70	0	191
" 0.01 %	40	196		60	0.75	302
E. brunetti		D + 7		D + 7	D + 6	
umui	39	252		0	0	0
umi	40	123.5		100	4	100
31,559 R.P. 0.01 %	39	201.7		60	0.25	14
" 0.00875 %	40	196.5		90	1.75	58
" 0.0075 %	39	208.7		100	2.75	44
monensin 0.0121 %	40	175.7		100	0.75	45
" 0.01 %	40	199.5		100	2	43

umui = unmedicated uninfected   umi = unmedicated infected
awg = average weight gain   D + = day postinoculation

E. maxima : the data substantiate the activity of 31,559 R.P.
(0.01 - 0.00875 and 0.0075 %) against an infection that caused a
weight gain reduction of 62 % in nonmedicated infected birds.
Weight gains of the 31,559 R.P. treated birds were about 90 % of
these for noninfected nonmedicated birds. These results compare
favorably with those obtained with monensin (0.0121 and 0.01 %).

E. brunetti : although 31,559 R.P. at the levels tested (0.01-
0.00875 - 0.0075 %) does not demonstrate the high level of activity
reported for other species of Eimeria, it is slightly more potent
than monensin at 0.0121 and 0.01 %.

Floor Pen Experiments

The first experiment was designed to evaluate the activity of
31,559 R.P. against a 5 species infection and also to evaluate the
ability of the compound to prevent or control the spread of
coccidiosis to birds whose pen mates were experimentally infected.
Day-old chicks were started on clean litter and medicated feed was
offered immediatly. On the 14th day 50 of 180 birds in each pen
were inoculated ; medication was continued until the birds were
8 weeks old. The results are summarized in table 3. The mortality
of inoculated chicks ranged from 79 % in the nonmedicated control
group to 0 % in the 0.009 % 31,559 R.P. medicated group. The
0.0063 % and 0.0045 % levels of 31,559 R.P. and the 0.0121 % level
of monensin also gave good protection against the severe infection
(mortalities of 1 - 5.6 and 0.5 % respectively).Sampling and
necropsy of pen mates of the inoculated birds revealed that a high
percentage of nonmedicated birds had contracted coccidial infection.
In contrast, those groups which received 31,559 R.P. and monensin
showed few, if any, gross lesions. The 0.009 and 0.0063 % levels
of 31,559 R.P. were as active as monensin at 0.0121 %.

In a second experiment recent field strains of coccidia were
used : 12 strains of 5 species ; most of which were resistant to
several coccidiostats. The "seeder bird" technique was employed.
Day-old chicks were again medicated up to 8 weeks of age. The
results are summarized in table 3. The 31,559 R.P. treatment
groups (0.009 - 0.0063 and 0.0045 %) showed weight gains superior
to those of the exposed basals and similar to the gains of the
nonexposed basals. The gains made by the 31,559 R.P. medicated
groups were equal or better than those for broilers medicated with
monensin at 0.0121 %.

ANTICOCCIDIAL ACTIVITY IN RABBITS

The activity of 31,559 R.P. on hepatic coccidiosis was
evaluated in battery trials against E. stiedae ; oocysts were
inoculated by gavage and medicated feed was initiated 48 hours

Table 3 - Floor pen evaluation against 5 species of coccidia

Treatment		No chicks	awg (g) D + 56	Mort. % (*)	Feed/ gain
umi		720	1995	79	
31,559 R.P.	0.009 %	720	2033	0	
"	0.0063 %	720	2056	1	
"	0.0045 %	720	2058	56	
monensin	0.0121 %	720	1948	0.5	
umui		200	1902	0	2.2
umi		200	1753	3	2.29
31,559 R.P.	0.009 %	200	1905	0	2.14
"	0.0063 %	200	1916	0	2.19
"	0.0045 %	200	1937	0	2.14
monensin	0.121 %	200	1884	0.5	2.18

(*) first experiment = dead x 100/inoculated

prior to inoculation and continued for 28 days. At 0.0025 % 31,559 R.P. suppressed mortality, hepatic lesions and oocyst production.

MODE OF ACTION

Cidal Effect of 31,559 R.P. on E. tenella

Infected birds were medicated tor 8 days commencing the day prior to inoculation. Oocyst counts were made from day 7 post inoculation to day 18. During the withdrawal period there were no signs of relapse or delayed E. tenella cycling. This observation demonstrates that 31,559 R.P. is coccidiocidal rather than coccidiostatic.

Stage of the Life Cycle of E. tenella on which 31,559 R.P. Acts

The medication (31,559 R.P. at 0.04 %) was initiated on the day of inoculation, or on the 1st, 2nd or 3rd day after and was continued until 7 days post exposure. The results showed that 31,559 R.P. had the greatest effect when initiated on the day of inoculation or on the 1st day after. The compound is therefore active against early stages of E. tenella.

Effect on the Development of Immunity

Those studies demonstrated that birds which have previously been infected and medicated with 31,559 R.P. or monensin showed little or no immunity when challenged after drug withdrawal and

therefore confirm that these compounds are active against the
parasites at a stage before the immune mechanisms are elicited.

RESISTANCE TO 31,559 R.P.

Effect on the Emergence of Drug Resistance

Following 10 passages of E. tenella through chicks medicated
with 0.02 and 0.01 % respectively, no increase in resistance to
31,559 R.P. was observed.

Cross-resistance studies

Species of Eimeria resistant to 4-hydroxyquinolines,
amprolium + ethopabate, robenidine, meticlorpindol, nicarbazin and
zoalene were susceptible to 31,559 R.P.

CONCLUSION

The new antibiotic 31,559 R.P. possesses high anticoccidial
activity in chickens and compares favorably with monensin. At
levels of 0.01 to 0.0063 % (dependent on species of Eimeria) in the
feed, it demonstrates an activity equal or superior to that of
monensin at 0.0121 %.

SUMMARY

Emericid (31,559 R.P.) is a new antibiotic belonging to the
cyclic polyether group. Its anticoccidial activity has been tested
against single and mixed infections using 5 species of Eimeria in
battery experiments and in floor pen trials in chicks. At levels
of 0.01 to 0.0063 % in the feed the compound showed a high degree
of activity, equal or superior to that of monensin at 0.0121 %.
The action is cidal rather than static and the compound affects
the early stages of coccidia. By passages through medicated
chicks, it does not induce resistance of Eimeria.

EFFICIENCY OF LEVAMISOLE "KETRAX"*ON SOME NEMATODE INFECTIONS IN
ASSIUT PROVINCE

A.M. Mandour and Laila A.M. Omran

Department of Parasitology, Faculty of Medicine

Assiut University, Egypt

INTRODUCTION

Intestinal helminthes have been known to constitute a major
public health problem in some localities in Egypt. Among those
helminthes are Ascaris, Ancylostoma, Enterobius and to a lesser
degree Trichuris and Strogyloides. In our country Ascaris and
and Enterobius are treated with piperazine compounds; Ancylostoma
is treated with Bephenium hydroxynaphthoate "Alcopar";Trichuris
is treated with Dithiazanine iodide "Telmid" and Strongyloides is
treated with "Telmid".

Recently some workers such as Lionel et al (1969), Laigert
et al (1969), Hall et al (1970) have claimed that a new drug
Levamisole "Ketrax" is very efficient against Ascaris infections.
Later Al Saffar et al (1971), Pene and Delmont (1973) have tried
the effect of this drug on Ancylostoma infections with excellent
results. The efficiency of "Ketrax" has been tested against mixed
infections by Bouyer (1970), Gatti et al (1972) and Farid et al
(1973). They all concluded that "Ketrax" is a safe and effective
treatment against Ascaris and hookworm infections. Moreover they
concluded that it is easy to be administered in mann treatment
without special care and minimum or no side effects.

These findings stimulated the interest of the present authors
to study the effect of this new drug on some nematode infections
in Assiut Province

* A Product of I.C.I. (England)

MATERIAL AND METHODS

Patients from different localities of Assiut Province were
examined for nematode infections. Some of them were treated as
in-patients, while others received the drug in the out-patient
clinic in Ahnoub Hospital and some patients were treated in a
private clinic. Some of the patients were co-operative and they
were followed up, while many were non-co-operative that they only
came on one occasion post-treatment.

Eight hundred sugar-coated tablets of "Ketrax" and 1000 ml
of the syrup were provided by the Scientific Division of I.C.I.
in Egypt. Each tablet contains 40 mg of levamisole (as hydrochloride), while the red raspberry-flavoured syrup contained
40 mg levamisole (as hydrochloride) in each 5 ml.

The positive cases were diagnosed by floatation method (using
saturated salt solution) in addition to routine direct smear
examination and sedimentation in normal saline solution. Diagnosis
of Enterobius needed in addition a peri-anal swab. Stoll's egg
count technique was made pre- and post-treatment in cases of
Ascaris and Ancylostoma to evaluate the effect of the drug. This
technique cannot be depended upon in Trichuris since the female
worm does not put a standard number of eggs (it is known that it
sometimes lays 1,000 eggs per day and sometimes 3,000 in another
day). Diagnosis of Strongyloides was based on the finding of larvae
in the stools using Baermann's technique.

The drug "Ketrax" was given as one or two doses and rarely
three doses were given, especially in infections with Enterobius.
The actual dosage regimes followed the pattern outlined below:-

Patient Age	No.of Tablets	Syrup
1-4 years	1	5 ml (1 spoonful)
5-15 years	2	10 ml (2 spoonful)
16 years and over	3	30 ml (3 spoonful)

The drug was given after a light breakfast without any purga-
tive post-treatment.

The patients selected for the present trial were grouped as
follows:-

Group 1 consisted of twenty patients (aged between 2.5 - 35 years)
infected with Ascaris lumbricoides. Diagnosis depended on the presence of Ascaris ova in their stools. Samples of stools were re-
examined 7-10 days after giving a single dose of the drug.

Group 2 consisted of sixty patients (aged between 12 - 32 years)
infected with Ancylostoma duodenale, who were given one dose
treatment, in addition to forty patients (aged from 9 - 20 years)
who were given two dose treatment with 24 hours interval. Stoll's
egg count was carried out in this group. Samples of stools were
re-examined 7-10 days after dosage was given.

Group 3 consisted of eighty patients (aged from 2 - 45 years)
infected with Enterobius vermicularis. Diagnosis depended upon
either finding of the pinworms in the stools, or the ova were
detected by floatation technique. Rarely a peri-anal swab was
resorted to before defaecation, so as to ascertain whether the
infection is present or not. The same technique was applied 7-10
days after giving one or multiple doses.

Group 4 consisted ot two patients (aged 20 and 25 years from a
locality 50 Km south Assiut calledEl-Ghourayeb). The infection
was detected on stools examination by direct smear. The first one
swallowed three tablets of "Ketrax" and the second one took two
doses with 24 hours interval.

Group 5 consisted of two patients (18 and 40 years). One is a
student from the suburbs of Cairo and the other was a female
living in a rural area beside Assiut. The female patient
received one dose of three tablets, then it was subjected to
stools examination 7 days later. The male student was given
another dose 7 days later and a third dose 24 hours after the
second dose.

RESULTS

1.   Trials on Ascaris infected patients:

     The worms were expelled 24 hours (on the second day) after
giving the drug. Re-examination of the stools 7-10 days later
proved negative. No side effects were reported. The percentage
of cure reached 100%. It is worth to mention here that a child
aged 2.5 years old passed 32 Ascaris worms at a time while another
child of 3 years old passed 20 worms. The latter has got nutritional oedema which improved much after expulsion of the worms.

2.   Trials on Ancylostoma infected patients:

     Could be illustrated in Table 1 as follows:

TABLE 1

THE EFFICIENCY OF LEVAMISOLE AGAINST ANCYLOSTOMA WHEN ONE
DOSE TREATMENT WAS APPLIED

Intensity of infection as shown by egg count	No.of treated patients	No. cured	% efficiency
Light infection: egg count 600 - 900/gm stools	30	27	90
Heavy infection: egg count 1300- 3200/gm stools	30	21	70
Total No.	60	48	average 80

TABLE 2

THE EFFICIENCY OF LEVAMISOL AGAINST ANCYLOSTOMA WHEN TWO
DOSES WERE GIVEN WITH 24 HOURS INTERVALS

Intensity of infection as shown by egg count	No.of treated patients	No. cured	% efficiency
Light infection: egg count 600 - 900/gm stools	20	18	90
Heavy infection: egg count 1300 - 2500/gm stools	20	17	85
Total No.	40	35	average 87.5

It is noticed that one dose treatment gave no side effects,
while two out of twenty who complained of heavy infection showed
loose stools and giddiness. The average percentage efficiency
was 87.5%.

3.   Trials on <u>Enterobius vermicularis</u> infected patients:

This could be illustrated in Table 3.

TABLE 3

THE EFFICIENCY OF LEVAMISOL ON ENTEROBIUS VERMICULARIS
WHEN ONE DOSE, TWO OR THREE DOSES WERE GIVEN

Intensity of infection	No. of Doses	No.of treated patients	No.cured	% efficiency
Light infection only the ova were detected	1	30	16	53
Heavy infection both worms and ova were detected	1	10	4	40
Light infection	2	20	18	90
Heavy infection	2	10	7	70
Heavy infection	3	10	8	80
Total No.	−	80	53	average 66.6

It is noticed that one dose treatment gave an average percentage efficiency of 46.5, two dose treatment gave 80% cure rate and three doses gave 80% cure. The overall average efficiency could be calculated as 66.6%. As regards side effects, they were mild and transient, being in the form of discomfortable belly (one case), giddiness (three cases), and diarrhoea (one case).

4.   Trials on <u>Trichuris trichura</u> infected patients:

One patient was cured as a result of one dose, while the other who received two doses passed a few eggs 7 days after giving the second dose. Thus the cure rate could be calculated as 50%. No side effects could be detected inboth cases.

5.   Trials on <u>Strongyloides stercoralis</u> infected patients:

Only reduction in the number of larvae passing with the stools was noticed in both patients when one dose was given. The stools of the infected student showed marked reduction in the number of

larvae, but it was not eradicated when two doses were given. Three
doses cured the student. The female patient was not co-operative
since she did not come back to attempt another trial. Accordingly
the cure rate is considered to be 50%.

DISCUSSION

Interpretation on the efficiency of levamisol against Ascaris

The present study has shown that levamisole"Ketrax" is the
drug of choice for the treatment of Ascaris infections when only
one dose was given. The absence of side effects made the drug
acceptable by both the patient and the physician. Moreover the
good taste of the syrup is attractive for children and babies.
However, the authors recommend a second dose if the patient still
has signs indicating the possible presence of male Ascaris infection. The 100% cure rate in Ascaris infection could be due to
the fact that these worms are living more or less free in the
lumen of the intestine, thus they could be expelled more rapidly
when being paralysed potentiated by the slight increase of the
peristaltic movements of the intestine produced by the drug.

Interpretation on the efficiency of levamisole against Ancylostoma

The present findings coincide much with those reported by
Bouher (1970) and Farid et al (1973). The cure rate rarely
exceeded 90%, a finding which might be explained on the fact that
these worms are firmly attached to the mucosa by their teeth and
buccal capsule. However, the very small number of worms being
left without being expelled might have been got rid of by the
effect of body defensive mechanism. Even if there will be a few
number (1-2) of worms it will not affect much the general health.
For this reason "Ketrax" is the drug of choice in mass treatment
campaigns, since it is free of side effects and easy to be administered. Second dose treatment did not affect much the cure rate
as shown in Table 2. It is worthwhile mentioning here that
anaemic patients with 50-60% haemoglobin showed no side effects.

Interpretation on the efficiency of "Ketrax" against Enterobius infections

It is difficult to assess exactly the effect of any drug
against this type of worm because of the following: 1) The
difficulty to diagnose the infection, since some laboratory methods
can fail to establish a definite diagnosis while the patients
insists that he saw worms by himself. This means that light
infection can be overlooked by experts.   2) Re-infection and
retrofection and auto-infection are all factors which make the
assessment of the drug difficult.   3) Scratching around the anus

or around the vulva does not mean in every case an <u>Enterobius</u>
infection. However, the present work has been done trying to avoid
these factors. The present results indicate that "Ketrax" is not
curative when one dose is relied upon. For this reasons the
authors recommend two or three doses to be given every 24 hours.
The failure of one dose treatment might be attributed to the
fact that <u>Enterobius</u> inhabits the caecum which is far from the
effect of such an absorbable drug. For this reason, the authors
suggest the production of enteric coated tablets to be given in
case of both <u>Enterobius</u> and <u>Trichuris</u> which inhabit the caecum.

Interpretation on the efficiency of "Ketrax" in Strongyloides infections

The life cycle of this worm is complicated and the infected
patient can be infected by the larvae before they leave the body,
and for this reason superinfection usually takes place. It is
difficult to assess the effect of "Ketrax" against this parasite
in only two patients. For this reason this work should be done
on a large scale which is difficult to be applied in the Assiut
locality.

CONCLUSION

It could be concluded that "Ketrax" is a safe drug to be
given for mixed infections with <u>Ascaris, Ancylostoma</u> and <u>Enterobius</u>.
In this respect it is excellent from the economy point of view
in addition to its ease of application, with minimal side effects.

REFERENCES

Al-Saffar, G., Al-Saleem, M. and Bakhdus, I.J. (1971)
    L-Tetramisole in the treatment of Ancylostomiaisis. Trans.
    Roy.Soc.Trop.med.Hyg., 65, 836-837.

Bouyer, C. (1970) Traitment des Parasitoses intestinales par
    le Levamisole (Levamisole in the treatment of intestinal
    worm infections) Bull.Soc.Path.exot., 63, 255-265.

Farid, Z., Bassily, S., Young, S.W. and Hassan, A. (1973)
    Tetramisole in the treatment of Ancylostoma duodenale and
    Ascaris lumbricoides infections in Egyptian farmers.
    Trans.Roy.Soc.Trop.med.Hyd., 67, 425-426.

Gatti, F., Krubwa, F., Vandepitte, J. and Thienpont. D. (1972)
    Control of intestinal nematodes in African schoolchildren by
    the trimestrial administration of levamisole. Ann.Soc.belg.
    Med.Trop., 52, 19-32.

Hall, S.A., Joseph, M.M., Saggar, S.N., Wood, C.H. and Gleisner, E.
    (1970) A trial of Ketrax (The laevo-isomer of tetramisole)
    in the treatment of Ascariasis. E.Afr.med.J., 47,8, 424-433.

Laigret, J., Tourres, M. and Doschi, S. (1969) Anthelmintic
    activity of the laevo-isomer of Tetramisole. Bull.Soc,
    Path.exot., 62, 4, 734-740.

Lionel, N.D.W., Mirando, B.H., Nanayakkara, J.C. and Soysa, P.E.
    (1969) Levamisole in the treatment of Ascariasis in children.
    Brit.Med.J., 4, 340-341.

Pene, P. and Delmont, J. (1973) Action of L-tetramisole in the
    treatment of Ancylostomiasis. Med.d'Afrique Noire, 20, 41-43.

REVIEW OF AMPHOTERICIN B

John E. Bennett

Clinical Mycology Section, Laboratory of Clinical
Investigation, National Institute of Allergy and
Infectious Diseases, Bethesda, Maryland 20014

Many of the important biologic properties of amphotericin B
may be ascribed to binding by certain sterols in fungal and
mammalian cell membranes. Avid binding to serum proteins,
probably coupled at least in part by cholesterol, makes
amphotericin B equilibrate slowly with infected exudates and
penetrate poorly into cerebrospinal fluid, urine and hemodialysis
baths. Despite toxicity and unfavorable pharmacokinetics, the
drug is still the most useful agent against most systemic mycoses.

CHEMOTHERAPEUTIC SPECTRUM

More than many antibiotics, the ability of amphotericin B to
influence the course of a given infection is profoundly
influenced by the severity of the infection and the defense
mechanisms of the patient. A beneficial chemotherapeutic effect
is also dependent upon the physician's expertise in managing
toxic reactions in such a way that they do not deter an adequate
dose or duration of therapy. With this caveat in mind, it is
still useful to catalogue in a general way the chemotherapeutic
effect of intravenous amphotericin B against the most common
susceptible systemic mycoses. The drug is very effective in deep
candidiasis, with a few notable exceptions. Candida endocarditis
and chronic mucocutaneous candidiasis can be controlled but rarely
cured with intravenous amphotericin B. Patients with disseminated
candidiasis who are seriously immunosuppressed often succumb
rapidly, despite a few days therapy with amphotericin B. Forms of
candidiasis responding well to amphotericin B include disseminated
infection in the non-immunosuppressed patient, meningitis,
endophthalmitis, arthritis and esophagitis. Equally gratifying

results are obtained in blastomycosis, with cure rates of 85% or
better usually being reported. In cryptococcosis, cure rates run
lower, usually about 70%. For histoplasmosis, rapid culture
conversion is the rule in chronic pulmonary and disseminated
infection. Relapse is infrequent in chronic pulmonary
histoplasmosis but is distressingly common in disseminated
histoplasmosis. Paracoccidioidomycosis, or South American
blastomycosis, responds very well but the relapse rate is
uncertain. In most progressive forms of coccidioidomycosis, it
is fairer to talk about disease control than cure with
amphotericin B. Sporotrichosis of the lungs or joints responds
slowly and to a variable degree during intravenous amphotericin B
therapy. The cure rate with a single course of therapy is
probably not much more than 50%. Invasive aspergillosis usually
occurs in the immunosuppressed host and is most often fatal
despite treatment. A few cures with amphotericin B have occurred,
generally in those patients who were the least compromised
originally or whose immunosuppression was decreased, such as a
leukemic who achieves remission or a renal transplant whose
Immuran and prednisone dose is markedly reduced. With craniofacial mucormycosis, a multifaceted approach with control of
acidosis, surgical debridement and intravenous amphotericin B
seems to be curing one-third to one-half the cases. Chromomycosis
has been treated with injections of amphotericin B into the lesion,
but therapy is painful, prolonged and not very effective.

STRUCTURE-ACTIVITY RELATIONSHIPS

The amphotericin B molecule contains seven conjugated double
bonds. These double bonds are probably responsible for the
ability of these drugs to bind certain sterols and, in turn,
sterol binding accounts for many major properties of these drugs.
Conjugation of water insoluble amphotericin B with desoxycholate
permits the intravenous preparation to be marketed as a clear
solution which in actuality is a colloidal sol. Once in the
bloodstream, unpublished studies in my laboratory have shown the
drug binds to beta-lipoprotein, presumably because of the
cholesterol content of the beta-lipoprotein. After leaving the
circulation, amphotericin B binds to sterols in fungal cytoplasmic
membranes, causing fungistatic activity. In all likelihood,
binding to human cytoplasmic membranes accounts for some of the
toxic reactions, particularly loss of intracellular potassium.
Although high concentrations of amphotericin B in vitro can lyse
human erythrocytes, there is good evidence that this does not
occur in man (Brandriss et al., 1964).

The conjugated double bonds may be the portion of the molecule
which accounts for loss of biologic activity in the presence of
light. This photosensitivity has been considerably overrated.

Studies have shown that covering the bottle to protect drugs from light during intravenous infusion is not necessary (Shadomy et al., 1973; Block and Bennett, 1973).

TOXICITY

Rapid intravenous infusions of amphotericin B can produce hyperkalemia and cardiotoxicity in dogs and rabbits. There are not well documented cases of ventricular arrhythmias in man from amphotericin B, but sudden deaths have been reported due to overdose or extremely rapid infusion. Infusions in man over the usual 3-4 hour interval do not cause hyperkalemia, but in one-fourth of the patients hypokalemia results. The mechanism is probably the same and that is chronic loss of intracellular potassium into the bloodstream and out of the kidney.

Other dose-related toxic reactions include nausea, emesis and headache. Early in therapy, drug-induced fever is usually the most pressing problem. Later on, nephrotoxicity becomes significant. Anemia is due to suppressed erythropoesis and usually stabilizes during therapy with a hematocrit between 20 and 30%. After therapy, anemia disappears in about 3 months. Transfusion is rarely indicated. Hypokalemia is usually correctable by oral potassium supplements. Two other reactions, neutropenia and thrombocytopenia, occur rarely and are less clearly dose dependent. Nephrotoxic reactions occur in nearly all patients and are a function of daily dose. Decreased glomerular filtration rate and its attendant azotemia probably contribute to nausea, vomiting, weakness and anemia. Decreased concentrating ability and decreased ability to excrete a water load make it necessary to watch for dehydration or over-hydration in these patients. Renal tubular acidosis rarely is pronounced enough to warrant correction. Not listed here is cylindruria which occurs in almost all patients. After treatment stops, most toxic reactions clear slowly but completely. In contrast, renal biopsy shows evidence of permanent renal tubular damage in almost all patients and some degree of decreased glomerular filtration rate usually persists. The loss becomes clinically significant if multiple courses of therapy are required or if renal function was seriously impaired prior to therapy.

There has been considerable interest in the observation that, in dogs, addition of mannitol to the infusion decreases amphotericin B nephrotoxicity without lowering serum amphotericin B levels (Hellebusch et al., 1972). In evaluating this procedure, I found that simultaneous administration of mannitol 25 gm with each amphotericin B infusion over 18-24 days did not alter established, stable amphotericin B induced azotemia in three patients.

DOSE

It is customary to begin therapy of adults with a 1 mg test dose of intravenous amphotericin B in order to assess the severity of the febrile reaction and to judge the necessity of adding 25-50 mg hydrocortisone to the infusion bottle. Daily doses are raised as rapidly as fever permits to approximately 0.4-0.6 mg/kg body weight. I prefer to adjust the dose so that the patient's blood urea nitrogen remains below 50 mg% and serum creatinine below 3.5 mg%. At higher levels of azotemia, it is often difficult to maintain the patient's hydration, electrolyte balance and nutrition. It is usual to treat the infections most refractory to amphotericin B with maximum tolerated doses. Examples of this would include disseminated coccidioidomycosis, invasive aspergillosis or craniofacial mucormycosis. To date, no one has shown that sensitivity tests on the infecting fungus help predict which patients will require a higher dose. This is true even in relapsed patients because secondary drug resistance is rare. Nor does determining blood level seem helpful to me in determining the dose. Amphotericin B blood levels are fairly predictable and are not influenced by kidney or liver function. The effect of renal function is easiest to see in the anephric patient, who has normal amphotericin B blood levels. Hemodialysis does not influence amphotericin B blood levels much at all. Amphotericin B is cleared by the artificial kidney at only 3 to 15% of the rate at which creatinine is cleared (Block et al., 1974). This low rate of clearance has no significant impact on the normal rate of fall of amphotericin B blood levels. Poor filtration by normal and artificial kidneys may be due in part to the fact that amphotericin B is 90-95% bound to plasma proteins. This protein binding may also interfere with penetration into certain body fluids. Amphotericin B penetrates the inflamed meninges so poorly that spinal fluid amphotericin B is rarely measurable. Drug levels in highly proteinaceous exudates in the peritoneum, joint and pleura have ranged in my laboratory from 0.22-0.66 µg/ml. Drug concentration in the exudate did not seem to rise during the transient peak blood levels but remained about two-thirds of the valley serum level. This same slow equilibration was seen in aqueous humor drug levels of rabbits with experimental uveitis following a single injection of intravenous amphotericin B. By 24 hours, the aqueous homor drug level was 43% of the serum level (Green et al., 1965). Cord blood from a mother receiving intravenous amphotericin B was 0.37 µg/ml, or half the valley blood level on the day of delivery.

LOCAL AMPHOTERICIN B

Limited penetration of amphotericin B sometimes warrants direct injection into the infected fluid. In the joint, local

injections may aid in the therapy of Coccidioides, Candida and
Sporothrix infections. The injection causes a temporary increase
in pain and swelling but little or no azotemia. Intrapleural
drug is rarely indicated. Intrathecal amphotericin B is very
helpful in coccidioidal meningitis. Occasionally, a refractory
case of cryptococcal meningitis seems to benefit from combined
intravenous and intrathecal drug. Lumbar intrathecal injections
have often caused severe asymmetrical radiculitis, presumably
from extradural leakage of drug. There is hope that injecting
the drug in hyperbaric glucose may help move the drug away from
the injection site and reduce extradural leakage of drug
(Alazraki et al., 1974). This may reduce reactions. Injection
of amphotericin B into the lateral cerebral ventricle by means of
a subcutaneous reservoir is fraught with problems. While
inserting 31 such reservoirs, we found that a third of the
reservoirs never could be used because of difficulties in
insertion (Diamond and Bennett, 1973). Of the 22 reservoirs
that could be used, a third became unusable because of leakage or
clogging. Infection was the usual reason for clogging. In the
aqueous humor even very small quantities of amphotericin B cause
inflammation, and this route is not clearly useful. Irrigation
of the bladder is very helpful in bladder thrush occurring in
catheterized patients. A solution of 50 µg/ml is not irritating.
Corneal baths with up to 1000 µg/ml are not irritating and are
helpful in corneal infections with some fungi.

BIBLIOGRAPHY

Alazracki, N.P., Fierer, J., Halpern, S.E. and Becker, R W.
    (1974). New Eng.J.Med., 290, 641.
Block, E.R. and Bennett, J.E. (1973). Antimicrob.Agents
    Chemother., 4, 648.
Block, E.R., Bennett, J.E., Livoti, L.G., Klein, W.J.,
    MacGregor, R.R. and Henderson, H. '1974). Ann.Intern.Med.,
    80, 613.
Brandriss, M., Wolff, S., Moores, R. and Stohlman, F. (1964).
    JAMA, 189, 663.
Diamond, R.D. and Bennett, J.E. (1973). New Eng.J.Med., 288, 186.
Green, W.R., Bennett, J.E. and Goos, R.D. (1965). Arch.
    Ophthalmol., 73, 769.
Hellebusch, A.A., Salama, F. and Eadie, E. (1972). Surg.Gynecol.
    Obstet., 134, 241.
Shadomy, S., Brummer, D.L. and Ingroff, A.V. (1973). Amer.Rev.
    Resp.Dis., 107, 303.

POLYENES: ACTIONS AND PROSPECTS

D. Kerridge & N. J. Russell

Sub-department of Chemical Microbiology
Department of Biochemistry
Tennis Court Road
Cambridge

The essential requirement for the successful treatment of a
microbial infection is that there should be at least one significant
difference between the host and the parasite to provide a site for
antibiotic action. This is clearly illustrated for bacterial
(prokaryotic) infections where, for example, peptidoglycan synthesis
and 70S ribosome-mediated protein synthesis are selectively
inhibited by penicillin and chloramphenicol respectively. The
situation for fungal infections is complicated by the fact that
both parasite and host are eukaryotic organisms and the metabolic
and structural differences which might provide a basis for
chemotherapeutic attack result from variations on the same basic
theme (Table 1).

Table 1. Major differences between Fungi and Man

Structural component	Fungus	Man
Cell Wall	Complex containing polysaccharide, protein and lipid	Absent
Membrane sterol	Ergosterol	Cholesterol

In spite of the major differences between host and fungal parasite
residing in the cell wall structure no clinically important
antibiotic acts at this site. Polyoxin D, an analogue of
UDP-N-acetyl glucosamine, is a competitive inhibitor of chitin
synthetase but the levels required to inhibit fungal growth in vivo

are frequently much greater than those required to inhibit in vitro
synthesis and reflect the presence of a permeability barrier
(Endo et al, 1970). Polyene antibiotics, although toxic to Man are
used clinically, and exert their effect by impairing the function
of the plasma membrane.

The polyenes constitute a group of about 300 complex macrolide
antibiotics characterised by a carbon ring possessing both a
conjugated double bond system and an hydrophilic region, and closed
by lactonisation (Reviewed by Hamilton-Miller, 1973).   X-ray
analysis by Mechlinski et al (1970) demonstrated that amphotericin B
is an elongated rigid molecule with both hydrophobic and
hydrophilic faces. Very few polyene antibiotics are used
clinically: these include, nystatin, candicidin, hamycin and
amphotericin B, and of these only amphotericin B is used for
treatment of systemic infections. These antibiotics exert their
effect by interacting with sterol-containing plasma membranes
causing an impairment of function, leakage of cellular constituents
and ultimately cell death. Prokaryotic organisms which lack
membrane sterols are unaffected (Lampen 1966). The extent of
membrane damage depends both on the nature of the membrane sterol
and the antibiotic. In general the smaller polyenes cause more
extensive damage than the larger ones. It is the difference in
the relative affinities for the membrane sterols, cholesterol and
ergosterol, that makes it possible to use these antibiotics for
the treatment of mycotic infections (Gale, 1973; Archer & Gale,
1975).

In vivo the presence of sterols in the plasma membrane appears
to be essential for the polyene action; however, in vitro studies
by HsuChen & Feingold (1974) using model membrane systems suggest
that the presence of sterols in the membrane is not essential,
and it is membrane fluidity that determines polyene sensitivity.
In natural membranes the fatty acid composition is such that the
presence of sterols affects the lipid mobility thus rendering them
sensitive. The mechanism by which polyenes disrupt the plasma
membranes of sensitive cells may differ from one polyene to another.
In the case of amphotericin B (a heptaene) the experimental data,
largely derived from model lipid membrane studies, support the
hypothesis that incorporation of the antibiotic into the membrane
results in the production of an aqueous pore (5A radius).
Crystallographic studies of amphotericin B and cholesterol have
provided a basis for a model of this aqueous pore which consists
of an annulus of amphotericin B and sterol in which the
hydrophilic region of the polyene faces the interior of the pore.
The length of the annulus is such that two "half-pores" are
required to span the lipid bilayer. This may explain why the
effect of the polyene antibiotics on black lipid membranes is
greater when the antibiotic is present on both sides (De Kruijff
&Demel 1974; Andreoli, 1974; Holz, 1974). How such pores are

created in natural membranes is not known. Furthermore, electron
microscopic studies reveal gross membrane disorganisation in the
presence of amphotericin B suggesting that its action is much
more drastic than only the creation of a pore (Verkleij et al 1973).
A particularly relevant study of the effect of amphotericin B on
Epidermatophyton floccosum by Nozawa et al (1974) demonstrates this.
Filipin, a "smaller" pentaene, which cannot span half the lipid
bilayer, may form aggregates with the membrane sterol within the
bilayer rather than across it so disrupting the membrane (De Kruijff
& Demel, 1974).

The interaction of the antibiotic with the plasma membrane is
influenced by a variety of factors some of which may be relevant
to polyene treatment of clinical infections. Polyene antibiotics
and sterols interact in vitro (Bittman & Fischkoff, 1972; Norman
et al 1972), although the significance of an interaction between
two water-insoluble compounds is difficult to assess. The addition
of sterols and other lipids together with the polyene can reduce
the effect of the antibiotic on growth and metabolism of sensitive
cells (Gottlieb et al, 1960). This apparent increase in the MIC
results from an effective lowering of the concentration of the
antibiotic. The failure to achieve serum levels $>$1-2 ug
amphotericin B/ml may result from an interaction of the antibiotic
with lipid constituents of the serum (blood cholesterol would be
particularly important in this respect), as well as with host
cellular membranes. The inhibitory effects of a number of polyene
antibiotics can be nullified by the addition to the growth medium
of K^+ and Mg^{++} ions at high concentrations (Liras & Lampen, 1974).
It is presumed that the antibiotic interacts with the plasma
membrane, but the presence of K^+ and Mg^{++} ions prevents the
internal concentration of these ions falling to such a low level
that growth ceases. The polyene treated yeast can give rise to
viable colonies in the presence of K^+ and Mg^{++} at high
concentrations if excess antibiotic is removed. It is likely that
continued membrane synthesis results in dilution of the membrane-
associated antibiotic to a sub-inhibitory level. However, if the
salts as well as excess antibiotic are removed from the growth
medium the cells rapidly become non-viable suggesting that once
the polyene is incorporated into the yeast membrane it cannot
easily be removed. This is in contrast to the findings with
erythrocytes (Cass & Dalmark 1973) and HeLa cells (Kumar et al
1974) where amphotericin B has been used to alter reversibly the
permeability of the plasma membrane to ions and DNA respectively.
This apparent reversibility of the polyene action on animal cells
may be important clinically and could reflect the differences in
envelope structure between the fungus and its host, with the
fungus having a complex cell wall covering the plasma membrane.

The role of the cell wall in influencing the interaction of

the polyene with the fungal plasma membrane has been further
emphasised by studies on the phenotypic variation in polyene
sensitivity of Candida albicans (Gale, 1974; Gale et al 1975).
In these studies polyene-mediated K^+ release was used to monitor
antibiotic sensitivity. When growth of C. albicans in defined
medium is limited by either the carbon or nitrogen source the
cells become increasingly resistant to amphotericin B methyl ester
(AME) once growth ceases. Sphaeroplasts derived from non-growing
cells are sensitive, so the increased antibiotic resistance
probably results from changes in the structure of the cell wall.
An analogous situation was observed in Aspergillus fumigatus;
dormant conidia are resistant to polyenes but rapidly become
sensitive during the early swelling stage of germination prior
to germ tube emergence (Russell et al 1975). However, if mycelial
growth in liquid culture is limited by nitrogen starvation, no
change in sensitivity to AME occurred during the incubation
(unpublished observations). This phenotypic variation in
antibiotic sensitivity in the opportunistic fungi may be of
clinical importance and could account for the persistence of
fungal infections, since the population of cells in any lesion
will be heterogeneous with both growing (antibiotic-sensitive)
and non-growing (antibiotic-resistant) cells present.

     What are the prospects for the future? The fundamental
problems in polyene therapy of systemic mycoses are:- insolubility
and instability of the antibiotic, and toxicity to the host.
Antibiotic resistance is not yet a problem, but since the maximum
serum levels are but marginally greater than the MIC's of
amphotericin B for Candida albicans (Hamilton-Miller, 1972) there
is no room for complacency in the use of nystatin and candicidin
in the treatment of superficial infections. Furthermore, in the
laboratory polyene-resistant mutants invariably show cross-
resistance to other antibiotics of this type.

     A greater understanding of the mechanism of the interaction
of the polyenes with both cholesterol- and ergosterol- containing
membranes could lead to an improvement in selectivity and a
reduction in toxicity but the complexity of the polyene structure
does pose problems. In this context it is a pity that so many of
the in vitro studies have been performed with cholesterol and
filipin, since ergosterol is the major fungal sterol and filipin
is too toxic to be used clinically. Hopefully, as in the case of
the synthetic penicillins, chemical modification of the
biosynthetically produced polyene might result in the development
of more effective antibiotics. Polyenes are large, complex and
unstable molecules and the possibilities of successful chemical
modification are correspondingly reduced: this should not, however,
preclude such an approach to the problem. The hydrophobic conjugated
double bond system is essential for the interaction of the
antibiotic with the sterol-containing membrane and is also

responsible for the instability of the molecule, so modifications of this region to improve stability and water solubility can at the most have only a limited success. Amino and carboxyl groups in certain polyenes have been modified by acetylation, methylation, etc., and although this may increase their apparent solubility and pharmaceutical acceptibility as antibiotics, it often decreases their antimycotic efficiency (reviewed by Hamilton-Miller 1973). A notable success is the synthesis of AME (Mechlinski & Schaffner, 1972; Schaffner & Mechlinski, 1972 Bonner, et al 1972, Keim et al, 1973) where methylation has reduced the toxicity and increased the apparent solubility of amphotericin B without reducing its antimycotic activity.

An alternative approach is that of biological modification. Since only one out of approximately 300 known polyenes can be used systemically the possibility of obtaining genetic variants of the polyene-producing strains capable of yielding a clinically useful derivative is worthwhile exploring. The polyenes are satisfactory for the treatment of superficial fungal infections. In fact their detergent-like properties probably increases their effectiveness in this role. In the future attention should be focussed on developing polyenes that are more effective in the treatment of systemic infections.

Acknowledgement

The authors wish to thank the Medical Research Council for financial support.

References

Andreoli, T. E. 1974 Annals of the New York Academy of Sciences
235, 448.
Archer, D. B. & Gale, E. F. 1975 Journal of General Microbiology,
in press.
Bittman, R. &. Fishkoff, S. A. 1972 Proceedings of the National
Academy of Sciences U.S.A. 69, 3795.
Bonner, D. P., Mechlinski, W. & Schaffner, C. P. 1972 Journal
of Antibiotics (Tokyo) 25, 261.
Cass, A. & Dalmark, M. 1973 Nature, New Biology 244, 47.
De Kruijff, B. & Demel, R. A. 1974 Biochimica et Biophysica Acta
339, 57.
Endo, A., Kakiki, K. & Misato, T. 1970 Journal of Bacteriology
104, 189.
Gale, E. F. 1973 British Medical Journal 4, 33.
Gale, E. F. 1974 Journal of General Microbiology 80, 451.
Gale, E. F.,Johnson, A., Kerridge, D. & Koh, T. Y. 1975 Journal
of General Microbiology 87, 20.
Gottlieb, D., Carter, H.E., Wu, L.C. & Sloneker, J. M. 1960
Phytopathology 50, 594.

Hamilton-Miller, J.M.T. 1972 Sabouraudia 10, 276.

Hamilton-Miller, J.M.T. 1973 Bacteriological Reviews 37, 166.

Holz, K. W. 1974 Annals of New York Academy of Sciences, 235, 469.

HsuChen, C-C. & Feingold, D. S. 1974 Biochemical and Biophysical
        Research Communications. 51, 972.

Keim, G.R.Jr., Poutsiaka, J.W., Kirpan, J. & Keysser, C.H. 1973
        Science 179, 584.

Kumar, B. V., Medoff, G., Kobayashi, G. & Schlessinger, D. 1974
        Nature, 250, 323.

Lampen, J. O. 1966 Symposium of the Society for General Microbiology
        16, 111.

Liras, P. & Lampen, J. O. 1974 Biochimica et Biophysica Acta 374, 159.

Mechlinski, W. & Schaffner, C. P., 1972 Journal of Antibiotics
        (Tokyo) 25, 256.

Mechlinski, W., Schaffner, C. P. Ganis, P. & Avitabile, G. 1970
        Polyhedron Letters 44, 3873.

Norman, A. W., Demel, R.A., De Kruyff, B., Geurts van Kessel, W.S.
        M. & Van Deenen, L.L.M. 1972 Biochimica et Biophysica
        Acta. 290, 1.

Nozawa, Y., Kitajima, Y., Sekiya, T. & Ito, Y. 1974 Biochimica et
        Biophysica Acta 367, 32.

Russell, N. J., Kerridge, D. & Gale, E. F. 1975 Journal of General
        Microbiology 87, 351.

Schaffner, C. P. & Mechlinski, W. 1972 Journal of Antibiotics
        (Tokyo) 25, 259.

Verkleij, A. J., De Kruijff, B., Gerritsen, W.G., Demel, R.A.,
        Van Deenen, L.L.M., & Ververgaert, P.H.J. 1973 Biochimica
        et Biophysica Acta 291, 577.

REVIEW OF IMIDAZOLE GROUP

R. J. HOLT

Department of Clinical Microbiology

Queen Mary's Hospital for Children, Carshalton, Surrey

Early indication of the antimicrobial potential of the imidazoles was given by Woolley (1944) in his report that benzimidazole and certain of its derivatives inhibited the growth of some fungi and bacteria. Woolley had noticed the close structural resemblance between benzimidazole and the purines and he showed that the inhibition of microbial growth was reversed by the aminopurines adenine and guanine, although other purines were ineffective.

CHLORMIDAZOLE

In 1952 Jerchel et al. pointed out that some substituted benzimidazoles had strong antifungal activity and this prompted a team at Chemie Grunenthal GmbH led by Herrling and Mückter to made a broad study of substituents of benzimidazole; they selected a chlorbenzyl imidazole (CHLORMIDAZOLE, H.115), inhibitory at concentrations below 50 µg/ml towards many fungi and active against some gram-positive cocci (Seeliger, 1958; Herrling et al., 1959; Holt, 1974). The compound was marketed as a topical cream (Myco-Polycid) containing 5% chlormidazol and has had many successful clinical trials (Ledig, 1958; Huriez, Agache and Souillart, 1962; Kejda, 1974). Chlormidazole was also shown to have high antihistaminic activity, and this property foreshadowed the biological versatility of many subsequent imidazoles, particularly as anthelminthics.

Almost simultaneously in 1969 two quite distinct imidazole derivatives with marked antimycotic activity entered laboratory and clinical trials: these were CLOTRIMAZOLE (Bayer AG) and MICONAZOLE (Janssen Pharmaceutica).

Table 1   Range of Activity of Some Imidazoles

	Protozoa	Helminths	Micro-organisms
Metronidazole 1959 and Tinidazole 1969	Trichomonas Giardia Trypanosomes Amoeba		Some anaerobic bacteria
Thiabendazole 1961		Nematodes	Trichophyton Microsporum Aspergillus
Mebendazole 1971		Nematodes	Trichophyton Aspergillus
Tetramisole 1966 Levamisole		Nematodes (also immuno-modulating activity)	
Niridazole 1966		Schistosoma Dracunculus	

CLOTRIMAZOLE

Büchel and his colleagues (1972) found that many tritylimidazoles had considerable antimycotic activity, both in-vitro and in animal experiments, and a tritylimidazole with chlorine substituted in one benzene ring was eventually selected, given the name CLOTRIMAZOLE, and marketed as CANESTEN. The drug is very active in-vitro against candida and cryptococci, aspergillus spp. and almost all dermato-phytes of medical and veterinary interest; concentrations below 2 µg/ml are usually adequate for growth inhibition, and fungicidal activity occurs almost always at below 10 µg/ml (Plempel et al., 1969; Holt, 1970). Most of these studies were made by liquid dilution methods, but clotrimidazole discs containing 10 and 50 µg/ml are suitable for routine screening procedures; in both systems pronounced inoculum effects are met, and it is necessary to use a standardised light initial inoculum (Holt, 1974).

Clotrimazole has limited activity against bacteria (Waitz, 1971; Holt and Newman, 1972); is amoebicidal towards Naegleria fowleri (Jamieson and Anderson, 1974); trichomonacidal (Plempel and Bartmann, 1972), and, on the basis of animal studies, the drug appears to have cidal action on toxoplasma (Schassan et al., 1974). Laboratory experiments have repeatedly failed to induce significant changes in the resistances of candida, aspergillus, cryptococcus and other fungal species (Holt and Newman, 1972), and these obser-vations are replicated in clinical studies (Clayton and Connor, 1973; Holt and Newman, 1972).

Iwata, Yamaguehi and Hiratani (1973) showed that the site of activity of clotrimazole is probably the cell membrane, in common with miconazole and the polyene antimycotic agents; the activity of the latter depends considerably on the membrane sterol content, but the imidazoles appear to be less dependent on this. These workers suggested that fungicidal concentrations of clotrimazole damaged the permeable membrane and that leakage of intracellular phosphorus compounds and potassium ions resulted, with consequent inhibition of macro-molecular synthesis. In 1974 Renz et al. reported elevated myeloperoxidase activity in a high proportion of infants on oral clotrimazole, and they postulated that the imidazole may stimulate leukocyte myeloperoxidase activity.

Pharmacokinetic studies on clotrimazole showed that absorption of the drug through intact skin was neglible when a 1% cream or solution was applied under occlusive dressings; and the systemic absorption of clotrimazole from vaginal tablets was estimated at 3% (Duhm et al., 1972). Peak serum levels are reached at about three hours after oral administration; following the maximal dose of 25 mg/kg body weight each six hours, these peak levels in adults rarely exceed 2 µg/ml of microbiologically active drug; a great excess of inactive drug metabolite is also present in serum (Plempel et al., 1969),and assays by photo-colorimetric or radiochemical methods therefore record much higher levels. ^{14}C labelled-clotrimazole studies showed that biliary excretion plays a major role in drug removal (Duhm et al., 1972), and it is known that the drug produces increases in liver enzyme activity (Tettenborn, 1974).

Clotrimazole has had a high success rate in many trials for the local treatment of vaginal candidiasis and for a variety of mycotic cutaneous and muco-cutaneous infections; several studies suggest that optimal therapy requires a longer course than the six days usually followed (Lohmeyer, 1974; Widholm, 1974). Clotrimazole tablets appear less successful for the treatment of vaginal tricho-moniasis; in a double-blind trial Schnell (1974) found a cure rate of 45%. Many clinical and mycological cures have been reported with clotrimazole cream in dermatophytosis and cutaneous conditions (Clayton and Connor, 1974; Comaish, 1974) and Male (1974) found clotrimazole cream and tolnaftate cream equally effective in the treatment of dermatophytoses. All topical preparations were well tolerated and local irritation was rarely severe.

A multi-centre European trial of oral clotrimazole therapy at a dosage of 60 mg/kg/day for at least one month produced clinical and mycological cures in a considerable proportion of 314 cases with systemic mycoses (Weuta, 1974), including septicaemia, pulmonary and urinary candidiasis and pulmonary aspergillosis (Table 2). Similar results have recently been collected by Good (personal communication, 1975) in the U.K. where 133 cases of pulmonary aspergillosis and 73 cases of systemic candidiasis received doses up to 100 mg/kg/day (Table 3). Successful treatment of urinary candidiasis in infants receiving 100 mg/kg/day of the drug (Holt and

Table 2   Systemic Clotrimazole Therapy (Weuta 1974)

	Pulmonary	Urinary Candidiasis	Septicaemic Candidiasis
No. of cases	203 { 101 Candida) (102 Asp.)	21	85
Cultural Results			
Elimination	60	17	62
Reduction	38	0	4
No Change	105	4	15
Clinical Results			
Cured	45	15	58
Improved	91	5	13
No Change	57	1	6
Died	10	0	8

Pulmonary Candidiasis showed 59% elimination or reduction on culture
Pulmonary Aspergillosis showed 37% elimination or reduction on culture

Newman, 1972), and in renal transplant cases (Bewick and Raper, 1974), has also been reported. Topical and systemic clotrimazole therapy was unsuccessful in patients with paranasal aspergillomas and madurella mycetomas (El Sheik Mahgoub) but Jones et al. (1974) reported the successful eradication of A. fumigatus in two cases of severe fungal corneal infection with preservation of sight by prolonged topical and oral treatment with the drug.

Systemic therapy with clotrimazole has met a major problem in the high incidence of gastro-intestinal disturbances. In Weuta's study (1974) 13% of the 314 patients complained of this, and Good (personal communication, 1975) noted that 57% of 115 cases in the United Kingdom had some degree of gastro-intestinal intolerance; relatively high doses appear to be well tolerated by children (Holt and Newman, 1972). Good also recorded mental effects in 35% of all patients, including depression, disorientation and hallucinations.

Table 3
Clinical and Cultural Assessment of Response to Therapy with Oral Clotrimazole in U.K. (Good, 1975)

	Clinical Cure/Improvement	Culture Positive Pre Rx	Culture Positive Post Rx
Aspergillus 133 cases	39%	87%	25%
Candida 73 cases	60%	84%	25%

MICONAZOLE

MICONAZOLE NITRATE is a phenethyl imidazole derivative synthesized by Janssen Pharmaceutica (Godefroi et al., 1969); its activity in-vitro against candida and other yeast-like fungi and against Aspergillus spp. and dermatophytes is comparable with clotrimazole, concentrations of 2 µg/ml being inhibitory for most species. Agar diffusion methods using impregnated paper discs containing 10 and 50 µg miconazole are satisfactory for routine sensitivity screening. No wild fungal resistance to miconazole has been reported, nor was emergent resistance of candida, aspergillus or dermatophytes induced during prolonged in-vitro studies with gradient plates (Holt, 1974). Miconazole exhibits considerable activity towards Gram-positive cocci, but enterobacteria and pseudomonads are virtually resistant (Holt, 1972). Van den Bossche (1974), using ^{3}H-miconazole, suggested that the activity of miconazole on cell membranes may include effects on microsomal membranes, resulting in decreased uptake of purines and glutamine. Brugmans et al. (1972) applied ^{3}H-miconazole cream topically and intravaginally to volunteers, and showed that virtually no systemic absorption occurred.

Topical therapy for vaginal candidiasis with 2% Miconazole cream and powder has resulted in clinical cure and cultural clearance in 85%-98% of patients in several studies (Alexander et al., 1972; Wheatley, 1974; etc.). Most of the patients received intravaginal insertion from 5 gm applicators each night for 10-14 days, and in one trial the sexual partner was also treated with miconazole cream (Peeters et al., 1973). Topical miconazole is effective in the treatment of fungal skin infections (Brugmans et al., 1970; De Barros and Belda, 1972; etc.) and of refractory fungal paronychia (Heinke, 1972).

Symoens (1975) has recently reviewed the oral and intravenous use of miconazole in 100 patients, many with severe candida infections, who received daily doses of up to 1000 mg I.V. and 1.5 gms orally; he noted some gastro-intestinal upsets, but even prolonged therapy appeared to have no adverse haematological or biochemical effects. In his view, the intravenous form is more effective and reliable for systemic mycoses. Intravenous miconazole, 200-400 mg at 8 hourly intervals for 5-30 days, was given to several patients by Scheef et al., (1974), and a solution of the drug was instilled directly into primary infection sites. Boelaert et al. (1975) reported peak plasma levels of 0.3 µg/ml after single oral doses of miconazole and after single I.V. injections they recorded initial plasma concentrations of 6 µg/ml, which decreased to 0.5 µg/ml in four hours. Cartwright (personal communication, 1975) has recorded serum levels up to 1.75 µg/ml in a patient receiving 1.5 g/day oral miconazole, and in a small healthy adult volunteer study I have found serum levels in the range 0.4-1.2 µg/ml and urine levels 1-5 µg/ml on a dose of 1 gm miconazole at 8 hourly intervals.

ECONAZOLE

A second phenethyl-imidazole, ECONAZOLE, (Peveryl, Cilag-Chemie) has recently entered clinical trials as a topical agent following extensive in-vitro and laboratory animal studies; it bears a close structural resemblance to miconazole and its activity against fungi is very similar, although it is more active against some Gram-positive bacteria (Thienpont et al., 1975). A number of carefully organised clinical trials have now been reported using topical cream and powder containing 1% econazole in the treatment of a wide range of dermatomycoses (Schmid, 1974; Quadripur and Bosse, 1974; etc.) with a success rate comparable to that anticipated from miconazole; no unacceptable side-effects were met. Thus far no studies with oral or intravenous econazole have been reported.

DISCUSSION

The imidazole derivatives in clinical use today are active against members of many genera of the plant and animal kingdoms other than fungi, and wild resistance of individual species is very rare. Chlormidazole, clotrimazole, miconazole and econazole are active in-vitro against almost all fungi of medical interest; wild resistance has not been reported nor has it been possible to induce the emergence of resistant mutants, and resistance has not appeared during prolonged therapy. All are highly effective topical agents, and give rise to few side-effects. Relatively high oral doses of clotrimazole or miconazole yield low body fluid concentrations, and side-effects with clotrimazole are common and sometimes severe; nevertheless, several workers have reported impressive success in the treatment of serious systemic infections with both imidazoles, and intravenous miconazole holds considerable promise.

The characteristics of the imidazoles in systemic therapy must be viewed against those of other drugs available, and Speller has well summarised their contrasting properties (Table 4). Amphotericin B has considerable antifungal activity over a wide spectrum of clinical interest, wild and emergent resistance is rare, but its intravenous administration is fraught with toxic hazards; fear of these should not cause amphotericin B to be withheld in progressive systemic mycosis (Symmers, 1973). 5-Fluorocytosine (5FC) is very active against most clinical isolates of candida and cryptococcus, but strains with wild resistance are met, and during therapy the emergence of mutants with virtually total resistance to 5FC has become distressingly common. Oral 5FC therapy results in high blood, urine, CSF and sputum concentrations, and the drug appears free from side-effects if not used to excess.

No faultless systemic antifungal agent is yet available, although the imidazoles come close to this in topical therapy; innumerable

Table 4
    Contrasting Properties of Imidazoles, 5 Fluorocytosine and
    Amphotericin B as Systemic Antifungal Agents (after Speller)

	Imidazoles	5FC	Amphotericin B
In-vitro			
Antifungal Range	+++	+	++
Degree of Activity	++	+++	+++
Wild Resistance	0	++	0
Clinical			
Ease of Administration	++	++	0
Frequency & Severity of Side-effects	0/++	++	0
High Body Fluid Levels	0	+++	0
Emergence of Resistance	0	+++	0

new imidazole derivatives are possible and it is among these that
the ideal agent may eventually be found.

REFERENCES

ALEXANDER, J., CORNELISSEN, J., DEBRABANDERE, L.,
TIMMERMANS, H.L., VANDEPUTTE, E., Van WAES, A. and Van
WAES-Van de VELDE, E. (1972). Miconazole in the treatment of
vaginal candidosis. Eur. J. Obst. Gyn., 2, 65-70.
BEWICK, M. and RAPER, D.A. (1974). The diagnosis of systemic
fungal infection in renal transplant patients and treatment with
clotrimazole. Postgrad. Med. J. 50 (Suppl. 1) 34-38.
BOELAERT, J., DANEELS, R., de MEYERE, R., Van LANDUYT, H.,
HEYKANTS, J.J.P. and LEWI, P.J. (1975). Plasma concentrations
obtained after a single dose of miconazole in man. This Congress.
BRUGMANS, J.P., Van CUTSEM, J.M. and THIENPONT, D.C.
(1970). Treatment of long term tinea pedis with miconazole.
Arch. Dermatol. 102, 428-432.
BRUGMANS, J.P., Van CUTSEM, J., HEYKANTS, J.,
SCHUERMANS, V. and THIENPONT, D (1972). Systemic antifungal
potential, safety, biotransport and transformation of miconazole
nitrate. Europ. J. Clin. Pharmacol. 5, 93-99.
BÜCHEL, K.H., DRABER, W., REGEL, E. and PLEMPEL, M. (1972).
Synthesis and properties of clotrimazole and other antimycotic
1-triphenylmethyl imidazoles. "Drugs made in Germany" Vol. 15,
79-94.
CLAYTON, Y.M. and CONNOR, B.L. (1974). Clinical trial of
clotrimazole in the treatment of superficial fungal infections.
Postgrad. Med. J. 50 (Suppl. 1) 66-68.
COMAISH, J.S. (1974). Double-blind comparisons of clotrimazole
with Whitfield's and nystatin ointments. Postgrad Med. J. 50
(Suppl. 1) 73-75.

DE BARROS, J.M. and BELDA, W. (1972). Treatment of tinea pedis with miconazole on an outpatient basis. Rev. Saude. Publica 6, 287-292.

DUHM, B., MAUL, W., MEDENWALD, H., PATZCHE, K., WAGNER, L.A. and OBERSTE-LEHN, H. (1972). Pharmacokinetics of topically applied bis phenyl-(2-chlorophenyl)-1-imidazole-methane- $[^{14}C]$. Drugs made in Germany 15, 99-103.

EL SHEIKH MAHGOUB (1972). Laboratory and clinical experience with clotrimazole. Sabouraudia 10, 210-213.

GODEFROI, E.F., HEERES, J., Van CUTSEM, J. and JANSSEN, P.A.J. (1969). The preparation and antimycotic properties of derivatives of 1-phenethylimidazole. J. Med. Chem. 12, 784-791.

HEINKE, E. (1972). Clinical experience with miconazole with special considerations of the conservative treatment of onychomycosis and paronychia. Mykosen, 15, 405-407.

HERRLING, S., SOUS, H., KRUPPE, W., OSTERLOH, G. and MÜCKTER, H. (1959). Experimentelle Untersuchungen uber eine neue gegen Pilze wirksame Verbindung. Arzneimittel-Forsch. 9, 489-494.

HOLT, R.J. (1970). Studies on the broad-spectrum antimycotic agent Bay b 5097 (Clotrimazole). Proc. of the 10th International Congress of Microbiology, Mexico City, 149.

HOLT, R.J. and NEWMAN, R.L. (1972). Laboratory assessment of the antimycotic drug clotrimazole. J. clin. Path. 25, 1089-1097.

HOLT, R.J. (1972). Laboratory and clinical studies on antifungal drugs of the imidazole series. Advances in antimicrobial and anti-neoplastic chemotherapy, 243-247.

HOLT, R.J. (1974). Recent developments in antimycotic chemo-therapy. Infection, 2, 2, 95-107.

HURIEŻ, P.C., AGACHE, P. and SOUILLIART, Mlle. (1962). Interet d'un derive du Benzimidazol en applications locales dans le traitement des Mycoses superficielles. Mouvement Therapeutique, 3, 1-11.

IWATA, K., YAMAGUCKI, H. and HIRATANI, T. (1973). The mode of action of clotrimazole. Sabouraudia, 11, 158-168.

JAMIESON, A. and ANDERSON, K. (1974). Primary amoebic meningoencephalitis. Lancet 1, 261-262.

JERCHEL, D., FISCHER, H. and KRACHT, M. (1952). Zur Darstel-lung der Benzimidazole. Liebigs Ann. Chem. 575, 162-173.

JONES, B.R., RICHARDS, A.B. and CLAYTON, Y.M. (1974). Clotrimazole in the treatment of ocular infection by aspergillus fumigatus. Postgrad. Med. J. 50 (Suppl. 1) 39-45.

KEJDA (1974). Die Behandlung von superfiziellen mykotischen Affektionen mit Myco-Polycid. Castellania, 2, 11.

LEDIG, R.(1958). Die Behandlung von Mykosen mit einem neuartigen Kombinationspraparat. Zeitschr. fur Haut-und Geschlechtskrank-heiten XXV, 190-192.

LOHMEYER, H. (1974). Treatment of candidiasis and trichomoniasis of the female genital tract. Postgrad. Med. J. 50 (Suppl. 1) 78-79

MALE, O. (1974). A double-blind comparison of clotrimazole and tolnaftate therapy of superficial dermatophytoses. Postgrad. Med.J.50, (Suppl. 1) 75-76.

PEETERS, F., SNAUWERJ, R., SEGERS, J., Van CUTSEM, J. and
AMERY, W. (1973). Treatment of candidal vaginitis with miconazole, a broad-spectrum antimycotic. Arzn.-Forsch. 23, 1107-1111.
PLEMPEL, M., BARTMANN, K., BÜCHEL, K.H. and REGEL, E.
(1969). Experimentelle Befunde über ein neues oral wirksames
Antimykotikum mit breiten Wirkungsspecktrum. Dtsch. med. Wschr.
94, 1356-1364.
PLEMPEL, M. and BARTMANN, K. (1972). Experimental studies
on the antimycotic action of clotrimazole (Canesten) in-vitro and
after local application in-vivo. Drugs made in Germany, 15, 103-120.
QADRIPUR, S.A. and BOSSE, K. (1974). Econazol, ein neues
Breitbandantimykoticum. Z. Hautkr. 49, 769-773.
RENZ, M., FARQUHAR, J.W., COHEN, M. and HARKNESS, R.A.
(1974). Elevation of myeloperoxidase activity in infants with oral
candidiasis treated with clotrimazole. Postgrad. Med. J.50
(Suppl. 1) 30-34.
SCHASSAN, H-H., MATZ, K., FREISENHAUSEN, H-D. and HARM,K.
(1974). Treatment of acute toxoplasmosis with clotrimazole.
Infection, 2, 7-11.
SCHEEF, W., SYMOENS, J., Von CAMP, K., DANEELS, R. and
DeLEEUW-DEVIGNE, C. (1974). Chemotherapy of candidiasis.
Brit. med. J. 1, 78.
SCHMID, P. (1974). Klinische Erfahrungen bei der Behandlung von
Hautmycosen mit Econazol-Creme und -Puder.Schweiz. Rundschau
Med. (PRAXIS) 63, 1156-1158.
SCHNELL, J.D. (1974). The incidence of vaginal candida and tricho-
monas infections and treatment of trichomonas vaginitis with
clotrimazole. Postgrad. Med.J. 50 (Suppl. 1) 79-81.
SEELIGER, H.P.R. (1958). Pilzemmende Wirkung eines neuen
Benzimidazol Derivates. Mykosen 1, 5, 162-171.
SYMMERS, W. St.C. (1973). Amphotericin pharmacophobia. Brit.
med. J. 4, 460-463.
SYMOENS, J. (1975). Miconazole for the treatment of systemic
mycoses : a review. This Congress.
TETTENBORN, D. (1974). Toxicity of clotrimazole. Postgrad. Med.
J. 50 (Suppl. 1) 17-20.
THIENPONT, D.,Van CUTSEM, J., Van NUETEN, J.M.,NIEMEGEERS,
C.J.E. and MARSBOOM, R.(1975). Biological and toxicological pro-
perties of econazole, a broad-spectrum antimycotic. Arzn.-Forsch.
VAN den BOSSCHE, H. (1974). Biochemical effects of miconazole
on fungi. Biochem. Pharmacol. 23, 887-899.
WAITZ, J.A., MOSS, E.C. and WEINSTEIN, M.J. (1971). Chemo-
therapeutic evaluation of clotrimazole. Appl. Microbiol.22,891-894.
WEUTA, H. (1974). Clinical studies with oral clotrimazole.
Postgrad. Med. J. 50 (Suppl. 1) 45-48.
WIDHOLM, O. (1974). An open trial of local therapy with clotrima-
zole for vaginal candidiasis. Postgrad. Med. J. (Suppl. 1) 85-86.
WOOLLEY, D.W. (1944). Some biological effects produced by benzimi-
dazole and their reversal by purines. J.Biol.Chem. 152, 225-232.
WHEATLEY, D. (1974). A new antimonilial drug. Pract.212, 254-257.

MODE OF ACTION AND RESISTANCE TO 5-FLUOROCYTOSINE

Jan Schönebeck, M.D.

Department of Surgery, Central Hospital, Norrköping,

S - 601 82 Sweden

5-Fluorocytosine (5-FC) (Fig.1) was synthesized in 1957 with
the expectation that, like 5-Fluorouracil (5-FU) (Fig.1), it
could be used as a cytotoxic agent in malignant diseases. It
proved complete to lack cytotoxic properties.

Luckily enough in animal experiments in 1964 it was
discovered that 5-FC heavily affected certain human pathogenic
fungi, e.g. Candida albicans and Cryptococcus neoformans. Later
it was shown that the drug also had an effect on other Candida
species, on Aspergillus species and on Chromomycosis.
Toxicologic studies on animals showed that 5-FC had a very low
toxicity. As a result of these discoveries the drug was used in
particular in infections caused by Cryptococcus neoformans and
Candida species in man.

5-FC only influences those cells which can absorb the drug
and transform it into 5-FU. Human cells lack this ability and
the drug is therefore non-toxic to man. In sensitive cells 5-FU
instead of uracil will be incorporated into RNA (Fig.2). The
cell then misinterprets the genetic code, makes the wrong protein
and the cell growth stops.

Thus 5-FC is a fungistatic agent and differs in this respect
from Amphotericin B and Nystatin which are fungicidal. This
biochemical difference is obvious also when the fungal surface is
examined. After treatment with Nystatin the fungi are collapsed
and cracked (Fig.3). When exposed to 5-FC the fungi are able to
grow for a while but finally succumb. As a result there are
many budding forms (Fig.4), but the cell wall is smooth and
without cracks.

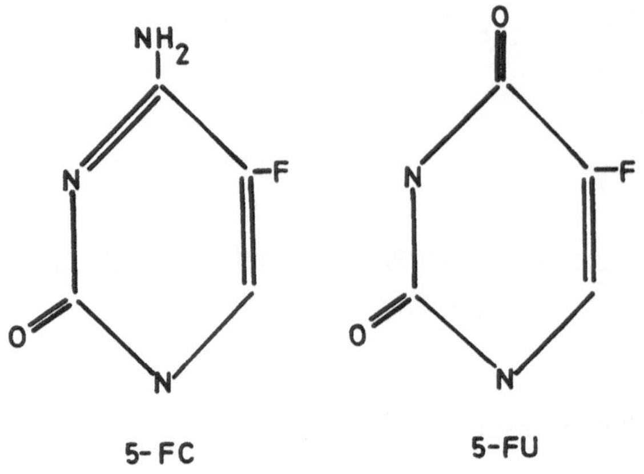

5-FC   **5-FU**

Fig.1   5-Fluorocytosine and 5-Fluorouracil

In man more than 90% of the drug is absorbed in unchanged
form in the gastro-intestinal tract. Of this, 98% in unchanged
form as well is excreted via the kidneys. No metabolism of 5-FC
into 5-FU seems to take place in man. If this happened, the drug
could not be used, as 5-FU is extremely toxic for human cells.
Theoretically it could be feared that 5-FU could be released from
killed fungi and be resorbed to human cells. In practice this
does not happen as no symptoms typical of 5-FU side-effects in
humans treated with 5-FC have been observed. If given orally
the maximal serum concentration is normally obtained within
1 - 2 hours (Fig.5). The drug is distributed rather uniformly
in the body fluids and therapeutic values are obtained, e.g. in
cerebrospinal fluid, intraocularly and in synovial fluid. As
5-FC is completely eliminated via the kidneys high urine
concentrations are reached and that even in cases with advanced
uremia.

In patients with normal renal function this elimination
happens quickly, as with patient C (Fig.5). Already after 12

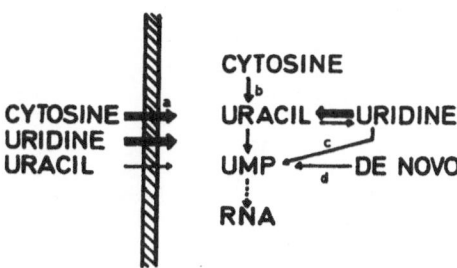

Fig.2   Presumptive scheme of uptake and utilization of 5-FC in
Candida albicans.   5-FC takes the same way as cytosine.   After
being taken up into the cell it is deaminated to 5-FU,
transformed to 5-F-uridine and incorporated into the RNA.   The
step 5-FU to 5-F-uridine is catalysed by the enzyme
UMP-pyrophosphorylase.

hours the serum concentration has decreased to a very low level.
In patients with impaired renal function the elimination is much
slower, as with patient B (Fig.5) with a serum-creatinin value
of 2.2 mg%.   Patient A (Fig.5) did not have any kidneys and the
serum level is unchanged for a very long time.

     If the patient is haemodialysed the drug is completely
eliminated.   A new dose of 5-FC should therefore be administered
after every dialysis.

     Normal fungistatic concentrations for Candida albicans are
0.1 - 1.0 μg/ml and for Cryptococcus neoformans 0.4 - 2.0 μg/ml.
Adequate therapeutic serum concentration is between 25 - 100 μg/ml.
Below 25 μg/ml the risk of selection of resistant strains increases,
above 100 μg/ml the risk of side effects appears to increase.

     Based on these facts and considering the renal function, the
following simple scheme can be used:

Creatinine clearance ml/min.	5-FC dose mg/kg	Dose interval, h
> 40		6
20 - 40	50	12
10 - 20		24
< 10		regular control of 5-FC serum concentration.

The drug is available as tablets of 500 mg, 10% ointment and 1% solution for infusion.

5-FC has proved teratogenic in the rat but the lowest teratogenic dose was 700 mg/kg body weight and therapeutic dose in man is only 200 mg/kg body weight per 24 hours. 5-FC has been used for treatment of Candida infection in two pregnant women, one for 11 weeks during the first part of the pregnancy and the other for a fortnight during the 3rd to 4th months of pregnancy. Both patients gave birth in due time to completely normal children.

In in vitro trials we found out that there were strains of Candida albicans, lacking the normal sensitivity to 5-FC. Therefore, we tested a number of Candida species to find out their susceptibility to 5-FC. We found a divergent sensibility to 5-FC in 10 out of 135 Candida albicans strains, 14 out of 48 other C ndida species and 3 out of 50 Torulopsis glabrata strains, i.e. 7.4%. 30% and 6% respectively.

When we studied the divergent strains we found that they in principal seemed to be of two types (Fig.6). Curve C indicates the growth of a normal C ndida albicans in the presence of 5-FC; it ceases rather rapidly. The completely resistant type of fungus which we called type A, was able to form colonies normal or nearly normal in appearance after 3 days of incubation at very high 5-FC concentrations. The other type, which we called type B, is markedly affected by even low concentrations of 5-FC, but is able to thrive at very high concentrations if the time of incubation is prolonged.

Some of these resistant strains we tested by incubating them together with C^{14} -labelled 5-FC. Their ability to grow in the presence of this C^{14}-labelled 5-FC is demonstrated by Fig.7. We then investigated how much of this was incorporated into their RNA (Fig.8). The completely resistant fungi did not incorporate

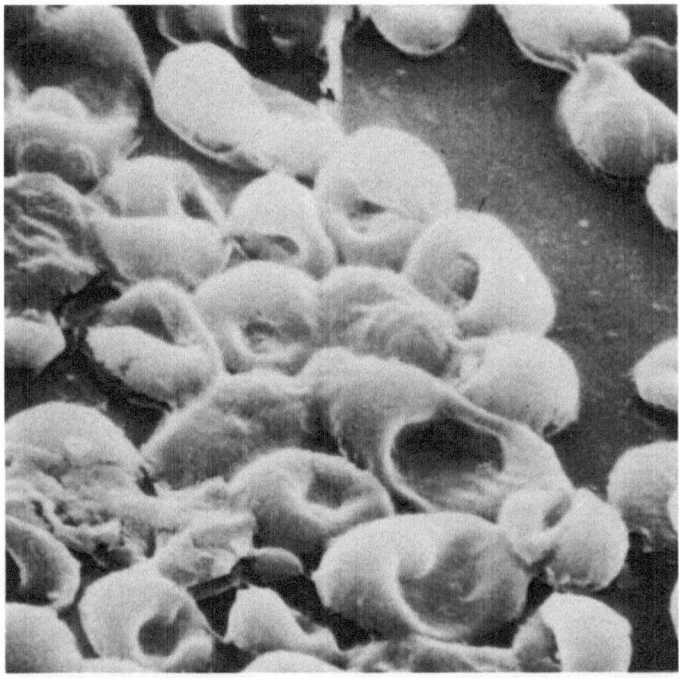

Fig.3   Scanning - electron microscopic appearance of Candida
albicans treated with Nystatin.

any 5-FC at all and their growth was unaffected. The sensitive
ones incorporated quite a lot and their growth was much retarded.
It is quite clear that the more 5-FC is incorporated into RNA the
more sensitive the fungus is to the drug.

     We were able to show that this type of resistance depends on
a mutation in the gene coding for UMP-phosphorylase (Fig.2).
Other types of resistance are of course possible and 5-FC-
resistance because of permease-deficiency has also been proved.

     I will now present my own material of fungal infections
treated with 5-FC. I was one of the first in Sweden to investigate
the drug. This resulted in many of my colleagues turning to me to
discuss the treatment of their patients. This is the reason why
rather varying kinds of diseases are represented.

     Out of 9 patients with asymptomatic candiduria 7 were cured.
One had a relapse with 5-FC sensitive strain and one with a 5-FC
resistant one. My further experiences have shown that patients

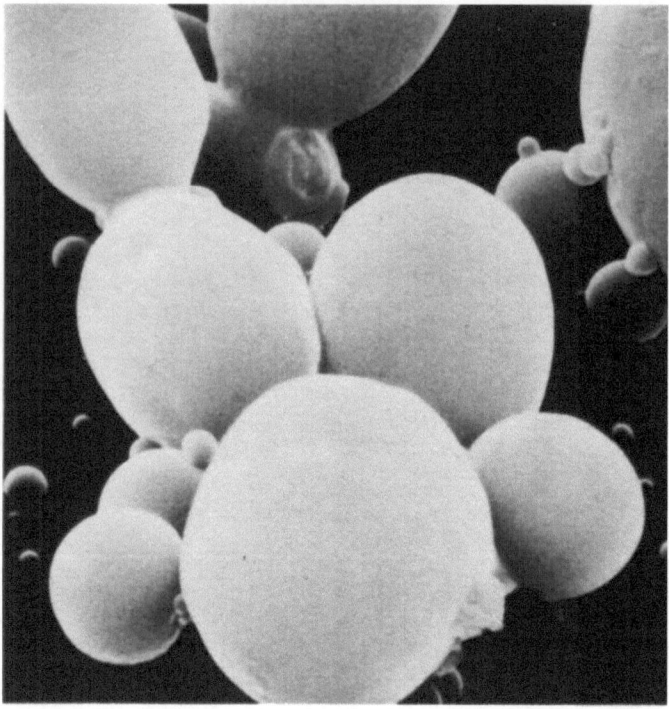

Fig.4   Scanning - electron microscopic appearance of Candida
albicans treated with 5-FC.

asymptomatic candiduria need no treatment.

        Thirteen patients with obvious urinary tract infection were
all cured.   Three patients with bezoar formation demanded a
surgical operation to remove the bezoar, the remaining funguria
then disappeared during 5-FC-treatment.

        Six out of 7 cases with Candida pharyngis were cured.   One
of the patients, who relapsed with a 5-FC sensitive strain had
no longer any problems when swallowing and this fungus must be
interpreted as saprophytic.

        Out of 4 cases of pulmonary candidosis 3 were cured.   The
4th patient had bronchiectasis with a lot of retained bronchial
secretion.   She relapsed with a 5-FC resistant strain.

        All of 6 patients with Candida septicemia were cured.   The
underlying reason for the septicemia was an infection after

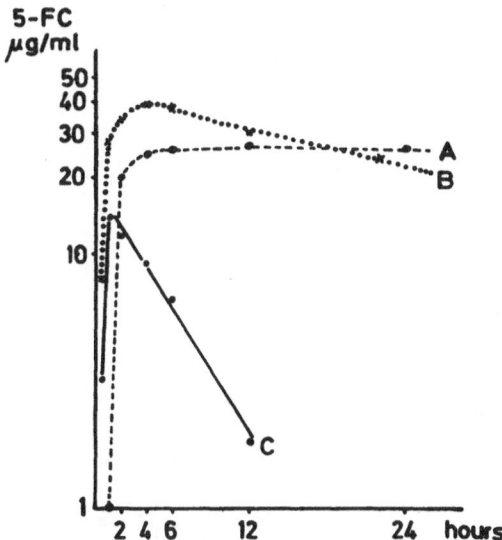

Fig.5   The concentration of 5-FC in serum at different times
in three typical subjects: an anuric patient (A), a patient
with a moderate degree of renal insufficiency (2.2 mg%) (B), and
a normal person (C).

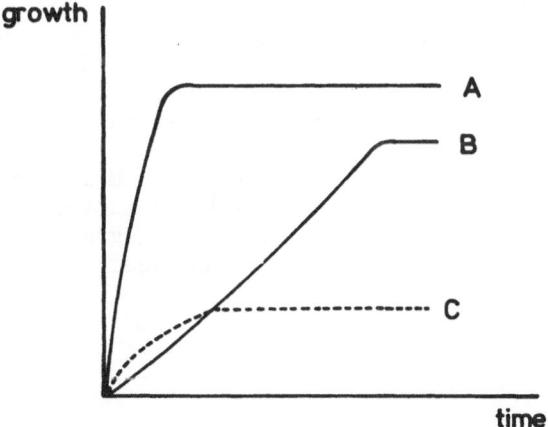

Fig.6   Growth in the presence of 5-FC of a type A mutant (A),
a type B mutant (B), and a Candida albicans strain with normal
sensitivity to 5-FC (C).

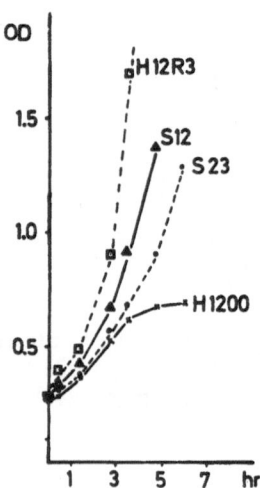

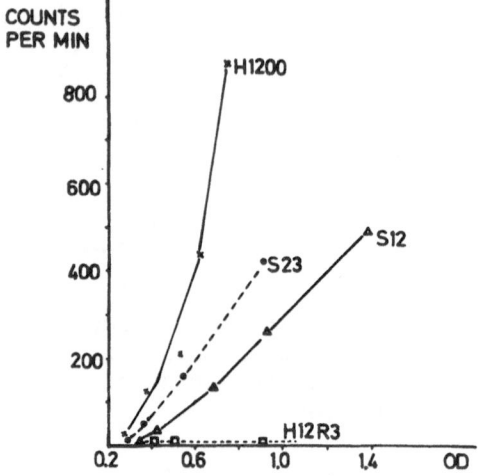

Fig.7   Growth of the wild
strain Candida albicans
(H 1200), the type A mutant
(H 12R3) and the two type B
mutants (S 12 and S 23) in
the presence of C^{14}-labelled
5-FC.

Fig.8   Correlation between the
uptake of C^{14}-labelled 5-FC into
the RNA and growth (OD) of the
wild strain Candida albicans
(H 1200) and the 5-FC-resistant
mutants (H 12R3, S 12 and S 23).
Note the close inverse
correlation between growth and
ability to incorporate 5-FC into
the RNA.   H 12R3 represents
type A-resistance, S 12 and S 23
varying degrees of type B-
resistance.

appendectomy, hyperemesis gravidarum, malabsorption, kidney transplantation, medulloblastoma and drug addiction.

Finally 11 cases of otomycosis treated with topical application of 5-FC cream should be mentioned. Several of these patients had earlier defied all treatment. Nine of them were cured after a couple of 5-FC treatments and the two who were not cured, were infected with penicillium fungi. These are obviously resistant to 5-FC.

My experiences with 5-FC treatment are thus very positive. Relapses caused by a selection of resistant strains have been few and I have in no case seen any side effects of importance. However, in the literature side effects are described, even fatal ones. The most frequent are leucopenia, thrombocytopenia and deterioration of hepatic function.

Even if the patients treated by me have been spared, side effects do exist. This, combined with the risk of selecting 5-FC resistant strains, makes me recommend the drug only on strict indications. In such cases 5-FC has proved to be an excellent antimycotic drug.

COMBINATION OF AMPHOTERICIN B AND 5-FLUOROCYTOSINE

Annemarie Polak and H.J. Scholer

Department of Experimental Medicine

F. Hoffmann-La Roche & Co. Ltd., Basle, Switzerland

SUMMARY

Moderate synergism of fungistasis was demonstrated in all normally sensitive <u>Cryptococcus neoformans</u> and in the partially 5-fluorocytosine (5-FC)-resistant <u>Candida albicans</u> strains. Synergism of the fungicidal effect was found throughout. It was more pronounced in Sabouraud broth than in an antagonist-free medium. In all strains the appearance of 5-FC-resistant mutants was significantly reduced by subinhibitory concentrations of amphotericin B (amph. B).

Survival rate of mice treated with a combination of the two drugs was increased in comparison to that of animals treated with each drug alone, viable fungus cells in the organs being reduced in number. Mycological cure was only achieved by combined therapy.

Attempts were also made to explain the mechanism of synergism. Addition of amph. B was shown to increase incorporation of fluorinated pyrimidine into RNA of the fungi. Decreased protein synthesis as produced by 5-FC alone was found more pronounced when amph. B was added in concentrations ineffective by themselves.

RESULTS AND DISCUSSION

Synergism between the polyene antibiotic amphotericin B (amph. B) and 5-fluorocytosine (5-FC) has been proved <u>in vitro</u> and in experimental animals (Shadomy and Davis, 1973; Block and Bennett, 1973; Medoff et al., 1971; Titsworth and Grunberg, 1973; Polak, 1974; Shaw et al., 1972) and seems to be confirmed also in human mycosis patients (Garriques et al., 1973; Halkin et al., 1974 and Kitahara et al., 1974).

The main practical interest of this synergism lies in the possibility to use smaller and, therefore, less toxic doses of amph. B than normally required, and in reducing the risk of 5-FC resistance.

In the present paper the synergism of amph. B and 5-FC was investigated in three in vitro models by measuring fungistatic and fungicidal activity as well as resistant frequency and in two animal models of acute candidiasis and cryptococcosis in mice. Further attempts were made to explain the mechanism of the synergism on a biochemical basis.

Fungistatic activity of 5-FC and amph. B alone and in combination was determined after a 3-day incubation at $37^{\circ}C$ in a chemically defined antagonist-free medium (Yeast Nitrogen Base Difco + 5% glucose, YNB). In three sensitive C. albicans strains, the MIC of the two drugs in combination was about the same as those of the drugs alone. This was also reflected by an FIC value (fractional inhibitory concentration index; Elion et al., 1954), greater than one indicating absence of synergism. However, in three C. albicans strains showing considerable but not complete resistance to 5-FC, the MICs' of the drugs in combination were lower than those of the drugs alone. The FIC ranged between 0.25 and 0.75 indicating slight synergism. A similar slight synergistic effect was found in three normally sensitive strains of Cryptococcus neoformans (FIC 0.125-0.75). Shadomy and Davis (1973) and Montgomerie et al. (1974) observed also the synergism most pronounced in 5-FC-resistant C. albicans strains.

In the fungicidal experiments definite numbers of yeast cells were incubated in YNB-medium and in Sabouraud broth containing various concentrations of 5-FC alone or in combination with 0.25 and $0.5\mu g/ml$ of amph. B. After a 3-day incubation at $37^{\circ}C$ the number of viable cells was determined by colony count on Sabouraud agar. In the Sabouraud medium which was used also by Medoff (1971) synergism was quite well distinguishable since 5-FC alone showed no fungicidal effect. For C. albicans the fractional fungicidal concentration index FFC (Elion et al., 1954) was <0.3-0.25, for Cryptococcus neoformans <0.25-0.37.

In the chemically defined medium in which 5-FC alone produced a moderate fungicidal effect, synergism was still present, but less pronounced (FFC for C. albicans = <0.625-1, for Cryptococcus neoformans = 0.375-0.75).

Interaction of amph. B with the development of 5-FC-resistant mutants was studied in 6 strains, each of C. albicans and Cryptococcus neoformans being normally sensitive to 5-FC. 10^8 cells

were incubated in yeast morphology agar containing 100µg/ml of
5-FC. After a 14-day incubation, the colonies indicating the number
of resistant mutants were counted. In all strains of both species,
the number of resistant mutants was markedly decreased by the addition of subinhibitory concentrations of amph. B. In C. albicans
a 50% reduction of resistant mutants was brought about by 0.2µg/ml
of amph. B and in Cryptococcus neoformans by 0.04µg/ml. By increasing the dose, a 100% reduction can be achieved.

For the in vivo studies mice were injected intravenously with
0.4×10^6 cells of C. albicans strain H12 or 2×10^6 cells of Cr.
neoformans H1281 and treated three times with 5-FC and/or amph. B,
namely at the time of the infection and after 6 and 24 h. Survival
time was recorded and the viable cells in the kidney and brain were
counted. In both candidiasis and cryptococcosis, survival time of
the animals treated with the combination of the two drugs was consistently longer than that of those receiving corresponding doses
of each drug alone.

Even more convincing were the differences in the number of
viable fungus cells in the organs of the surviving animals. 20 days
after the infection with C. albicans the number of viable cells in
the two kidneys was 2×10^4 in the animals treated with 25mg/kg of
5-FC alone, and $2.5 \times 10^5 - 3.6 \times 10^6$ in those treated with 0.06,
0.12 or 0.25mg/kg of amph. B alone. With the same doses of these
two drugs given in combination, the cell number was $2.5 - 5 \times 10^2$
only. Among the animals treated with the combination 25% were cured
completely, i.e., free of viable cells. This complete cure was
never observed in animals treated with either of the two drugs
alone.

In another experiment the mice infected with Cr. neoformans
were killed after 5 days and the viable fungus cells in the brain
counted. Again, the cell number was significantly lower in mice
treated with the combination ($0.4 \times 10^2 \pm 0.25 \times 10^2$) than in those
treated with amph. B ($2.36 \times 10^2 \pm 2 \times 10^2$) or 5-FC ($2.8 \times 10^4 \pm 1.4$
$\times 10^4$) alone.

Our in vitro and in vivo results are in agreement with the
findings of Block and Bennett (1973) and Shadomy and Davis (1973).
Moreover, the last found that the synergism in vivo is partially
attributed to the reduction of resistant mutants. Besides several
reports on synergism in vitro and in vivo (Titsworth and Grunberg,
1973; Medoff et al., 1971; Montgomerie et al., 1974 and Rabinovich
et al., 1974), there exists one report on antagonism (Hamilton,
1975) and several others claiming no effect at all (Beggs et al.,
1974; Shadomy and Davis, 1973 and Fields et al., 1974).

Therefore, the demonstration of synergism between amph. B and 5-FC seems to be dependent on methodology and the strains used.

When treating animals with the combination of 5-FC and amph. B, the following points should be considered: It may well be that the enhancement of the chemotherapeutic effect which is observed in vivo is not only due to the synergistic effect shown in vitro, but also to the impaired kidney function. We proved in fact that biologic half-life of 5-FC is prolonged when mice are treated with 3 doses of amph. B, thus synergism might be just simulated by higher 5-FC levels in serum and tissues. We also found that, when given alone, 5-FC was excreted less rapidly in candida-infected mice than in healthy ones because of numerous abscesses developing in the kidney. For assuring a correct interpretation an in vivo model was chosen where the effect of the drugs was investigated before any impairment of kidney function, either by amph. B or by the renal foci of candidiasis, was produced. Treatment was started 6 h after infection, i.e., at the time when candida cells have just settled down in the kidney and are beginning to grow. Amph. B was given in a single dose of 0.5mg/kg and 5-FC was administered in 4 doses of 50mg/kg each at one-hour intervals. This dosage schedule is analogous to that used in man when one takes into account that in mice the biological half-lives of both drugs are 4 to 6 times shorter than in healthy humans. Two hours after the last 5-FC treatment, i.e., 11 hours after infection, the mice were killed and the viable candida cells in both kidneys counted. The mean cell number found in the untreated control group ($6.2 \times 10^4 \pm 4.2 \times 10^4$) was significantly reduced by 5-FC ($3.7 \times 10^4 \pm 1.6 \times 10^4$) but not by amph. B ($6.8 \times 10^4 \pm 4.8 \times 10^4$). When the drugs were given in combination, the number of viable cells was reduced to $1.2 \times 10^4 \pm 1 \times 10^4$. The difference in the number compared with both the 5-FC and amph. B groups was statistically significant ($p < 0.05$).

In further experiments an attempt was made to explain the mechanism of this synergism. Confirming the observations first made by Medoff et al. (1972), we found that 0.05 and 0.1µg/ml of amph. B increased significantly the incorporation of fluorinated pyrimidine into the RNA of Candida albicans, incubated with 100µg/ml of 5-FC. After a 6-hour incubation, 382 ng of 5-FU/mg dry weight were incorporated by the cells treated with 5-FC alone. In the presence of 0.01 or 0.05µg/ml of amph. B 528 ng of 5-FU/mg dry weight and 678 ng of 5-FU/µmg dry weight, respectively, were incorporated.

These findings are in agreement with our in vitro observations that the potentiation with 5-FC and amph. B was most pronounced in a cytosine-permease-negative strain of Sacharomyces cerevisiae. However, synergism was also found in strains which are not lacking cytosine permease activity but another enzyme.

In order to find out whether an increased incorporation of 5-FU into RNA caused by amph. B may also have a stronger influence on the utilization of amino acids, uptake and distribution of radio-labelled amino acids in the yeast cells were investigated in the presence of 5-FC, amph. B and of the combination of these two drugs.

Reduction in the uptake of phenylalanine (-15%), histidine (-6%) and alanine (-28%) as produced by 100μg/ml of 5-FC alone was significantly enhanced (-42%, -69%, -56%,respectively)at a concentration of 0.05μg/ml of amph. B which was ineffective by itself. With 5-FC alone, a reduced incorporation of histidine and alanine in the proteins and a relative accumulation in the pool were observed, whereas the distribution of phenylalanine remained the same as in the untreated controls. There was no additional influence of amph. B on the intracellular distribution of the three amino acids.

The activity of polyene antibiotics is well-known to be connected with the release of substances such as potassium, phosphate and amino acids from treated cells (Gosh and Gosh, 1963). In our experiments a dose-dependent release of amino acids caused by amph. B was observed during one hour at 37°C. The release was consistently more pronounced from cells pretreated with 100μg/ml of 5-FC for 4 h, e.g., 10μg/ml of amph. B caused in 5-FC-pretreated cells a release of 18.9μg/ml amino acids in comparison to 12.5μg/ml in unpretreated cells.

The enhanced incorporation of the deaminated 5-FC into the RNA may be attributable to the enhanced permeability of the cell membrane caused by amph. B. The amino acid release, however, points to the fact that 5-FC has an effect on the specific amph. B activity. Yet, it was not possible to demonstrate a significant increase in the phosphate and potassium release as a result of 5-FC treatment.

REFERENCES

Beggs, W.H., Sarosi, G.A. and Andrews, F.A. (1974), Res. Comm. chem. Path. Pharm. 8, 559.

Block, E.R. and Bennett, J.E. (1973), Proc. exp. Biol. 142, 476.

Elion, G.B., Singer, S.and Hichtings, G.H. (1954), J. biol. Chem. 208, 477.

Fields, B.T., Meredith, W.R., Galbraith, J.E. and Hardin, H.F. (1974), Clin. Res. 22, 32A.

Garriques, I.L., Sande, M.A., Utz, J.P., Mandell, G.L., Warner, J. F., McGehee, R.F. and Shadomy, S. Abstract presented at the 13th Int. Conference on Antimicrobial Agents and Chemotherapy, Washington, September, 1973.

Gosh, A.J. and Gosh, J. (1963), Ann. Biochem. 13, 611.

Halkin, H., Ravid, M., Zulman, J. and Reichert, N. (1974), Israel J. med. Sci. 10, 1148.

Hamilton, J.D.and Elliot, D.M. (1975), J. infect. Dis. 131, 129.

Kitahara, M., Medoff, G. and Kobayashi, G.S. Abstract presented at the 14th Interscience Conference on Antimicrobial Agents and Chemotherapy, San Francisco, September, 1974.

Medoff, G., Kobayashi, G.S., Kwan, C.N., Schlesinger, D. and Venkov, P. (1972), Proc. nat. Acad. Sci. USA 69, 196.

Medoff, G., Comfort, M. and Kobayahi, G.S. (1971), Proc. Soc. exp. Biol. Med. 138, 571.

Montgomerie, J.Z., Edwards, J.E. and Guze, L.B. (1974), Clin. Res. 22, 450A.
Polak, A. (1974), Bull. Soc. fr. Mycol. Méd. 3, 175.

Shadomy, S. and Davis, B. Abstract presented at the Annual Meeting of the American Society of Microbiology, Miami Beach, May, 1973.

Shaw, D.B., Rabinovich, S. and Donta, S.T. Abstract presented at the Annual Meeting of the American Society of Microbiology, Ann Arbor, 1972.

Rabinovich, S., Shaw, B.D., Bryant, T. and Donta, S.T. (1974), J. infect. Dis. 130, 28.

Titsworth, E. and Grunberg, E. (1973), Antimicrob. Ag. Chemother. 4, 306.

COMBINED FLUCYTOSINE - AMPHOTERICIN B TREATMENT OF

CRYPTOCOCCOSIS

J.P.Utz*,M.D., I.L. Garriques,M.D., M.A. Sande,M.D.,
J.F. Warner,M.D., G.L. Mandell,M.D., R.F.McGehee,M.D.,
R.J. Duma,M.D. and S. Shadomy,Ph.D.

Divisions of Immunology and Infectious Diseases,
Departments of Medicine, Medical College of Virginia,
Virginia Commonwealth University and McGuire Veterans
Administration Hospital, Richmond and University of
Virginia School of Medicine, Charlottesville, Virginia

*School of Medicine, Georgetown University,
Washington, D.C. 20007

SUMMARY

In a prospective study from May 1971 to November 1973, 20
consecutive patients with a diagnosis of disseminated cryptococcosis were treated for six weeks with a combination of amphotericin B (20 mg/d) intravenously and flucytosine (5-FC) (150
mg/kg/d) orally. Fifteen patients had culturally documented
Cryptococcus neoformans meningitis, and three died of infection
early in therapy. Of the remaining 12 patients, eight were alive
and well eight to 34 months following therapy, and four died of
other causes. None of the surviving patients has relapsed.

Hematologic complications developed in nine patients, three
of whom had no underlying lymphoreticular disorder or therapy
with known cytotoxic agents. Renal insufficiency of mild degree
occurred in only six patients.

A shorter period of hospitalisation and reduction in amphotericin B toxicity suggest that combined therapy is a safe and
efficacious alternative to other regimens.

143

INTRODUCTION

Prior to 1956 no effective therapy existed for Cryptococcus
neoformans meningitis. Following the introduction of amphotericin
B, 69 to 87% of patients responded to therapy in terms of clinical
improvement and failure to culture the fungus (1,2). These figures
are a dramatic improvement from the previous universally fatal
outcome. Yet amphotericin B can hardly be considered ideal therapy,
since 13 to 31% of patients failed to respond and an additional 18
to 25% relapsed following completion of therapy (1,2). As importantly, in greater than 80% of patients treated, nephrotoxicity
was an irreversible and often serious complication (3,4).

In 1964 flucytosine (5-FC), a fluoro-pyrmidine evaluated
earlier as an antineoplastic agent, was reported therapeutically
active in yeast infections in mice (5) and in 1968 in man (6,7).
However, 5-FC can not be considered ideal·therapy for cryptococcosis, as only 80% of patients treated responded, and of those
responding 20% relapsed following completion of therapy. In
addition scattered reports expressed concern about hematopoietic
toxicity (6,7,8).

Combinations of antimicrobial agents have been used successfully in several diseases, e.g. enterococcal endocarditis and
tuberculosis. Theoretically, a combination of amphotericin B and
5-FC might act additively or synergistically by virtue of ampho-
tericin.B increasing the permeability of yeast cell membranes to
5-FC (9). In 1971 Medoff et al (10) reported synergism of amphotericin B and 5-FC in vitro against three isolates of C.neoformans.
In other studies (Shadomy, S., unpublished data), additive fungicidal activity was shown in 6 of 21 isolates. Thus, in 1971 a
co-operative prospective study of a combination of 5-FC and amphotericin B in the treatment of human cryptococcosis was initiated.
Objectives of the study were to (a) achieve a therapeutic response
better than that which might be realised with either drug alone,
(b) utilise lower doses (11) of amphotericin B in order to reduce
toxicity and (c) treat for a period of time (6 weeks) shorter than
that (10 weeks) of previous studies (11) thus decreasing the period
of hospitalisation.

MATERIALS AND METHODS

From May 1971 to November 1973 patients with a diagnosis of
disseminated cryptococcosis were treated by the Infectious
Disease Services of the University of Virginia, Medical College of
Virginia, and McGuire Veterans Administration Hospitals. No
patients with cryptococcosis admitted to the hospital during the
30 month period were excluded from the study. Prior treatment
did not exclude patients from the study, provided there was clear

cut (cultural) evidence of failure or relapse. According to protocol, cerebrospinal fluid, blood, bone marrow, sputum, urine, and
all biopsy specimens were examined microscopically and cultured
for C.neoformans. Specimens from sites initially positive were
re-examined at 2 week intervals during therapy and at each visit
following completion of therapy. During treatment each patient
had hematologic, renal and hepatic function studies twice weekly.
Following completion of therapy, the same studies were repeated
during each visit. Additional studies performed initially on all
patients included electroencephalograms, radioiodinated serum
albumin (RISA) scan, glucose tolerance, skull films, serum electrophoresis, and quantitative serum immunoglobulins.

C.neoformans was identified (a) by demonstration of encapsulated budding yeasts microscopically, (b) by growth at 30°C and
37°C on Sabouraud's agar, (c) by urease production on Christian's
urea media and (d) by in vitro assimilation of galactitol, glucose,
inositol, maltose, sucrose, trehalose, but not lactose, melibiose,
or nitrate. In vitro susceptibility studies to amphotericin B and
5-FC were performed as previously described (12,13). Resistance
was defined as a minimal inhibitory concentration (MIC) > 25 ug/ml
for 5-FC or > 1.0 ug/ml for amphotericin B. To assay amphotericin
B in the presence of 5-FC in serum and cerebrospinal fluid as previously described (14,1-) cylinder plate bioassay was modified by
supplementing the basic medium with 10 ug/ml of cytosine and
employing an isolate of Crysosporium pruinosum resistant to 5-FC
but sensitive to amphotericin B. Bioassays for 5-FC were performed
using a standard bioassay for this drug (15).

At the completion of initial diagnostic and protocol studies,
or sooner if clinical conditions dictated, each patient received
5-FC 150 mg/kg/d orally in 4 equally divided doses and amphotericin
B intravenously beginning with 1 mg on day 1, 5 mg day 2, 10 mg
day 3, 15 mg day 4, and 20 mg day 5 and thereafter. The combined
treatment was continued for a total of 6 weeks, after which patients were re-evaluated for evidence of relapse 3 months, 6 months,
1 year, and yearly thereafter. During therapy other drugs, such
as immunosuppressants and antineoplastic agents, were continued
at the discretion of the attending physician.

For the purpose of this study, a patient was considered cured
if he or she was free of disease clinically and by laboratory
examination 12 months or more following completion of therapy.
Patients were considered improved if they were free of disease for
a period of less than 12 months after completing therapy, or if
they died of other causes within 12 months of completing therapy
and were free of cryptococcal disease at the last follow-up visit
or at necropsy.

TABLE 1

COMBINED FLUCYTOSINE – AMPHOTERICIN B THERAPY: CLINICAL FEATURES

I. Documented cryptococcosis
A. Meningeal

Patient Race/ Sex/Age	Associated Conditions	C.neoformans Cultured from:	Therapeutic Results	Complications during therapy	Length of Follow-Up Months
WK W/M/47	Lymphopenia hepatospleno-megaly, predni-sone therapy	CSF[1], bone marrow, urine, sputum, pleural fluid	Alive, free of cryptoccoccosis	Hypokalemia, anemia, elevated alka-line phosphatase, leukopenia.	34
DS B/F/54	Pulmonary tuber-culosis, alcoho-lism, chronic lymphocytic leukemia	CSF	Died of other causes	Azotemia, anemia, elevated alkaline phosphatase.	11
MB W/F/68	Lymphosarcoma, prednisone therapy	CSF	Alive, free of disease	Thrombocytopenia, leukopenia	24
RL B/M/62	Lymphosarcoma	CSF	Died with crypto-coccosis, day 5 of therapy	None	0
MH W/F/70	None	CSF	Alive, free of disease	Anorexia, nausea, vomiting, anemia, renal tubular acidosis	23

TABLE 1 (contd)

Patient Race/ Sex/Age	Associated Conditions	C.neoformans Cultured from:	Therapeutic Results	Complications during therapy	Length of follow up Months
JG W/M/49	Chronic active hepatitis, prednisone therapy	CSF, kidney (at autopsy)	Died with cryptococcosis day 11 of therapy	Azotemia	0
BM W/M/48	Chronic glomer-ulonephritis, prednisone therapy	CSF, blood, urine, peri-toneal fluid	Died with cryptococcosis, day 10 of therapy	None	0
SM W/M/50	Chronic aggres-sive hepatitis, prednisone therapy	CSF, blood, urine, bone marrow	Alive, free of cryptococcosis	Thrombocytopenia, anorexia, elevated alkaline phosphatase and $SGOT^2$	20
HT W/M/63	Chronic obstruc-tive pulmonary disease, predni-sone therapy	CSF	Died, free of cryptococcosis	None	5
SD W/M/63	Lymphosarcoma, macroglobulinemia, prednisone therapy	CSF	Died, free of cryptococcosis	Leukopenia	1/6
HL W/M/72	Lymphosarcoma, prednisone therapy	CSF, blood	Died, free of cryptococcosis	Thrombocytopenia, hypokalemia	3

TABLE 1 (contd)

Patient Race/ Sex/Age	Associated Conditions	C.neoformans cultured from:	Therapeutic Results	Complications during therapy	Length of follow-up Months
WC W/M/31	None	CSF	Alive, free of disease	Azotemia	12
RJ B/M/19	Lympho- sarcoma	CSF, blood, bone marrow	Died with cryptococcosis prior to beginning 5-FC	Not evaluated	0
JGK W/M/22	None	CSF	Alive, free of disease	None	10
HH B/M/23	Sarcoidosis	CSF, urine, skin, sub- cutaneous abscess	Alive, free of cryptococcosis	Fever, chills	8
EC W/M/55	Diabetes mellitus	CSF	Alive, free of cryptococcosis	Azotemia, fever, chills, phlebitis	8
B. Non-meningeal					
AB W/M/75	Organic brain syndrome	Blood, urine	Alive, free of cryptococcosis	Azotemia, anemia, leukopenia.	16

TABLE 1 (contd)

II. Suspected, not culturally documented, meningitis

Patient Race/ Sex/Age	Associated Conditions	C.neoformans Cultured from:	Therapeutic Results	Complications during therapy	Length of follow-up Months
NK W/M/43	None	0	Alive, free of cryptococcosis	Azotemia, fever, chills, thrombo-cytopenia, phlebitis	13
CO W/M/54	None	0	Alive, free of cryptococcosis	None	12
DPD W/M/22	Drug addiction	0	Alive, free of cryptococcosis	None	11

1 Cerebrospinal fluid

2 Serum glutamic oxaloacetic transaminase

RESULTS

Twenty patients were treated for disseminated cryptococcosis
with a combination of 5-FC and amphotericin B. Pertinent clinical
data, course, and outcome on all treated patients are presented
in Table 1. Middle-aged white men predominated. Eleven patients
either had associated lymphoreticular disorder or were receiving
adrenalcorticoid therapy. In 7 patients C.neoformans was cultured from several body sites in addition to the cerebrospinal
fluid.

One patient with cryptococcosis and lymphosarcoma (RJ) died
12 hours after receiving the first dose of amphotericin B and
without receiving 5-FC. A second patient (AB) with fungemia and
funguria but without clinical or laboratory evidence of meningitis received 6 weeks of 5-FC (50 mg/kg/d) plus amphotericin B
(20 mg/d). Three additional patients (NK, CO and DPD) received
6 weeks of combined therapy with a diagnosis of cryptococcal
meningitis based on the presence of antigen in the cerebrospinal
fluid. These 5 patients are excluded from therapeutic evaluation,
though they are included in toxicity evaluation.

Of the 15 patients with meningitis, 12 completed 6 weeks of
treatment. The remaining 3 patients died with active cryptococcosis early during the course of therapy. All 3 had fatal
underlying diseases. Of the remaining 12 patients, 4 died of
other causes one week to 11 months post therapy. Two were free
of disease at necropsy, the other 2 had no evidence of cryptococcosis at the last follow up visit prior to death. The remaining 8 patients were alive with no evidence of cryptococcosis 8
to 34 months following completion of therapy. The mean duration
of follow up was 17 months.

Complications of therapy (Table 2) included decreased renal
function in 6 patients. The maximal serum creatinine recorded,
3.8 mg/dl, occurred terminally in a hypotensive patient, JG, who
at autopsy had C.neoformans renal involvement. Patient WC
received several large doses of amphotericin B with a concomitant
rise in creatinine to 3.3 mg/dl prior to being admitted and placed
on combined treatment protocol. His serum creatinine returned
toward normal and was 1.6 mg/dl at discharge. In no patient was
it deemed necessary to reduce or discontinue drugs by virtue of
decreased renal function. However, in view of more recent information (16) it now seems prudent to adjust interval between doses
of flucytosine according to degree of azotemia or, specifically,
creatinine clearance.

TABLE 2

COMBINED FLUCYTOSINE - AMPHOTERICIN B THERAPY:
COMPLICATIONS OF THERAPY

Complications	No. of Patients
Azotemia	6
Leukopenia	4
Anemia	4
Thrombocytopenia	4
Elevated alkaline phosphatase	3
Fever, chills	3
Hypokalemia	2
Nausea, vomiting, anorexia	2

Hematologic complications were encountered in 9 patients. Singly or in combination, leukopenia (white cell count < 2500 cell/mm^3) developed in 4, thrombocytopenia (platelets $< 50,000$/mm^3) in 4, and anemia (hemoglobin <11.0 gm/dl) in 4 patients. Of these 9 patients, 4 had underlying lymphoproliferative disorders or were receiving agents potentially toxic to hematopoiesis. Two additional patients receiving adrenalcorticoids during therapy developed anemia, leucopenia, and thrombocytopenia. Three patients had no associated diseases or known cytotoxic drugs.

In in vitro susceptibility studies on 14 pretreatment isolates, 11 had an MIC of ≤ 25 ug/ml of 5-FC, and 5 had minimal fungicidal concentrations of less than 100 ug/ml. In 2 patients (SD, HL) isolates recovered prior to treatment were resistant to 100 ug/ml of 5-FC. Both patients improved on therapy and were culturally free of infection prior to death 5 days and 3 months after completing therapy. Resistance to 5-FC did not develop in 4 isolates obtained during therapy. One one isolate, from patient DS, was resistant to amphotericin B. That patient improved, but died of other causes 11 months later.

Eight patients had sufficient specimens to compare serum and cerebrospinal fluid drug concentrations and renal function (Table 3). Concentrations of 5-FC in the cerebrospinal fluid approximated serum levels and exceeded the MIC of the patient's fungus in all cases except patient SD. Serum concentrations of amphotericin B were approximately twice the MIC of the infecting fungus. However, the drug was not detected in the cerebrospinal fluid of 4 patients, and was less than 10% of serum values in an additional 3 patients. As samples were randomly collected, no correlation could be made between the degree of renal impairment and the levels of 5-FC attained in either serum or cerebrospinal fluid specimens.

TABLE 3

COMBINED FLUCYTOSINE - AMPHOTERICIN B THERAPY: RENAL FUNCTION AND DRUG LEVELS

Patient	Max. serum creatinine (mg/dl)	Concentrations or ranges 5-FC (ug/ml)		Concentrations Amphotericin B ug/ml		Susceptibility ug/ml	
		Serum	CSF	Serum	CSF	5-FC	Am. B
DS	2.0	66-155	68-390	0.25-1.6	0	MIC 1.56 MFC >100	1.56 3.1
MB	Normal	29-150	53-74	0.22-2.3	0	MIC 12.5 MFC 50	0.5 >1.0
MH	Normal	60-150	74-80	0.29-1.2	0	MIC 12.5 MFC 2.5	0.78
HT	2.2	113-180	123-218	0.22-0.69	0-0.31	MIC 6.25 MFC 12.5	0.39 0.39
SD	1.6	48-96	36-65	0.26-1.65	0.13-0.56	MIC >100 MFC >100	0.2 0.78
HL	3.3	87	62	0.3	<0.03	MIC 25 MFC >100	0.1 0.5
HH	1.2	54-56	51	0.32-0.75	0.0	MIC 50 MFC >100	0.78 1.56
EC	2.8	43-108	43-84	0.14-0.46	0-0.06	MIC 0.1 MFC 0.1	0.35 0.78

MFC Minimal fungicidal concentration

DISCUSSION

The patients with documented C.neoformans meningitis comprising the present study are comparable in age, race, sex, and
underlying disease to those of previous studies (2,17). Again,
20% of patients died early in the course of therapy. In each
case death was associated with a serious underlying illness.
Of the 12 patients who completed combined, antifungal therapy,
none relapsed after a mean duration of follow up of 17 months.
This compares favourable to an 18 to 25% relapse rate following
other treatment regimens (1,2).

Notable rises in serum creatinine occurred in 6 patients.
The values returned to or nearly to pretreatment values in the
4 surviving patients. These results are similar to those reported
by Drutz et al (11).

In the 9 patients with hematologic complications most had
underlying lymphoreticular disorders or were receiving antineoplastic or cytotoxic drugs. In only 3 patients was the antifungal therapy considered the most likely cause of the complication. Since 2 of these 3 had concomitant rises in serum
creatinine, and since 5-FC is excreted almost exclusively by the
kidneys (7), it is possible that each accumulated excessively
high serum concentrations. Thrombocytopenia was the most pro-
found hematologic complication, with counts occasionally in the
range of 10 - 20,000/mm^3 and with epistaxis, petechiae, and
ecchymosis in one patient. Although platelet counts increased
promptly on withholding 5-FC for from 48 to 72 hours, this toxicity may limit the usefulness of combined or single 5-FC therapy
in patients with underlying lymphoreticular disorders and with
only limited bone marrow reserve.

The 3 patients with abnormal liver function tests during
therapy had pre-existing liver disease. These tests returned
to the pretreatment values following completion of therapy.

Though recently devised experimental models have demonstrated
in vivo potentiation of chemotherapeutic activity with combinations of amphotericin B and 5-FC (18,19), this phenomenon is not
readily proved in the treatment of humans. Nevertheless, it
appears from this study that a lower dose of amphotericin B for
a shorter period of time combined with 5-FC spares the patient
nephrotoxicity and excessive costs, and appears to be at least as
safe and efficacious as alternative single drug regimens. However,
definitive answers to the question of efficacy and safety await
a controlled, randomised study presently under way in a co-operative fashion. The failures occurring early in the course of
therapy suggest that earlier diagnosis and institution of treatment would be more helpful than higher doses of drug or longer

courses of therapy. The problem of earlier treatment is exem-
plified by the 3 patients in our study who risked 6 weeks of combined therapy for probable but culturally unproved C.neoformans
meningitis.

REFERENCES

1. Sarosi, G.A., Parker, J.D., Doto, I.L., Tosh, F.E.
    Amphotericin B in cryptococcal meningitis: long term
    results of treatment. Ann.Intern.Med., 71, 1079-1087,
    (1969).

2. Utz, J.P. Histoplasma and Cryptococcus meningitis. In
    Infections of the Nervous System, Proceedings of the
    Association for Research in Nervous and Mental Disease,
    44, 378-392 (1968).

3. Butler, W.T., Bennett, J.E., Alling, D.W., Westlake, P.T.,
    Utz, J.P., Hill, G.J.II. Nephrotoxicity of amphotericin
    B: early and late effects in 81 patients. Ann.Intern.
    Med., 61, 175-187 (1964).

4. Miller, R.P., Bates, J.H. Amphotericin B toxicity, a follow
    up report of 53 patients. Ann.Intern.Med., 71, 1089-
    1095 (1969).

5. Grunberg, E., Titsworth, E., Bennet, M. Chemotherapeutic
    activity of 5-fluorocytosine. Antimicrob.Agents Chemother.
    1963. American Society for Microbiology, Ann Arbor, 1964,
    pp.566-568.

6. Tassel, D., Madoff, M.A. Treatment of Candida sepsis and
    Cryptococcus meningitis with 5-fluorocytosine. JAMA,
    206, 830-832 (1968).

7. Utz, J.P., Tynes, B.S., Shadomy, H.J., Duma, R.J., Kannan, M.M.,
    Mason, K.N. 5-Fluorocytosine in human cryptococcosis-
    Antimicrob.Agents Chemother., 1968, American Society for
    Microbiology, Ann Arbor, 1969, pp.344-346.

8. Clinical data sheet on 5-fluorocytosine. Hoffman-La Roche,
    Inc., Nutley, N.J. (1969).

9. Gale, E.F., Cundliffe, E., Reynolds, P.E., Richmond, M.H.,
    Waring, M.J. The molecular basis of antibiotic action.
    John Wiley and Sons, New York (1972), pp.140-146.

10. Medoff, G., Comfort, M., Kobayashi, G.S., Synergistic action
    of amphotericin and 5-fluorocytosine against yeast-like
    organisms. Proc.Soc.Exp.Biol.Med., 138, 571-574 (1971).

11. Drutz, D.J., Spickard, A., Rogers, D.E., Koenig, M.G.
     Treatment of disseminated mycotic infections: a new
     approach to amphotericin B therapy. Am.J.Med., 45,
     405-418 (1968).

12. Shadomy, S. In vitro studies with 5-fluorocytosine. Appl.
     Microbiol., 17, 871-877 (1969).

13. Shadomy, S., Shadomy, H.J., McCay, J.A., Utz, J.P. In vitro
     susceptibility of Cryptococcus neoformans to amphotericin
     B, hamycin, and flucytosine. Antimicrob.Agents Chemother.,
     1968. American Society for Microbiology, Ann Arbor, 1969
     pp.452-460.

14. Shadomy, S., McCay, J.A., Schwartz, S.I. Bioassay for
     hamycin and amphotericin B in serum and other biological
     fluids. Appl.Microbiol., 17, 497-503 (1969).

15. Shadomy, S. Techniques for bioassay and sensitivity tests:
     amphotericin B and 5-fluorocytosine. In Laboratory
     methods in medical mycology. 3rd ed. CDC, PHS, USDHEW,
     Atlanta.

16. Schonebeck, J., Polak, A., Fernez, M., Sholer, H.J.
     Pharmaco-kinetic studies on the oral antimycotic agent
     5- fluorocytosine in individuals with normal and impaired
     kidney function. Chemotherapy, 18, 321-336 (1973).

17. Utz, J.P., Duma, R.J., McGehee, R.F., Warner, J.F. Chemo-
     therapy of the systemic mycoses: recent clinical observa-
     tions. In The Proceedings of the Fifth International
     Congress of the International Society for Human and
     Animal Mycology, 1971, pp.295-296.

18. Block, E.R., Bennett, J.E. Combined effect of 5-fluorocyto-
     sine and amphotericin B in the therapy of murine crypto-
     coccosis. Proc.Soc.Exp.Biol.Med., 142, 476-480 (1973).

19. Titsworth, E., Grunberg, E. Chemotherapeutic activity of
     5-fluorocytosine and amphotericin B against Candida
     albicans in mice. Antimicrob.Agents Chemother., 4,
     306-308 (1973).

THE TISSUE CULTURE STUDY OF ANTIFUNGAL AGENTS AND THEIR

MORPHOLOGICAL CHANGES ON YEAST AND YEAST-LIKE FUNGI

A. UETSUKA, S. SATOH, M. ITOH, N. OKAZAKI, Y. OHNO
AND K. YOSHIMURA
LABORATORY OF MEDICAL MYCOLOGY, DEPT OF INFECTIOUS

DISEASES, INSTITUTE OF MEDICAL SCIENCE, UNIV.OF TOKYO
JAPAN

Compared with virus and bacteria, there are few reports on the use of tissue culture techniques for the study of pathogenic fungi. Randall et al 1) used this method for studying Histoplasma capsulatum, while Larsh et al 2) reported on the diphasic fungi-Coccidioides immitis, Histoplasma capsulatum, Blastomyces dermatitis and Sporotrichum schenkii.

We 3) have studied the morphological changes in tissue culture of Candida species and Cryptococcus species. We found that with Candida albicans the pseudomycelium rapidly increased in length. In the case of Cryptococcus neoformans, the enlargement of the fungus body and thickening of the capsule could be seen in tissue culture.

In the fermentation industry, Candida, Cryptococcus and Saccharomyces species are widely used, and it is important that their pathogenicity is checked by every available method, including animal experiments.

In the present work, we have studied Candida tropicalis, Candida utilis and Saccharomyces cerevisiae, yeasts widely used in the fermentation industry, especially for single cell protein. We have compared their morphological changes in tissue culture and their pathogenicity to experimental animals.

As for the study of pathogenic fungi Randall 1) reported his several studies using tissue for Histoplasma capsulatum, while Larsh reported his studies on diphasic fungi of Coccidioides immitis and of Histoplasma capsulatum, Blastomyces dermatitidis, and Sporotrichum schenkii. In their numbers such studies are

remarkably few when compared with the studies made by applying
tissue culture of virus and bacteria. 3) We have studied the
morphological changes in the tissue culture of Candida species
and Cryptococcus species.

We reported that in the case of Candida albicans, its pseudomycelium became elongated longer in a very short time.

In the case of Cryptococcus neoformans the enlargement of
fungus body and thickening of the capsule could be seen in tissue
culture.

In fermentation industry, Candida species, Cryptocuccus species
and Saccharomyces species are widely used.

In this time now pathogenicity of those yeast and yeastlike
fungi must be checked carefully by every available method. Talking
about the pathogenicity of the yeast and yeastlike fungi, it is
natural that we should prove it by the animal experiments. But in
order to compare the morphological changes in tissue culture and
its pathogenicity to experimental animals, we experimented using
Candida tropicalis, Candida utilis and Saccharomyces cerevisiae
which are now widely used in the fermentation industry especially
for single cell protein.

Materials and methods

The following experiments were made by means of the Toplin's
plastic panel technique (a method generally used for screening
cytotoxicity) in the study of morphological changes and growth of
C. neoformans (Yoshida strain), Candida tropicalis (ATCC-750),
Candida utilis (IFO-0639) and Saccharomyces cerevisiae (IFO 0209)

1) 1×10^4 fungus cells/ml of each yeast was inoculated into
the L-929 cells or HeLa S T cells, which were then incubated
in an atmosphere of 5% CO_2.

2) As the control, 1×10^4 fungus cells/ml of each strain was
inoculated into 10%CS MEM (10% calf serum added to Maintenance Essential Medium) which is used for cell culture. The
incubation was done likewise under the same condition of 5%
CO_2.

3) After three days' incubation the content was taken out and
centrifuged at 1,000 r.p.m. for five minutes. Then the sediment was observed under the phase contrast microscope and
also in Indian ink preparation, Alcian blue staining, PAS
staining and fluorescent antibody staining. The cells of the
host were observed in HE staining and under scanning electron

microscope (Model JSM-S1 by Nippon Denshi).

4) Experiments were made to study the effect of various
antifungal agents upon HeLa ST cells and fungus strains
during cultivation. IxIO^4 cells/ml of fungi and antifungal
agents at various concentrations-Amphotericin B 0.03-I
microgram/ml, BAY B 5097, 5-FC and Mycostatin were
administered to the cells at the same time and their
incubation was made as before.

Pathogenicty tests were made in mice, using intravenous inoculation with yeast cells - 10^7 cells per mouse of C.tropicalis
and 2 x 10^8 cells per mouse of C.utilis and S.cerevisiae. The
mortality rate, histopathological examination and culture of organs
of weekly sacrificed mice were studied.

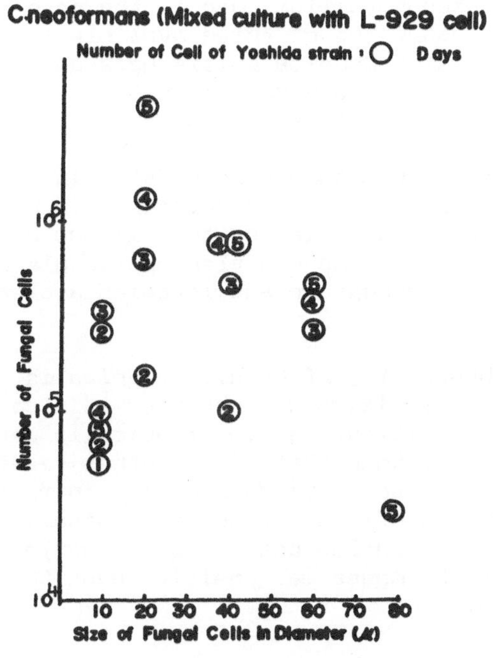

FIG 1.

Result

In experiments with Cryptococcus neoformans, when observed
each day under the microscope, a medium-size enlargement of the
yeast was observed the second day after inoculation. A remarkable
enlargement in size was found in 70-80% of the total number of
cells in Yoshida strain. The contrast had revealed an average of
5-10 micron in diameter, while the captioned fungi grew to 40
microns as shown in Fig. 1. The results were almost the same in
Indian ink preparations, alcian blue staining, fluorescent antibody
staining and observations under the scanning electron microscope .
When incubation was continued, some even grew up to 80 micron
ten-fold increase. Similar growth was also observed in HeLa ST
cells.

In the HeLa cells Candida tropicalis underwent elongation of
pseudomycelium from inside the cell, which after 24 hours
penetrated both the interior and surface of the cell and caused
the cell to degenerate owing to its very rapid growth of
pseudomycelium. Also in the macrophage strain (Kyoto University,
Department of Pathology) the elongation of pseudomycelium could be
observed on the phagocytyzed Candida tropicalis.

Candida utilis revealed far less transformation from
blastospore into pseudomycelium than in the case of Candida
tropicalis; it had only two or three oval blastospores in a chain.
Macrophage phagocytized Candida utilis were partly digested
and became vacuolated. The vacuoles in the macrophage were clearly
seen by fluorescent antibody staining.

Saccharomyces cerevisiae was inoculated in HeLa cells or
in the L-cells. Unlike Candida tropicalis, it was first
phagocytized in the HeLa cells and then showed a tendency to
become vacuolated. The same was also applicable when it was
phagocytized in the macrophage and revealed a clear tendency to
become vacuolated.

When the pathogenicity of Candida tropicalis, Candida utilis
and Saccharomyces cerevisiae was observed in mice by intravenous
injection, the mortality of Candida tropicalis was found to be
overwhelmingly higher than that of the other yeast strains. (See
Table 1). When we injected Candida utilis intravenously, a
slight pyelitis was confirmed histopathologically, and cultures
were positive. Also, in the case of Saccharomyces cerevisiae,
kidney culture of the mouse was positive even three or four weeks
after inoculation.

Table 1

Pathogenicity of Candida tropicalis, Candida utilis
and Saccharomyces cerevisiae in mice

	Sacrificed at (Weeks)	Mortality (died/used) (Range of days of death)	Pathology (Found/Examined)			Culture	
			Renal parenchymal Abscess	Pyelitis	Encephalitis	Kidney	Lung
Candida tropicalis ATCC-750 2x10^7 i.v.	1	3/10 (4-6)	Y~+++(4/7)	M+~+++(1/2)	Y+++(6/7)	+++(9/10)	+++(10/10)
	2	5/10 (3-9)	Y+ (2/5)	M+ ++(2/4)	Y+(2/5)	+++(7/10)	+++(9/10)
	3	7/10 (3-9)	Y++ (2/3)	M+ ++(2/3)	— (0/3)	+++(9/10)	+(9/10)
	4	9/10 (7-19)	— (0/1)	— (0/1)	— (0/1)	+++(9/10)	+++(9/10)
Candida utilis 2x10^8 i.v.	1	0/10	—	± (3/10)	± (2/10)	0	0
	2	0/10	—	± (2/6)	—	+(7/10)	0
	3	0/10	—	± (1/9)	—	0	0
	4	0/10	—	± (3/9)	±(1/10)	+(1/10)	+(1/10)
Sacch. cerevisiae IFO-0209 2x10^8 i.v.	1	0/10	—	—	—	+(6/10)	0
	2	0/10	—	—	—	+(3/10)	0
	3	0/10	—	—	—	(1/10)	0
	4	0/10	—	—	—	0	0

Y= Yeast form   M= Mycelial form

When C. tropicalis was inoculated a pathological change of
pyelitis was observed in a wide range; many pseudomycelium
were also observed in the tissues. With Candida utilis, the
histopathological finding of pyelitis was light, but both
blastospores and a few pseudomycelia were observed.

Fig 2 shows a table of growth curves of 3 stains, whereby
10% calf serum was added to Maintenance Essential Medium.
Candida tropicalis shows a rapid growth rate followed by Candida
utilis; the growth speed of Saccharomyces cerevisiae was much
slower by comparison.

Fig 3 shows the susceptibility of C. tropicalis after 24
hours in tissue culture against 4 antifungal agents. Inhibition
of growth in 0.11 microgrammes per mililiter concentration of
Amphoterin B was recorded; the growth of pseudomycelium was
subdued.

In the case of C. Utilis (Fig. 4) similar growth inhibition
was observed with Amphotericin B in 0.11 microngrammes per
mililiter concentration, and also with 5-FC in 1.7 microgrammes
per mililiter concentration.

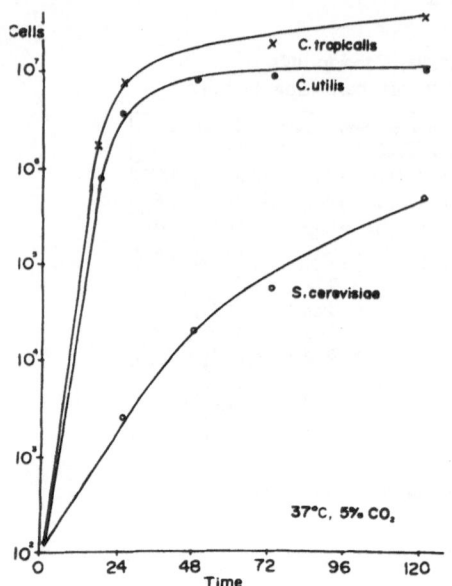

Fig. 2. Growth rates of C. tropicalis, C. utilis and S. cerevisiae in M.E.Medium + 10% Serum

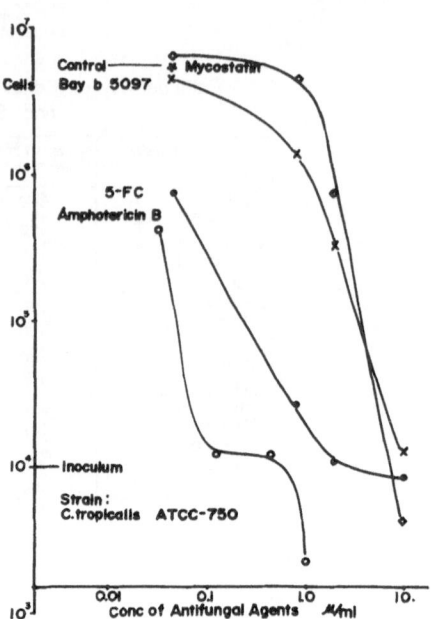

Fig. 3. Susceptibility of C. tropicalis to Antifungal Agents in Tissue Culture 24 hrs.

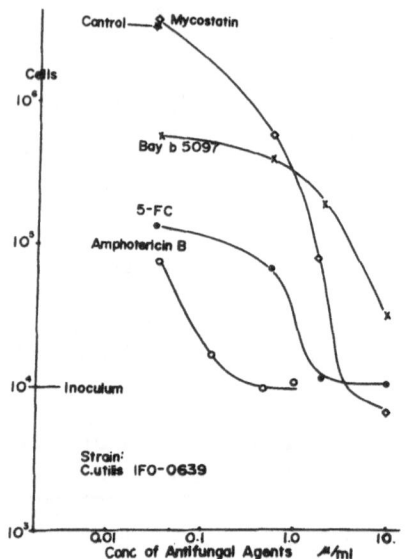

Fig. 4. Susceptibility of C. utilis to Antifungal Agents in Tissue Culture 24 hrs.

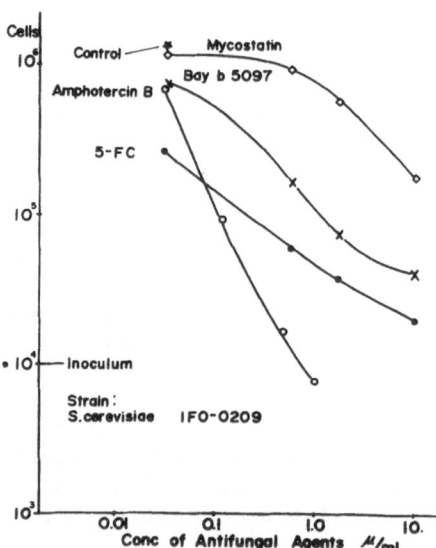

Fig. 5. Susceptibiltiy of S. cerevisiae to Antifungal Agents in Tissue Culture 72 hrs.

In tissue culture, Candida utilis still grew up in the HeLa cell even when 0.028 microgrammes per mililiter concentration of Mycostatin was used.

In Fig 5 no appreciable difference was observed in the susceptibility of Saccharomyces cerevisiae, when compared with the two aforementioned strains. When we observed HeLa cells by Gimsa staining, Saccharomyces cerevisiae was digested in the cell even with 0.025 microgrammes per mililiter concentration of 5-FC. They revealed outstanding vacuoles which differed from other strains.

In conclusion, it was observed that Candida tropicalis showed a transformation of pseudomycelium in a short time in the HeLa cell and in the macrophage. In the case of Candida utilis or Saccharomyces cerevisiae, the growth (transformation) in the tissue culture was far less and it had little morphological transformation. It was partly digested, and showed a tendency of slight morphological change. This means that when an antifungal agent was added in a given concentration, an outstanding difference was confirmed between the Pathogenic intracellular growth strain and the non-pathogenic extracellular growth strains.

References

1) Randall, C.C. & McVieker, D.L.: Proc. Sec. Exp. Biel & Met., 77 150-153, 1951

2) Larsh, H.W., Hinton A., Silbery, S.L.: Proc. Sec. Exp. Biel, Med. 93, 612-615 1956.

3) Akira Uetsuka: The Journal of the Japanese Association for Infectious Diseases. 33, 4, 336-363, 1969

MICONAZOLE PLASMA LEVELS IN HEALTHY SUBJECTS

AND IN PATIENTS WITH IMPAIRED RENAL FUNCTION

J. Boelaert, R. Daneels, H. Van Landuyt
  St. Jans Hospital
  Departments of Nephrology and Bacteriology
  B-8000 Brugge, Belgium

J. Symoens
  Janssen Pharmaceutica
  B 2340 Beerse, Belgium

INTRODUCTION

Systemic mycoses are increasingly recognized in association with various clinical situations. The paucity and toxicity of available drugs and drug resistance of yeasts all contribute to making the treatment of these infections problematic. It is therefore essential to have new, potentially useful antifungal drugs thoroughly explored. One of these, miconazole, an imidazole-derivate, has been shown to have potent fungistatic activity and few side-effects (Brugmans et al., 1972).

This study was undertaken:

1. To compare the effects of the oral and the parenteral routes of administration on the plasma concentration of the drug; and
2. To see whether renal failure alters the plasma concentration of micronazole and necessitates adaptation of the dosage.

METHODS

Twelve adult subjects participated in the study. Four were normal healthy subjects (group A) and served as controls. Four had chronic renal insufficiency with a serum creatinine of 2.1, 3.7, 4.8 and 7.8% (group B). Four had end-stage chronic renal disease and were undergoing intermittent haemodialysis: their residual glomerular filtration (endogenous creatinine clearance) was less than 3 ml/min., but none of them was anephric (group C).

In order to compare the plasma concentrations of miconazole, obtained after parenteral and oral administration, the four healthy subjects first received 522 mg of tritiated miconazole base (total radioactivity: 200 μC) as a single intravenous infusion over a 15 minute period; 9 months later they received a single oral dose of 522 mg, and four months later another single dose of 1000 mg of the drug. Venous blood samples were collected before and at scheduled intervals during a 72-hour period. Plasma was separated and deep frozen until analysis. The samples were assayed for miconazole by a gas chromatographic- and, for total radioactivity, by a radiochemical method (Heykants et al., 1974; Wynants et al., 1975).

To evaluate the effect of renal insufficiency and haemodialysis on the plasma concentrations of the drug, a single dose of 522 mg tritiated miconazole was infused intravenously in the subjects of groups B and C. The procedure was the same as for the subjects of group A. In the patients of group C, the infusion of the drug immediately preceded the start of a 6-hour haemodialysis with a disposable hollow fibre artificial kidney of the HFAK 4 type. A single pass technique was used. Dialysate samples were collected at regular intervals and assayed for total radioactivity. In the three groups, total urine was collected for 72 hours after miconazole infusion and assayed for total radioactivity and for unchanged miconazole.

For intravenous administration, a buffered and isotonic solution of miconazole base in 10% cremophor EL was used; for oral administration, miconazole base was provided as a 5% microsuspension.

RESULTS

Plasma miconazole concentrations obtained in group A after the infusion of 522 mg and after the oral administration of 522 and 1000 mg of the drug are shown in Figure 1. The mean initial plasma concentration reached 15 minutes after the start of the infusion was 6.18 µg/ml (extremes: 2.02 and 9.10). It dropped to 1.90 and 0.44 µg/ml after 1 and 4 hours respectively. After the oral administration of 522 and 1000 mg, peak plasma concentrations of 0.37, resp. 1.16 µg/ml were reached after 2 to 4 hours. The gastro-intestinal absorption of the drug was found to be 27%, as calculated from the ratio of the areas under the plasma concentration curve after intravenous and oral administration of 522 mg.

Mean initial (15 minute) plasma concentrations after intravenous administration of 522 mg micronazole in groups B and C were 21.85 µg/ml (extremes: 3.28 and 32.95) and 13.98 µg/ml (extremes: 2.36 and 31.78). The mean 1 and 4 hour values were 6.76 and 0.90 µg/ml for group B and 4.55 and 0.77 µg/ml for group C respectively. Plasma concentrations did not differ statistically between groups A, B and C.

Total radioactivity, recovered in the dailysis fluid during a 6-hour haemodialysis (group C) was only 2.80% of the total administered dose. Total radioactivity recovered from the 72-hour urine was 21.46 to 23.19% in controls and 11.63 to 17.06% in renal insufficiency patients (group B). Total radioactivity in urine consisted for 99.9% of metabolites.

DISCUSSION

This study confirms the existing data on miconazole metabolism (Brugmans et al., 1972): its moderate intestinal absorption, its rapid, probably hepatic, breakdown into various metabolites and its poor urinary excretion. The pharmacokinetic profile of miconazole in the subjects of the three groups has been described in detail elsewhere (Lewi et al., 1975) and was shown to be compatible with a 3-compartment open model. Biological half life was 24 hours in each of the groups.

The clinical significance of the plasma concentrations has to be interpreted in the light of MIC determinations on yeasts, e.g. Candida albicans. Holt (1974) used the tube dilution technique to demonstrate that the growth of 121 of 134 strains of C. albicans was inhibited by concentrations lower than 0.5 µg/ml. We also determined MIC by the tube dilution technique on 93 clinical isolates of C. albicans and found, after 48 hours incubation, that 100% of these were inhibited at 3.2 µg/ml, 98% at 1.6 µg/ml. 67% at 0.8 µg/ml, 33% at 0.4 µg/ml and 10% at 0.2 µg/ml (Van Landuyt, 1975).

Plasma levels exceeding the MIC for C. albicans last for only a few hours after a single intravenous infusion with 522 mg miconazole. Previous work (Brugmans et al., 1972; Heykants, 1975) has shown that after repeated administration of miconazole, peak plasma levels remain constant. Despite these relatively low and short-lasting blood levels, definite clinical efficacy has been shown in systemic candidosis, using a single or divided daily intravenous infusion of 522 mg miconazole (Symoens and Amery, 1975). Continuous miconazole blood levels in excess of MIC appear not to be needed to control yeast invasion.

After oral administration of 1000 mg, peak blood levels resemble blood levels found one hour after intravenous infusion of 522 mg but the initial peak of the intravenous infusion is not seen. This might explain why after oral administration of 1 gram three times daily, clinical efficacy in systemic candidosis has been less consistent than after intravenous treatment (Symoens and Amery, 1975).

Neither the initial plasma concentration nor the biological plasma half-life of miconazole are significantly affected by various degrees of renal insufficiency, so that dosage needs not be reduced in patients with renal failure. This is of practical importance, since systemic mycoses often appear in patients with underlying diseases that may include renal failure. Similarly, dosage should not be altered when the patient is treated by intermittent haemodialysis, as dialysis only removes minute amounts of the drug. In vitro, approximately 98% of miconazole is bound to plasma proteins (Heykants, 1975); this is consistent with its very poor dialysability.

Since only traces of unchanges miconazole can be detected in the urine, intravenous or oral miconazole
should not be used in the treatment of yeast infection
of the lower urinary tract (Fransen and Van Camp, 1974).

In conclusion, our data nave shown that after intravenous administration of miconazole, at a dose level
that is well tolerated (Symoens and Amery, 1975), therapeutic plasma concentrations are obtained.

ACKNOWLEDGEMENTS

We would like to thank J. Heykants and J. Wynants
for the miconazole determinations and P. Lewi for re-
viewing the manuscript.

REFERENCES

Brugmans, J., Van Cutsem, J., Heykants, J., Schuermans,
    V. and Thienpont, D. (1972), European Journal of
    Clinical Pharmacology, 5, 93.
Fransen, G. and Van Camp, K. (1974), Acta Urologica
    Belgica, 42, 452.
Heykants, J., Michiels, M., Knaeps, A. and Brugmans, J.
    (1974), Arzneimittel-Forschung, 24, 1649.
Heykants, J. (1975), unpublished data.
Holt, R.J. (1974), Infection, 2, 95.
Lewi, P.J., Boelaert, J., Daneels, R., De Meyere, R.,
    Van Landuyt, H., Heykants, J.J.P., Symoens, J. and
    Wynants, J. (1975), European Journal of Clinical
    Pharmacology, in press.
Symoens, J. and Amery, W. (July 1975), presented at the
    9th International Congress of Chemotherapy, London.
Van Landuyt, H. (1975), unpublished data.
Wynants, J., Woestenborghs, R. and Heykants, J. (1975),
    in preparation.

IN VITRO STUDIES WITH MICONAZOLE AND MICONAZOLE NITRATE

Smith Shadomy and Larry Paxton

Division of Infectious Diseases, Dept. of Medicine,
School of Medicine, Medical College of Virginia,
Virginia Commonwealth University, Richmond,
Virginia, U.S.A.

SUMMARY

The in vitro activity of miconazole and miconazole nitrate
against a variety of pathogenic and saprophytic fungi was studied
using an agar dilution procedure. 28 dimorphic pathogens were
tested: Histoplasma capsulatum and Blastomyces dermatitidis were
the most susceptible with inhibition of all strains at 0.5 ug/ml
of either compound. Coccidioides immitis was somewhat more resistant requiring 1 or 2 ug/ml for inhibition, while 4 isolates of
Sporothrix schenckii required 2 to 4 ug/ml for complete inhibition.
All strains of Cryptococcus neuformans were susceptible to 1 ug/ml
or less. Most strains of Candida albicans were resistant to less
than 16 ug/ml; other species of Candida were inhibited by 4 ug/ml
or less. Torulopsis isolates gave a range of MIC's from 0.5 ug/ml
to 16 ug/ml for inhibition. Of 15 dematiaceous isolates tested,
all but two were inhibited at 4 ug/ml or less. A brief discussion
of the possible clinical usefulness of miconazole is given.

Chemotherapy of the human mycoses is restricted to only a few
agents. Amphotericin B, although highly toxic, has proven itself
in the treatment of systemic and opportunistic infections. 5-
Fluorocytosine, although limited in its potential usefulness
because of the emergency of resistant organisms, has been proven of
value in the treatment of infections caused by pathogenic yeasts.
Thus, while both drugs are effective, neither is without serious
drawbacks. More importantly, neither drug has proven widely useful
in the treatment of other mycotic infections such as chromomycosis
although recent reports indicate that 5-fluorocytosine (Mauceri
et al, 1974) may be of value in treatment of this particular disease

which until now has lacked specific chemotherapy. Thus, it is
apparent that there continues to exist a significant need for new,
effective and nontoxic antifungal agents.

    The entry of miconazole, an imidazole antifungal agent, into
the arena of antifungal chemotherapy has generated much interest
(Van Cutsem and Thienpont, 1972). We were particularly interested in the potential usefulness of the intravenous form of this
drug in treatment of systemic fungal disease. Thus, a series
of in vitro investigations was undertaken to better define the
antifungal spectrum and level of activity of miconazole.

MATERIALS AND METHODS

    An agar dilution procedure was employed in most of the studies
being reported here. Media were either Sabouraud's agar or yeast
morphology agar. Drug concentrations ranged from 0.063 to 126
ug/ml. In the case of dimorphic organisms, only mycelial phase
cultures were tested. Incubation was at 30°C; time of incubation
was determined by the appearance of growth on drug-free control
plates. Two substances were tested. These were miconazole base
and miconazole nitrate. Drug solutions were first prepared in
dimethylsulfoxide, diluted and then added to molten media. Inocula
were applied to the surfaces of prepared plates with a replica
inoculator. The minimal inhibitory concentration was defined as
the lowest concentration which completely inhibited growth. 112
isolates of a variety of pathogenic and opportunistic fungi were
tested.

RESULTS

    Twenty eight dimorphic pathogens were tested (Table 1). All
were inhibited by miconazole and its nitrate salt. Histoplasma
capsulatum was the most susceptible with 6 of 6 isolates being
inhibited by 0.5 ug/ml of the base and 0.25 ug/ml of the salt.
Blastomyces dermatitidis was similarly susceptible. Coccidioides
immitis was somewhat more resistant than most isolates requiring
1 or 2 ug/ml for inhibition. The highest MIC for C.immitis was
2 ug/ml. Results with Sprothrix schenckii were not as encouraging;
4 of 5 isolates required 2 to 4 ug/ml for complete inhibition.

    These data reflect complete inhibition end points even though
many isolates were partially inhibited at much lower concentrations. The trend of somewhat lower MIC values for miconazole
nitrate as compared with the base was seen with many of the isolates tested. Differences in MIC end points for the two preparations were significant for B.dermatitidis but not for any
other species.

Table 1.   In Vitro Inhibitory Activity of Miconazole and Miconazole Nitrate
           for Dimorphic Fungal Pathogens

ORGANISM (No. tested)	Concn., µg/ml and Per Cent Inhibited													
	MICONAZOLE						MICONAZOLE NITRATE						
	0.13	0.25	0.50	1.0	G		0.13	0.25	0.50	1.0	G*		
Blastomyces dermatitidis (5)	20	60	100	-	0.29		60	100	-	-	0.17		
Histoplasma capsulatum (6)	33	67	100	-	0.25		33	100	-	-	0.19		
Coccidioides immitis (12)	17	17	25	75	0.78		17	17	25	92	0.67		
Sporothrix schenckii (5)	80% at 2.0 µg/ml				2.64		100% at 4 µg/ml				2.64		

*Geometric mean MIC values

Table 2 In Vitro Inhibitory Activity of Miconazole and Miconazole Nitrate for
         Pathogenic Yeasts

| ORGANISM (No. tested) | Concn., µg/ml and Per Cent Inhibited | | | | | | | | | | | |
| | MICONAZOLE | | | | | MICONAZOLE NITRATE | | | | | |
	1.0	2.0	4.0	>4.0	G	1.0	2.0	4.0	>4.0	G
Candida albicans (16)	6	–	–	94	13.5	6	–	13	87	11.8
Candida species (11)	46	64	73	100	3.07	not determined				–
Cryptococcus neoformans (12)	100	–	–	–	0.94	100	–	–	–	0.75
Torulopsis glabrata (6)	50	–	–	100	3.17	67	–	–	100	1.59

Table 3. In Vitro Inhibitory Activity of Miconazole and Miconazole Nitrate for Dematiaceous Fungi

Concn., μg/ml and Per Cent Inhibited

ORGANISM (No. tested)	MICONAZOLE						MICONAZOLE NITRATE					
	0.5	1.0	2.0	4.0	>4.0	G	0.5	1.0	2.0	4.0	>4.0	G
Phialophora sp. (2)	-	50	100	-	-	1.4	-	-	100	-	-	2.0
Fonsecaea sp. (6)	-	33	67	-	100	5.04	33	50	-	67	100	4.0
Cladosporium sp. (7)	43	57	-	100	-	1.35	29	57	-	71	100	1.81
All (15)	20	47	67	87	100	2.30	27	47	60	73	100	2.52

Table 4. In Vitro Inhibitory Activity of Miconazole and Miconazole Nitrate for Opportunistic Fungi

ORGANISM (No. tested)		MICONAZOLE					MICONAZOLE NITRATE				
		1.0	2.0	4.0	>4.0	G	1.0	2.0	4.0	>4.0	G
Aspergillus flavus	(5)	40	–	100	–	2.30	40	60	100	–	1.15
Aspergillus fumigatus	(5)	–	–	80	100	5.28	–	–	80	100	5.28
Aspergillus niger	(5)	–	40	100	–	3.03	20	40	100	–	2.64
All Aspergilli	(15)	13	27	93	100	3.33	20	33	93	100	2.52
Fusarium sp.	(7)	–	–	–	100	78	–	–	–	100	78
Mucor sp.	(2)	–	–	–	100	23	–	–	–	100	23

Concn., µg/ml and Per Cent Inhibited

Somewhat diverse results were obtained when pathogenic yeasts were tested (Table 2). Cryptococcus neoformans proved the most susceptible with all strains being inhibited by ug/ml or less. Three of 6 isolates of Torulopsis glabrata were inhibited by 1 ug/ml of the base and two were inhibited by 0.5 ug/ml of the nitrate salt; however, a nearly equal number required 8 to 16 ug/ml for inhibition. Most strains of Candida albicans were resistant to less than 16 ug/ml while nearly 75 per cent of Candida species other than C.albicans were inhibited by 4 ug/ml or less.

Fifteen isolates of the dematiaceous organisms were tested (Table 3). Most of these were of clinical or pathologic origin coming from such diverse clinical conditions as chromomycosis, cerebral cladosporiosis, endocarditis and pneumonitis in a penguin. All but two of the 15 dematiaceous isolates tested were susceptible to both forms of the drug at concentrations of 4 ug/ml or less. Two isolates of Fonsecaea required 64 ug/ml for complete inhibition but were partially inhibited at 16 ug/ml. The nitrate form was slightly less active than the case against Cladosporium species.

Many isolates of Aspergillus species were susceptible to 4 ug/ml or less of both compounds (Table 4). Aspergillus flavus was the most susceptible with several isolates being inhibited by 1 ug/ml. Aspergillus fumigatus was the least susceptible with 4 of 5 isolates being resistant to less than 4 ug/ml and one resistant to less than 16 ug/ml of either compound. Results with 2 isolates of Mucor and 7 of Fusarium were disappointing as none of these latter organisms were susceptible to less than 4 ug/ml.

DISCUSSION

These results are in agreement with previously published reports. Hoeprich and Huston (1975) recently reported that the clinical preparation of miconazole was inhibitory for C.immitis and C.albicans at concentrations as low as 0.6 ug/ml but was not fungicidal for either at less than 16 ug/ml.

Van Cutsem and Thienpont (1972) reported that miconazole was inhibitory for an unspecified number of isolates of pathogenic yeasts at concentrations of from 1 to 10 ug/ml. We differ somewhat from these latter authors in that most of our isolates of C.albicans were completely inhibited by not less than 16 ug/ml although partial inhibition was seen at lower concentrations. This difference probably reflects the more exacting end points obtainable with agar dilution than with broth dilution testing. In contrast to these authors, we found most isolates of Candida parapsilosis and Candida tropicalis susceptible to less than 10 ug/ml of drug. We also found most isolates of T.glabrata susceptible to less

than 10 ug/ml. Our results and those of Van Cutsem and Thienpont
also are in good agreement for the dimorphic fungi and Aspergillus
species.

DISCUSSION

A true assessment of the possible clinical usefulness of
miconazole must be based in part on in vitro susceptibility data,
and, in part, upon data regarding pharmacology of the drug in man.
Data regarding serum levels of miconazole are limited. Information
from Janssen Pharmaceutica indicates maximum plasma levels in the
range of 0.5 to 1 ug/ml following oral administration of a 1 gm
dose and of 1.6 ug/ml following intravenous injection of a 200mg
dose. In one patient treated at our hospital with the 200mg intravenous dose, we alsl found an average peak level of 1.6 ug/ml
1 hr post infusion. Hoeprich (Hoeprich and Goldstein, 1974) has
tried higher dosages and achieved a maximum of 5 ug/ml in one
patient receiving 1 gram per dose intravenously. Unfortun ately,
neither we nor Hoeprich have recorded CSF levels greater than
01. to 0.2 ug/ml.

Using a projected serum level of 2 to 4 ug/ml as the upper
limit of probable clinical susceptibility, most strains of
B.dermatitidis and H.capsulatum should be susceptible to the drug.
Thus, miconazole may have a place in treatment of human infections
caused by these organisms. The situation is less clear with
C.immitis and S.schenckii as many of these organisms are resistant
to less than 1 ug/ml. Systemic infections caused by Candida
species may prove susceptible. Pulmonary cryptococcosis should
also be treated with intravenous miconazole but the poor penetration of drug into the CSF will limit the usefulness of the drug
in treatment of cryptococcal meningitis. Few isolates of
Aspergillus species were susceptible to 2 ug/ml and usefulness
of the drug in infections caused by these organisms is uncertain.
With many isolates of Cladosporium being susceptible to 2 ug/ml
intravenous miconazole may be of value in treatment of chromomycosis.

REFERENCES

Hoeprich, P.D. and Goldstein, E. (1974) JAMA, 230.

Hoeprich, P.D. and Huston, A.C. (1975) Absts., 75th Ann. Meeting,
     Soc. Microbiol., Abst. A42.

Mauceri, A.A., Cullen, S.F., Vandevelde, A.G. and Johnson, J.E. (1974)
     Arch. Dermatol., 109, 843.

Van Cutsem, J.M. and Thienpont, D. (1972) Chemotherapy, 17, 392.

CLINICAL STUDIES WITH CLOTRIMAZOLE:

PHARMACOKINETICS, EFFICACY, TOLERANCE

H. WEUTA

Ressort Medizin, Bayer AG

Leverkusen, Germany

Clotrimazole is absorbed by the gastrointestinal tract and can therefore be given orally.

All studies which are reviewed were carried out using Canesten(R) tablets each containing o,5 g Clotrimazole.

PHARMACOKINETICS

The serum peak concentrations are reached after 2-4 hours. The concentration curves are distributed over a wide range. Increasing the dose from 2o mg/kg to 4o mg/kg body weight increases the level by a factor of 1,5 or even more as shown by PUETTER - Clotrimazole is nearly 1oo % bound to serum albumin and completely metabolised in the body.

During the course of treatment Clotrimazole induces the enzyme which metabolises the drug. For all these reasons dosing of Clotrimazole cannot be planned but must be adjusted to suit the demanded clinical efficacy and tolerance if there is no possibility to determine serum concentrations. - It is recommended that adults receive 2o mg/kg three times per day to begin with and then if the clinical picture requires, to increase the dose after three weeks up to 4o mg/kg three times per day.

During the perinatal stage, excretion of Clotrimazole
is delayed. Thus it can be given to premature and
newborn babies as a single daily dose. Depending on
the tolerance a daily dose of 6o-1oo mg/kg is recommended which can be increased to 15o mg/kg, if
the clinical picture requires it.

CLINICAL EFFICACY

We compiled all clinical results which were suffi-
ciently documented or published. - The results come
from Germany, Scandinavia, Great Britain, Japan and
Switzerland. - The mycological and clinical findings
were evaluated separately as shown in Tab. 1. It is
to be seen that in 14o from the 314 cases (= 6o %)
the fungi were eliminated. The clinical effectiveness
has been proven by 118 patients with cure and 11o
with improvement, i.e. 7o %.

Table 1:   Clotrimazole-Therapy

Fungus infections of	Fungi			
	n	elim.	red	not tested/ un- changed
Respiratory tract	203	60	38	105
Urinary tract.	21	17	—	4
Septicaemia	85	62	8	15
Endocarditis	5	1	—	4
	314	140	46	128
			~ 60%	

Fungus infections of	Clinics				
	n	cured	im- proved	not im- proved	✠
Respiratory tract	203	45	91	57	10
Urinary tract.	21	15	5	1	—
Septicaemia	85	58	13	6	8
Endocarditis	5	—	1	—	4
	314	118	110	64	22
		~ 70%			

TOLERANCE

Any drug like Clotrimazole deserves special attention as far as tolerance is concerned.

Volunteers received a therapeutic dose of the drug for 28 and 14 days respectively. The laboratory values fluctuated in the normal range with the following tendencies:

Erythrocytes	reduction
Haemoglobin	reduction
Hb/Ery ratio	increase
Leucocytes	reduction
Bilirubin	increase
Alkal. phosphatase	increase
Transaminases	increase
Total lipids	increase
Esterised fatty acids	increase
Total cholesterol	reduction, later increase
Urea in the serum	increase
Total proteins	reduction

Clotrimazole shows a mild sedative effect and reduces traffic-fitness as consequence of the sedative effect.

Side effects during Clotrimazole therapy are compiled in Table 2.

Table 2:   Side Effects During Clotrimazole Therapy

	n	stomac disorders	nausea vomiting	Pollaki-uria	Oliguria	vegetative disorders	Ageusia	loss of hair	Exan-thema
Resp. tract	203	25	6	14	2	2	—	—	6
Urinary tract	21	1	3	—	—	1	—	—	—
Septicaemia	90	1	5	—	—	—	—	1	1
	314	27	14	14	2	3	—	1	7
%		8.6	4.4	4.4					2.2
Dermatophytosis	37	8	3	6	—	—	1	—	5
Candidosis of the skin	42	4	—	—	—	—	—	—	2
Onychomycosis	20	7	6	6	—	1	—	—	1
	413	46	23	26	2	4	1	1	15
%		11	5.5	6	0.5	1	0.25	0.25	4

The general assessment of the tolerability judged
by the physicians is shown in Table 3.

Table 3: Tolerance of Clotrimazole

	n	good	moder-ate	bad without inter-ruption,	bad inter-rupted	not assess-ed
Resp. tract	203	106	52	21	15	9
Urinary tract	21	14	3	2	2	0
Septicaemia	90	80	3	2	3	2
	314	200	58	25	20	11
%		64	18,4	8	6,4	
Dermatophytosis	37	19	8	2	6	2
Candidosis of the skin	42	24	12	1	2	1
Onychomycosis	20	2	10	4	4	0
	413	245	88	32	32	14
%		59	21	8	8	3

For systemic application, Clotrimazole is still a
test preparation.

This drug represents a glimmer of hope for such
severely ill patients, but there is no reason for
overemphasizing.

ORAL CLOTRIMAZOLE IN THE TREATMENT OF FUNGAL INFECTION

R.Y. Cartwright

M.B., M.R.C. Path.

Pub. Hlth. Lab., Guildford, Surrey, U.K.

INTRODUCTION

For many years, griseofulvin was the only antifungal antibiotic which was administered orally. Its usefulness was limited
however, by its relative narrow spectrum of activity - effective
against the dermatophytes but not against yeasts and systemic
mycotic infections. The synthesis of imidazole derivatives has
produced compounds which have a wide antifungal activity, are
effective topically and are absorbed from the gastro intestinal
tract.

This paper describes the effects of oral administration
of one derivative, clotrimazole, to thirteen patients.

PATIENTS

Urinary Candidiasis

Two male patients who were recipients of renal transplants,
developed significant candiduria - > 10^5 Colony forming units/ml. on
more than one occasion - during the post-operative period. As
they were receiving both immuno-suppressive drugs and corticosteriods they were considered to be at risk for developing
systemic candidiasis. One patient was given a course of oral
5 fluorocytosine but the infecting candida became resistant
(Cartwright, Shaldon and Hall, 1972). Clotrimazole was given
1.5 grams. 6 hrly (approx. 100 mg/kg/24 hrs) and the candidura
cleared within 3 days. Treatment was continued for 7 days when

he became mildly disorientated, a symptom which cleared within
24 hrs. of stopping clotrimazole.

The candiduria in the other patient also cleared within 3
days. The clotrimazole was continued for 10 days. No side
effects were experienced.

Perinephric Abscess

A 65 year-old man with a perinephric abscess had received
multiple course of antibiotics. At operation a pure growth of
C. albicans was cultured from the pus obtained. He was given
clotrimazole 2 grams. 6 hrly. (approx. 100 mg/kg/24 hrs) but it
was discontinued after 24 hrs. owing to severe nausea and
vomiting.

Candida Oesophagitis

Hodgkins disease in a 34 year-old man was being treated
with an intensive course of cytotoxic agents and corticosteroids.
The patient developed a sore mouth and throat and could swallow
only fluids. C. albicans was isolated from white plaques in the
oropharynx. As only minimal relief was obtained from nystatin
lozenges clotrimazole, 1.5 grams. 6 hrly. (approx. 100 mg/kg/
24 hrs) was given - the tablets were crushed and suspended in
a small volume of water. Relief was obtained in 48 hours. No
side effects were experienced and treatment continued for 16 days.

Candida in a Bronchiectatic Lung

C. albicans was repeatedly isolated in pure culture from
the sputum of a 34 year-old man with lung cavities and bronchie-
ctatic changes. The significance of the candida was unclear
but as his pulmonary function was diminishing he was given a
three month course of clotrimazole 1 gram. 6 hrly. (approx. 100
mg/kg/24 hrs). Although there was a diminution in the amount of
yeast in the sputum there was no change in the pulmonary function
tests. The patient was given prophylactic prochlorperazine
25 mg. ½ hour prior to each dose of clotrimazole to prevent
nausea. There was no nausea, vomiting nor any other side effects.

Vulvo-vaginal Candidiasis

Six women who had "treatment resistant" yeast infections -
5 C. albicans, 1 Torulopsis glabrata - were given oral clotrimazole in addition to local clotrimazole. Four were given 1.5

grams. 6 hrly. (approx. 100 mg/kg/24 hrs) and the other two 1
gram 8 hrly. (approx. 50 mg/kg/24 hrs). All the patients
became nauseated and three vomited. One patient experienced
mild disorientation.   The symptoms occurred within the first
48 hrs. and cleared within 24 hrs. of stopping clotrimazole.

One patient continued with the tablets and the nausea
passed in 48 hrs.

Pulmonary Aspergillosis

a) Aspergillus fumigatus was repeatedly isolated from the
sputum of a 34 year-old man. He had a three month history of
fatigue, night sweats and weight loss. A chest X-ray showed
opacities in both upper lobes and a cavity containing a solid
opacity in the apical segment of the left lower lobe. His total
leucocyte count was 9.8×10^6/L, 13% were eosinophils. The
upper lobes cleared when the patient was given prednisolone.
He developed, however, a left sided spontaneous pneumothorax.
An exploratory thoracotomy was performed and an aspergilloma
was removed from the cavity in left lower lobe.

The patient was given oral clotrimazole 2 grams. 6 hrly.
(approx. 150 mg/kg/day) commencing the day before the operation
and continuing for 2 weeks. Prochlorperazine 25 mg. was given
$\frac{1}{2}$ hr. prior to each dose of clotrimazole. No side effects were
noted.

The pleural cavity was irrigated with 100 ml.of normal
saline containing 10 mg/L. clotrimazole during the operation, to
control any spread of the aspergillus on the outside of the lung.
The patient made an uneventful recovery. It is doubtful whether
the clotrimazole altered the course of the disease.

b) A 32 year-old man with chronic lung damage due to
sarcoidosis produced purulent sputum containing A. fumigatus.
Tomograms of the lungs showed widespread bronchiectasis.
Clotrimazole 1.5 mg. 6 hrly. (approx. 100 mg/kg/day) was given
for 2 weeks then the dose doubled for a further 6 weeks.
Prochlorperazine 25 mg. was given $\frac{1}{2}$ hr. prior to each dose of
clotrimazole. No side effects were experienced.

The treatment made no difference on either the volume of
sputum or the presence of A. fumigatus.

COMMENT

The results of treatment with oral clotrimazole are

disappointing. Gastrointestinal intolerance caused treatment to
be stopped in six patients although it was shown later that the
symptoms could be largely controlled with prochlorperazine.
This side effect appeared to be independant of the dosage.

Mental disturbances were seen in two patients.

In all the patients regular assessment was made of bone
marrow, kidney and liver function. No abnormalities were detected.
It is known, however, that clotrimazole has enzyme inducing
activity (Tettenborn, 1970) necessitating increased dosage to
maintain serum levels.

The favourable response of patients with yeast infections
who were able to tolerate the clotrimazole contrasts to the two
with pulmonary aspergillosis. This may, in part, be due to the
higher levels required to inhibit the growth of A. fumigatus and
partly due to the inability of the clotrimazole to penetrate into
the sputum. The poor response of patients with pulmonary aspergillosis supports the findings of Crompton and Milne, 1973. The
antifungal drug of choice for the treatment of aspergillosis
remains amphotericin B despite its' well documented side effects

The strains of A. fumigatus isolated were inhibited by 1-2
mg/L of clotrimazole; levels similar to those of Crompton and Milne,
1973. Microbiological assays showed serum levels up to 0.1 mg/L
in patients receiving 100 mg/kg/day. The sputum of the second
patient with pulmonary aspergillosis was examined for antifungal
activity but none was detected.

In none of the patients treated was there any evidence of
the emergence of strains showing an increased resistance to
clotrimazole.

Oral clotrimazole should be considered for the treatment of
patients with systemic candidosis and also prophylactically for
patients with depressed immunological mechanisms who require
antibiotic therapy. The use of oral clotrimazole for vulvovaginal
candidiasis can no longer be supported as it has been shown that
intensive local therapy with clotrimazole is effective.
(Cartwright, 1974).

SUMMARY

Thirteen patients with infections due to C. albicans,
T. glabrata and A. fumigatus were treated with oral clotrimazole.
A high incidence of sude effects mainly gastrointestinal were
found.

The treatment was of value in patients with candida infections.

REFERENCES

Cartwright, R.Y.   Clotrimazole in the treatment of acute and "resistant" vaginal candidiasis. Postgraduate Medical Journal. (Supplement 1) 50; 90-92 (1974)

Cartwright, R.Y., Shaldon, C. and Hall, G.H.   Urinary candiasis after renal transplantation. British Medical Journal. 2; 351 (1972)

Crompton, G.K. and Milne, L.J.R.   Treatment of bronchopulmonary aspergillosis with clotrimazole. British Journal of Diseases of the Chest. 67; 301-307 (1973)

Tettenborn, D.   Toxicity and enzyme inducing activity of clotrimazole. Naunyn-Schmiedebergs Archiv fur experimentelle Pathologie und Pharmakilogie. 266; 468-469 (1970).

CLOTRIMAZOLE (CANESTEN) THERAPY OF FUNGAL KERATITIS

Dan B. Jones, M.D.*, Barrie R. Jones, F.R.C.S.**, and
Nettie M. Robinson*

*Baylor College of Medicine, Houston, Texas
**Institute of Ophthalmology, London

Fungal keratitis is no longer an ophthalmic rarity in many
parts of the world. In the southeastern and southwestern United
States and in several South American countries, it is a significant
cause of microbial keratitis with consequent visual loss. The
principal responsible organisms are Aspergillus, Fusarium, and
Candida. As in other forms of microbial keratitis, preservation of
visual function requires early recognition and initiation of
effective medical therapy. Despite substantial advances in clinical
and laboratory diagnosis during the past decade, antifungal therapy
remains problematical outside of a few medical centers with special
experience in oculomycosis. There is no universally available
ophthalmic antifungal agent.

The antifungal activity of thiabendazole prompted one of us
(B.R.J.) in 1968 to search for a safe, broadly effective agent
among the imidazole compounds. The in vitro activity, stability,
non-toxicity, and simplicity of clotrimazole (Canesten) suggested
that it may be a valuable agent in the management of fungal
keratitis. Clotrimazole is a chlorinated tritylimidazole synthesized
in 1967 at the Research Laboratories of Farbenfabriken Bayer AG,
Germany. It is a colorless, crystalline substance with a molecular
weight of 344.8 and reacts as a weak base to form stable salts with
organic and inorganic acids. Although insoluble in water, clotrimazole is readily soluble in acetone, chloroform, dimethylformamide,
and ether. It is relatively resistant to light, hydrolysis, and
extremes of pH.

ANTIFUNGAL ACTIVITY

The minimal inhibitory concentration (MIC) for antibiotics against ocular isolates of Aspergillus, Fusarium, and Candida was determined by the tube dilution method. Amphotericin B methyl ester and flucytosine were dissolved in water; the remaining polyene and imidazole compounds in dimethylsulfoxide. Two-fold dilutions of the antibiotic were prepared in 1.0 ml of yeast nitrogen base medium (Difco) with L-asparginine and dextrose to which the fungal inoculum was added. The MIC was read at the time of first detectable growth in the control tubes after incubation at 25° C. The minimal fungicidal concentration (MFC) for eight antibiotics against Candida isolates was determined by subculturing the broth of clear tubes with a 0.01 ml calibrated loop onto blood agar plates. The MCF was read as the lowest antibiotic concentration which yielded no detectable growth after incubation at 35° C for 48 hours.

Figures 1-3 depict the cumulative percent of organisms sensitive to the various antifungal agents. Clotrimazole was the most active compound against Aspergillus (Figure 1). The geometric mean MIC for 5 species (A.flavipes 4; A.candidus 2; A.wentii 2; A.terreus 1; A.flavus 1) and 2 unidentified isolates was 1.6 μg/ml. No consistent antibiogram could be detected among the species. Clotrimazole was the least active compound against Fusarium, 3 of 11 isolates being resistant to 50 μg/ml (Figure 2). Among 20 strains

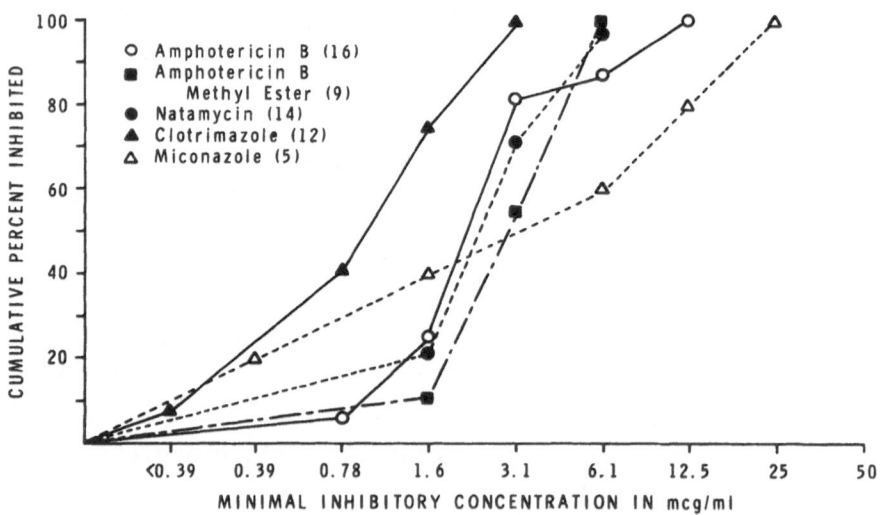

Figure 1. Activity of five antifungal agents against ocular isolates of Aspergillus. Bracketed number indicates strains tested.

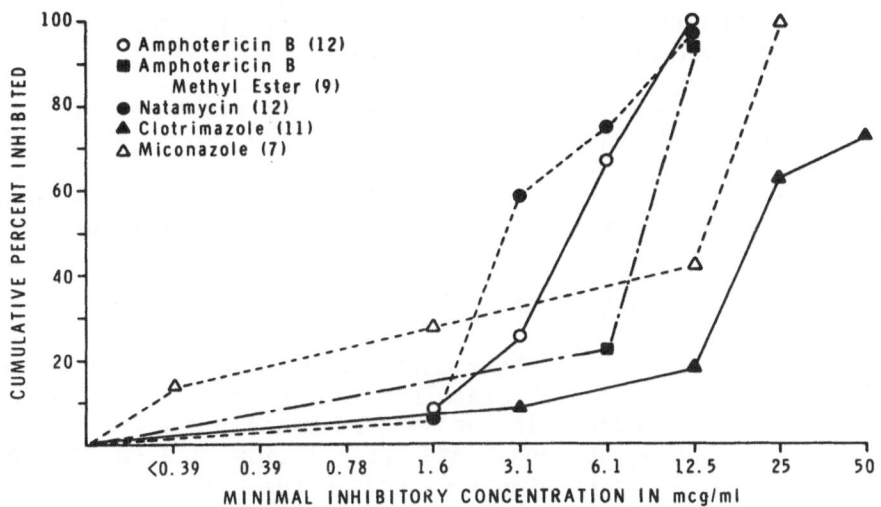

Figure 2.   Activity of five antifungal agents against <u>Fusarium</u>.

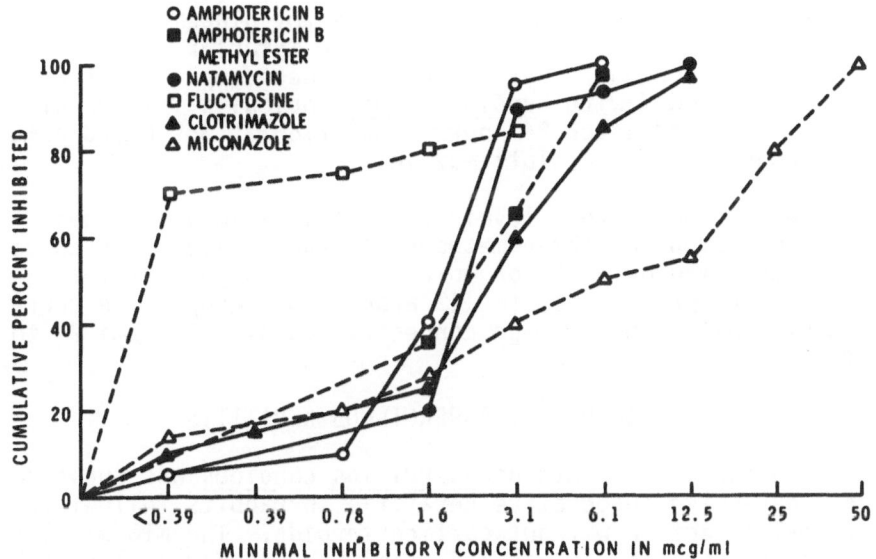

Figure 3.   Activity of six antifungal agents against 20 ocular
isolates of <u>Candida</u>.

of Candida (C.albicans 14; C.tropicalis 4; C.veronae 1; C.guillier-
mondii 1), clotrimazole was slightly less active than the polyene
antibiotics (amphotericin B, amphotericin B methyl ester, and
natamycin) but more active than miconazole (Figure 3).

Figures 4 and 5 compare the MIC and MFC of eight antibiotics
against Candida isolates. The MFC was generally two or three tubes
higher than the MIC for the four polyene antibiotics (Figure 4).
There was marked disparity between inhibitory and fungicidal concentrations of the three imidazole compounds and the pyrimidine,
flucytosine (Figure 5).

CONCENTRATION OF CLOTRIMAZOLE IN TEARS

Tear concentrations of clotrimazole were determined in rabbits
following application of a 1% arachis oil drop (Moorfields Eye
Hospital Pharmacy, London), 1% lanolin and mineral oil ointment
(Bayer AG, Leverkusen, Germany), and instillation of a continuous
drug delivery device (Alza Research, Palo Alto, California). The
device is an elliptically shaped unit which releases 10 μg of
clotrimazole per hour after placement into the rabbit cul-de-sac.
Two doses of drops (50 microliters) or ointment (50 mg) were
applied 15 minutes apart to the superior bulbar conjunctiva of 64
rabbit eyes and the lids held closed for 5 seconds. Therapeutic
devices were placed in the upper fornix of 16 eyes without anesthesia
or suture fixation. Control eyes received drug vehicles and placebo
insert devices. Tear samples were obtained by placement of a
standard paper disc (6.35 mm, 20 μl) in the inferior fornix for
approximately 60 seconds. Saturated discs were applied directly to
agarose plates seeded with Candida pseudotropicalis. Zones of
inhibition were read after 24 hours incubation at 35° C and compared
with a standard curve for clotrimazole.

Figure 6 compares tear levels of clotrimazole at various
intervals following the three methods of drug delivery. Each value
represents the mean of eight or more samples. Highest levels
(137 μg/ml) were produced by the 1% arachis oil drop. The therapeutic device maintained a mean concentration of 4.5 μg/ml 24 to 72
hours following instillation.

EFFICACY IN RABBIT ASPERGILLUS KERATITIS

A human corneal isolate of Apergillus candidus was found to
produce progressive suppurative keratitis in rabbits following
intrastromal injection without corticosteroids. The MIC of clotrimazole against this strain was 1.6 μg/ml. White New Zealand rabbits
weighing 2 to 3 kg were anesthetized with 0.4 ml intramuscular
Innovar-Vet. One-tenth ml of a suspension containing 860,000 A.
candidus spores per ml was injected with a #30 needle and tuberculin
syringe into the corneal stroma of 48 eyes. The eyes were examined

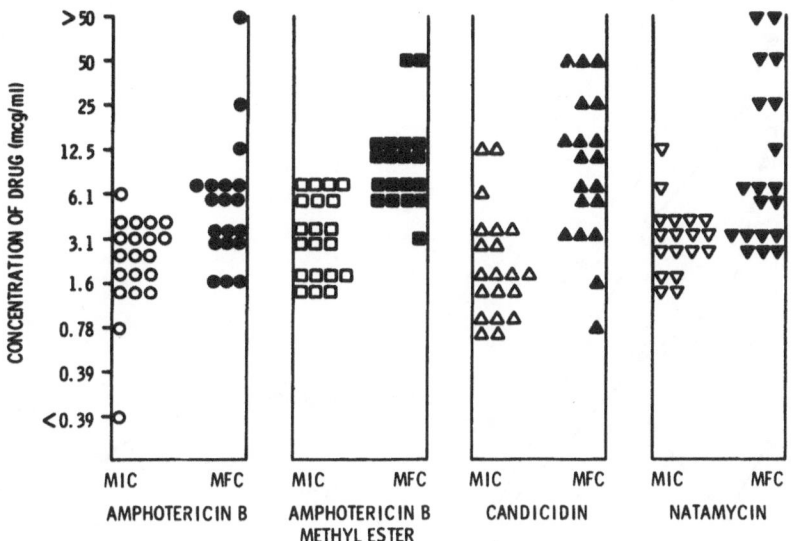

Figure 4. Comparative minimal inhibitory concentration (MIC) and minimal fungicidal concentration (MFC) of polyene antibiotics against Candida isolates.

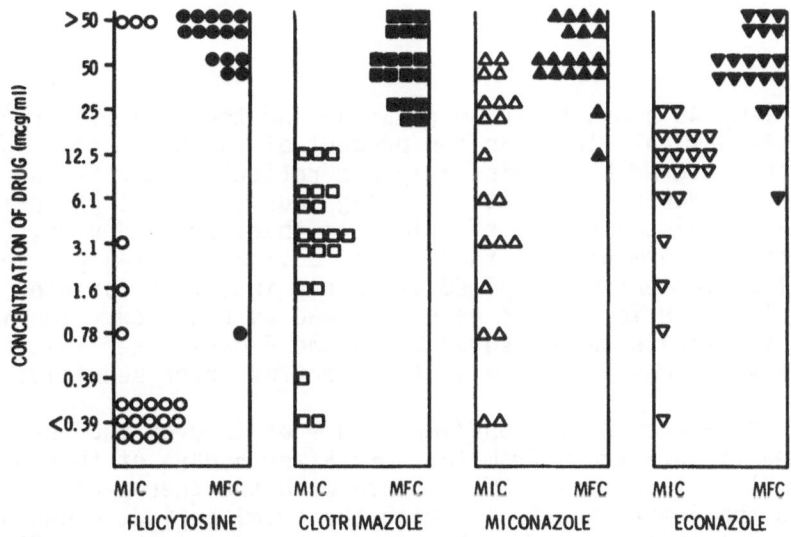

Figure 5. Comparative minimal inhibitory concentration (MIC) and minimal fungicidal concentration (MFC) of flucytosine and imidazole compounds against Candida.

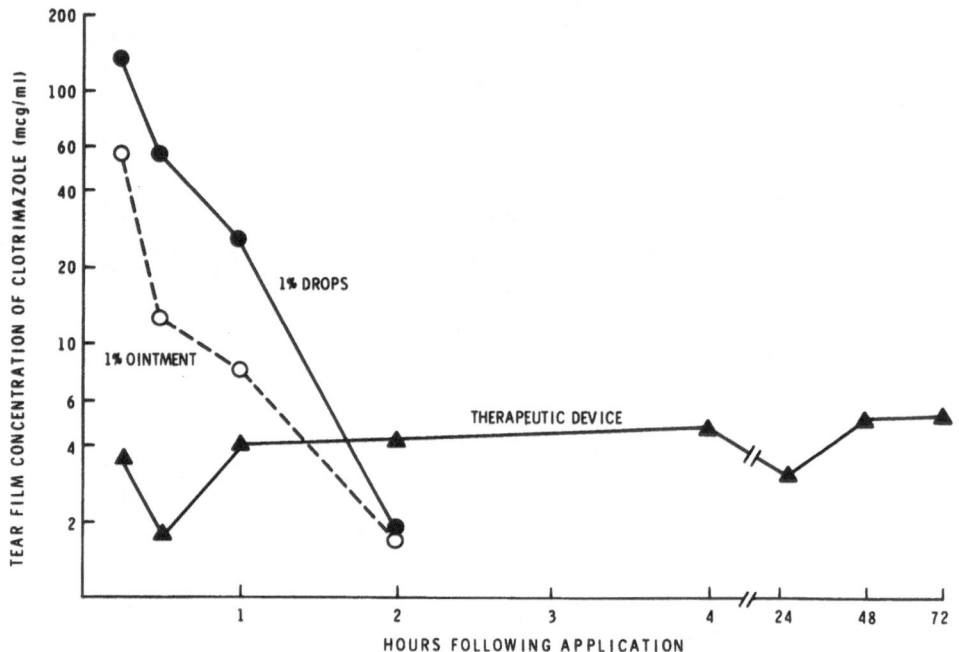

Figure 6. Concentration of clotrimazole in rabbit tears following application of 1% drops, 1% ointment, and insertion of a therapeutic device.

by slit lamp 48 hours after inoculation and the area of corneal infiltrate was calculated as the product of the greatest length and the width measured by a Zeiss eyepiece reticule. Rabbits were divided by severity of keratitis among four treatment groups: (1) 1% clotrimazole ointment, (2) clotrimazole therapeutic device, (3) 1% clotrimazole ointment plus therapeutic device, and (4) placebo ointment. Ointment was applied at hourly intervals for nine doses daily. Therapeutic devices were replaced as required. The area of corneal infiltrate was measured 2, 4, and 5 days after initiation of therapy without knowledge of treatment or prior sensitivity.

Clotrimazole 1% ointment improved 9 of 12 eyes and reduced the mean area of infiltrate from 16.7 mm^2 after 5 days of therapy (Figure 7). Clotrimazole 1% combined with the therapeutic device produced the greatest effect during the trial period, reducing the mean area of infiltrate from 16.9 mm^2 to 13.2 mm^2 (Figure 7). Suppuration increased in only one eye in this group.

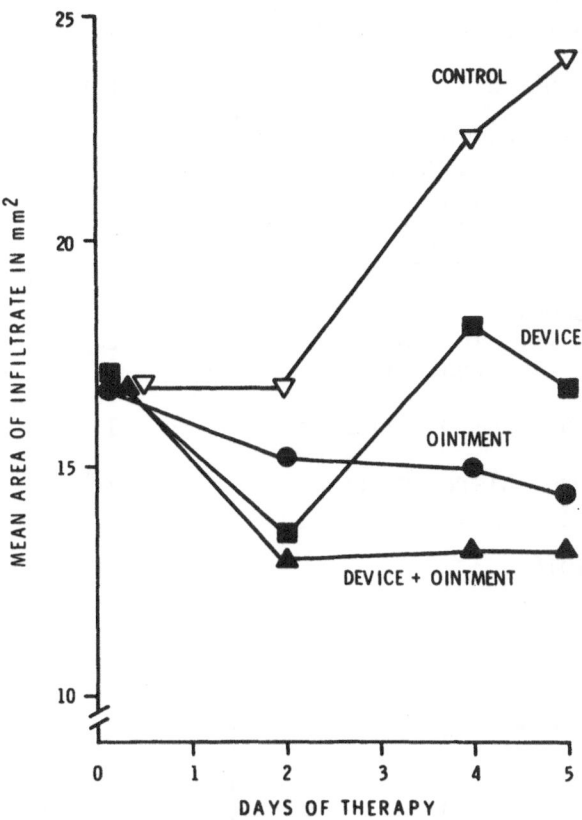

Figure 7. Severity of rabbit <u>Aspergillus</u> <u>candidus</u> keratitis by
mean area of corneal infiltrate following treatment by 1% clotrimazole ointment, therapeutic device, and 1% ointment plus device.

TREATMENT OF HUMAN KERATITIS

        Clotrimazole 1% oily drops and ointment have been used success-
fully in 13 cases of fungal keratitis caused by <u>Aspergillus</u>, <u>Candida</u>,
<u>Fusarium</u> <u>moniliforme</u>, and <u>Dreschlera</u> <u>rostrata</u> (Table 1). The
detailed histories of these cases have been previously reported
(Jones, 1975). Nine of the 13 had failed on prior antifungal
therapy. Six patients achieved vision of 20/60 or better. In five
of the remaining cases, the final vision was limited by pre-existing
ocular abnormalities. The effectiveness of clotrimazole permitted
the addition of topical corticosteroids to control late corneal

Table 1. Fungal keratitis treated successfully with clotrimazole 1%.

ORGANISM	NUMBER OF CASES
Aspergillus	
A. fumigatus	5
A. flavipes	1
A. wentii	1
A. species	1
Candida	
C. albicans	2
C. tropicalis	1
Fusarium moniliforme	1
Dreschlera rostrata	1
TOTAL	13

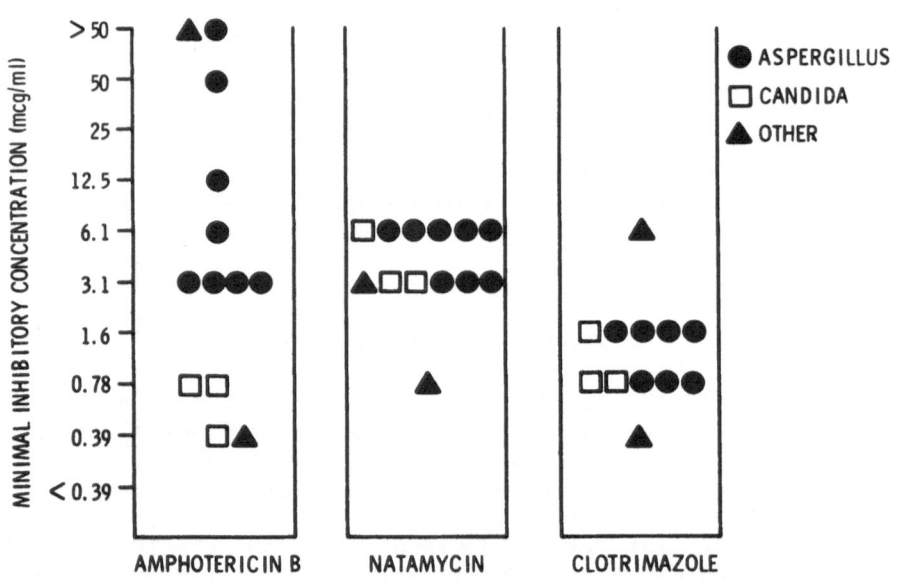

Figure 8. Activity of three antifungal agents against corneal isolates from human keratitis successfully treated with 1% clotrimazole.

inflammation in three cases. No allergic or toxic reaction developed during periods ranging from 15 to 91 days of topical therapy. The MIC of three antibiotics against the corneal isolates from these cases is compared in Figure 8. Clotrimazole was more active than amphotericin B and natamycin against the strains of Aspergillus and approximated the activity of amphotericin B against three Candida isolates.

DISCUSSION

The criteria for an ideal ocular antifungal agent are: (1) broad activity against the common varieties of yeast and filamentous ocular pathogens; (2) absence of naturally occurring and induced resistant strains; (3) solubility in water or organic solvents; (4) stability in a topical vehicle; (5) lack of toxicity; (6) corneal and intra-ocular penetration by topical, periocular, or systemic administration; and (7) efficacy in human infections. Our experience suggests that clotrimazole satisfies many of these criteria and is a valuable agent in fungal keratitis. It should be the drug of choice in Aspergillus keratitis and may be the initial form of therapy prior to definitive mycological determinations if there is no likelihood of Fusarium infection. The disparity between inhibitory and fungicidal concentrations of clotrimazole against Candida isolates suggests that combined therapy with a polyene antibiotic may be efficacious in candida keratitis. The development of a sustained release therapeutic device may expand our capabilities in the medical therapy of fungal keratitis.

REFERENCE

Jones, B.R. (1975), The American Journal of Ophthalmology, 79, 719.

REPLICATION OF PICORNAVIRUSES

DR. F. BROWN

ANIMAL VIRUS RESEARCH INSTITUTE

PIRBRIGHT, SURREY

The group of picornaviruses infecting animals contains agents
which cause some of our more important contemporary diseases, for
example those causing polio and the common cold in man and foot-
and mouth disease in animals. With the discomfort inflicted on us
two or three times each year when we are invaded by one of the many
serotypes of the rhinovirus group, there is an obvious need for a
chemotherapeutic approach to the problem of the common cold. Of
far more critical importance, this time in the supply of food, is
the problem of foot-and-mouth disease. Since more than 1000 million
doses of vaccine are inoculated annually in the control of this
disease, there is a large potential market for a chemotherapeutic
agent which will inhibit the growth of the virus.

The picornaviruses have a relatively simple structure. They
are spherical particles with a diameter of 25 to 30 nm and contain
30% RNA and 70% protein. The RNA is in the form of a single strand
of molecular weight 2.5×10^6 whereas there are 60 copies of each
of four polypeptides VP1, VP2, VP3 and VP4. The first three of
these have molecular weights of about 30×10^3 and the fourth is
about 10×10^3 giving a total molecular weight for the virus particle
of about 8.5×10^6. The polypeptides are arranged as a capsid
surrounding the RNA but the exact arrangement is not known.

Studies on the replication of the picornaviruses have been made
almost entirely with tissue culture cell systems in which the virus
will grow in high yield. Suitable systems are available for most of
the picornaviruses which have been described but most of the detailed
work has been done with a few examples, notably polio, encephalomyo-
carditis, the common cold and foot-and-mouth disease viruses.

The following steps in replication have been recognised:
adsorption, penetration, release of the RNA, translation of the RNA,
replication of the RNA and assembly of the progeny RNA and protein.
Interaction between a virus and the cellular receptors is specific.
For example, poliovirus will not attach to baby hamster kidney cells,
which are an excellent cell system for foot-and-mouth disease virus
and the latter virus will not attach to HeLa cells, which is the
most efficient system for growing poliovirus. In those instances
where two viruses grow in the same cell system, the interaction
between the viruses and cells is so specific that even closely
related viruses bind to different receptor sites.

The binding of the virion is followed by its engulfment,
probably by pinocytosis. The RNA is then released from its protein
coat and enters the cytoplasm. How this transfer is accomplished
is not known.

Picornaviruses replicate in the cytoplasm of the cell. The
process is independent of (1) DNA-dependent RNA synthesis, since it
occurs unimpaired in the presence of Actinomycin D and (2) DNA
replication as shown by the fact that it is not inhibited by
aminopterin or 5-bromouracil or 5-fluorodeoxyuridine. More recently
it has also been shown that the viruses can replicate in enucleate
cells.

The injected virus RNA fulfils two basic requirements in
initiating infection. In the first place it acts as its own
messenger RNA, which is translated into virus protein. The virus
induced protein includes an enzyme (a virus RNA dependent RNA
polymerase) for replicating the RNA since there is no evidence for
such an enzyme in uninfected cells. In the second place the virus
RNA must act as template for the synthesis by the polymerase of the
new RNA. This RNA is complementary to the virus RNA and serves in
turn as the template for the synthesis of new copies of virus RNA.
Each new molecule of virus RNA has three possible destinies: (1) it
can serve as a template for translation into protein, (2) it can
serve as a template for the transcription of a negative strand or
(3) it can become associated with virus protein to form new virus.

The translation step has now been worked out in some detail.
The virus RNA becomes attached at its 5^1 - end to several ribosomes
which proceed along the RNA molecule to the 3^1 - end, forming a
single giant protein (or polyprotein) with a molecular weight of
about 250×10^3. This polyprotein is then systematically cleaved
by proteolytic enzymes into three primary products. The products
at the 5^1 and 3^1 - ends are cleaved into smaller products but that
translated from the centre of the genome remains intact. The
structural proteins are translated from the 5^1 - end of the virus
RNA and this primary product is then cleaved into two of the polypeptides found in the virus particles, namely VP1 and VP3, together

with VPO, which is the precursor of VP2 and VP4. Polypeptides VP1, VP3 and VPO appear to remain as a single structural unit which aggregates into pentamers containing five of these units. Twelve of these pentamers then come together to form a shell, the procapsid, which combines with a molecule of progeny RNA to form a provirion. Finally VPO is cleaved into VP2 and VP4. Some difficulty arises in deciding whether this pattern of morphogenesis is identical in all the picornaviruses because, in two examples, VP4 seems to be present in the virus particles in half molar quantity compared with VP1, VP2 and VP3. If these analyses are confirmed, it would necessitate the loss of half the VP4 molecules when VPO is cleaved at the final stage of morphogenesis.

Interference with one or more of the steps in the replication process should, at least in theory, lead to inhibition of virus growth. Since the processes of replication are so closely bound up with the metabolism of the host cell, it is difficult to devise compounds which distinguish between the virus induced and normal cellular processes. However, two compounds, guanidine and 2 - ($\propto$- hydroxybenzyl) benzimidazole (HBB), have been found to inhibit the multiplication of several picornaviruses without affecting host cell metabolism. HBB prevents the replication of the virus RNA, probably by inhibiting the development of RNA polymerase activity, but the precise mechanism is unknown. The mode of action of guanidine is also not known with any certainty. It seems that the viral RNA polymerase is the principal target but Cooper's genetic analysis suggests that the site of guanidine action is located in the coat protein region of the genome.

One of the most intriguing features of the experiments with HBB and guanidine is that the different picornaviruses do not respond uniformly to the inhibitors. For example, the multiplication of three of the seven immunological types of foot and mouth disease virus is not affected by guanidine whereas the other four are greatly inhibited. The sensitive viruses also develop drug resistance very rapidly and some strains become dependent on the presence of the drug for growth. These observations emphasize that the molecular basis of the inhibitory activity of the drugs is still obscure.

Other specific targets may be worthy of attention. In the last three years, homopolymeric regions have been found in the genomes of the picornaviruses. It now seems certain that all the picornaviruses have a tract of about 50 adenylic acid residues at the 3^1 - end of the genome. Several of the picornaviruses also have long tracts which are rich in cytidylic acid residues. Baltimore has provided evidence which suggests that the poly (A) tract is necessary for the infectivity of poliovirus RNA but no role has been found so far for the poly (C) tract. If these homopolymers are found to have a role in the replication of the virus RNA, this would provide a new approach to the chemotherapy of picornaviruses.

Molecular biology of influenza virus

replication and points of action of inhibitors

J. S. Oxford

Division of Virology, National Institute for Medical

Research, Mill Hill, London NW7, England

Knowledge of the details of replication of the virus should
lead to more logical approaches for the selection of virus inhibitory compounds. The influenza virus exists as irregularly shaped
particles some 75 to 190 nm in diameter bounded by an outer lipid
membrane. The two envelope proteins haemagglutinin (HA) and
neuraminidase (NA) take the form of spikes covering the virus
surface and attached by one end at the lipid membrane. Internally
the particle contains several other components of which the two
major ones are the ribonucleoprotein (NP) which is closely associated with the helical RNA genome of the virus and the matrix
protein (MP) which underlies the lipid membrane and may form a
matrix surrounding the ribonucleoprotein-RNA complex. The polypeptide composition of highly purified influenza virus preparations
has now been established by polyacrylamide gel electrophoresis
studies. Seven polypeptides have been identified in the virus particle with molecular weights ranging from 25,000 to 94,000 daltons.

The genetic code of the virus is contained in the form of
single-stranded RNA with a molecular weight of approximately 4×10^6
daltons. A transcript of this genome acts as the genetic message
(complementary strand mRNA) to the invaded cell, which translates
the virus message into virus structural proteins and nonstructural
proteins including enzymes, such as the RNA dependent RNA polymerase
enzyme, necessary for the replication of the virus RNA (Fig. 1). An
interesting feature of the influenza genome is that it exists in fragments of varying size and each most likely acts as a monocistronic
message and codes for a particular virus specified protein (Skehel,
1972).

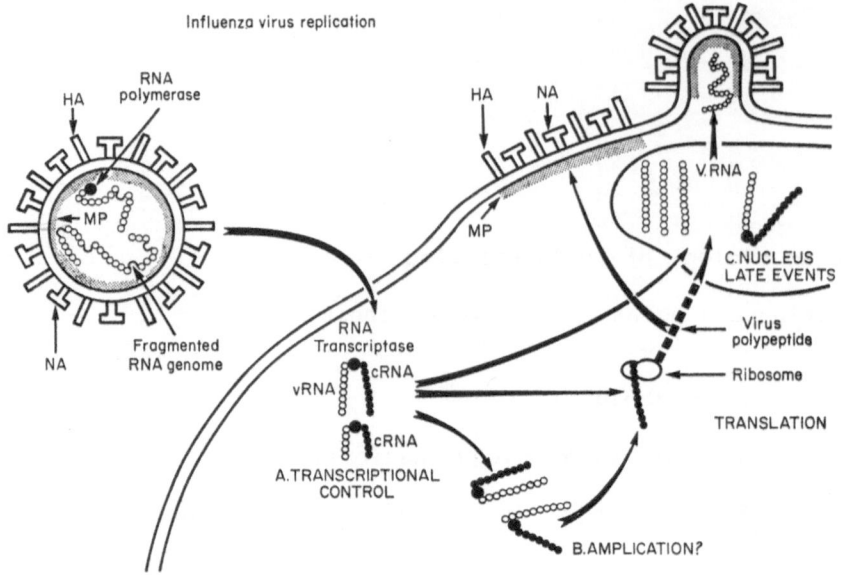

Influenza virus replication

As a first stage in the replication cycle the influenza virion
binds by its haemagglutinin projections to sialic acid residue containing receptors on the plasma membrane of the cell and probably
enters the cell by pinocytosis (Dourmaskin & Tyrrell, 1974).
Influenza virus adsorption may result in a spatial rearrangement of
membrane components such as glycoproteins or glycolipids (Aoyagi
et al., 1974). Investigation of the precise chemical structure of
the binding sites could lead to the synthesis of defined inhibitors
of virus attachment.

Little data are available about the next stage of uncoating
which takes place in the cytoplasm but cytoplasmic proteases and
lipases may disrupt the virus envelope and activate the virion
transcriptase enzyme. The latter enzyme is known to transcribe a
copy (complementary strand RNA) of the virus RNA which is then used
as a virus message (Pons, 1972). Obviously specific inhibition of
the transcriptase enzyme would act at a theoretically important stage
of the life cycle of the virus and this will be considered in more
detail below. At a later stage the complementary RNA enters the
nucleus to become the template for the synthesis of virion RNA. It
is not clear if a further "replicase" enzyme is required or whether
the existing transcriptase can be modified. Again inhibition of this
stage by an inhibitor would presumably inhibit the replication of the
virus in the cell. Chemicals binding with the enzyme itself rather
than the virus RNA would appear more useful because of the previously
demonstrated lack of specificity of antibiotics binding to nucleic
acid. A reservation of this approach is the recent demonstration of
an RNA dependent RNA polymerase in rabbit reticulocytes (Downey,
Byrnes, Jurmark & So, 1974). Although of unknown function, this cell
enzyme might be inhibited by chemicals blocking the virus enzyme.

An additional complication is that the replicase of phage QB has several subunits and the host bacterium contributes to these (Kuo & August, 1970). A similar cell dependence of the influenza RNA polymerase would lessen the chance of developing virus enzyme specific inhibitors.

An interesting point of action of an inhibitor would be to stop the binding of virus messenger RNA to the cell ribosomes, so preventing translation of virus message but allowing translation of cell mRNA's. It was speculated earlier that the virus induced non-structural polypeptide NS1 might act as a ribosome initiator factor so ensuring recognition and translation of virus messenger RNA. Blockage of such a factor would inhibit virus replication. However, although the polypeptide associates with ribosomes the attachment is loose and the function of NS1 is at present unknown (Krug & Etkind, 1973).

If virus specific tRNA's containing for example unusual bases are required at the stage of translation this would be another point of action for inhibitors. Inhibitors of virus replication control factors, such as the postulated "equestron" of polio virus (Cooper, Steiner-Pryor & Wright, 1973) would be expected to interfere specifically with virus multiplication.

Influenza virus is released by budding from the plasma membrane of the cell. It is conceivable that compounds could interrupt and inhibit the process. It is known that influenza virus release is inhibited by antibody directed against the neuraminidase of the virus and that antibody molecules may act stereochemically by crosslinking neuraminidase projections exposed on the outisde of the plasma membrane (Dowdle, Downie & Laver, 1974). Nevertheless, the precise function of neuraminidase in the replication of influenza is at present unclear, although it may be concerned with virus release from cells. Certainly synthetic analogues of neuraminic acid acting by competition with the substrate have been synthesized, such as 2-deoxy-2, 3-dehydro-N-trifluoroacetyl neuraminic acid (FANA), and reduce the yield of influenza virus in a multicycle system of replication (Palese, Schulman, Bodo & Meindl, 1974), and this may be a very important point of action for future inhibitors.

Of practical importance from the point of view of control of influenza by immunization or chemoprophylaxis is the fragmented genome of influenza virus which probably contributes to the high frequency of recombination or reassortment occurring between different influenza virus particles. Recombination between different human influenza A viruses or between human and animal viruses may explain the periodic appearance of completely new influenza virus subtypes, some able to cause pandemics such as the 1918, 1957 and 1968 viruses (antigenic "shift"). In addition, influenza viruses undergo more gradual changes in the antigenicity of their external proteins, the haemagglutinin and neuraminidase (antigenic "drift"). Control of influenza by vaccination is made extremely difficult by the changing HA and NA antigens.

Therefore, studies of possible virus inhibitory compounds as an alternative approach to immunization are important. It should be realized, however, that the same property of mutability and possibly recombination of influenza virus which makes control by vaccination so difficult may present problems in the use of chemoprophylactic agents. Thus, it might be expected that drug resistant virus mutants might occur and be selected; this has been demonstrated under laboratory conditions with amantadine (Oxford, Potter & Logan, 1970) and with other viruses and inhibitory agents (Subak-Sharpe, Timbury & Williams, 1969). The most effective inhibitor of influenza virus would be independent for its mode of action on the rapidly changing surface HA and NA antigens of the virus, would inhibit both type A and B viruses and would allow development, but without overt clinical signs, of influenza. Persons would thus develop protective antibody so preventing later re-infection with the same subtype. At present no single inhibitory compound has been described in the literature with all these properties.

Antiviral activity of amantadine. Amantadine is particularly active against influenza A viruses but has little or no inhibitory activity against influenza B or C viruses. The first point of interest is the great variability shown when different influenza A strains are tested under similar conditions. Thus influenza A/PR8 (H0N1), an old subtype of influenza A, is only marginally inhibited whereas A/Scotland/49/57 (H2N2) an "Asian" influenza virus is very significantly inhibited by the same concentration of amantadine. Fortunately, viruses having HA and NA of the H2N2 and H3N2 eras (that is recent and current influenza viruses) are very susceptible to inhibition by amantadine in tissue culture. Because of the frequency of antigenic "drift" noted earlier it is of great importance to investigate the inhibition or otherwise, by amantadine of influenza variants of epidemiological importance. Our studies (Table 1) have indicated that all recent variants of influenza A tested are inhibited by amantadine.

Virus		Log_{10} reduction in virus titre
A/HK/1/68	(H3 N2)	$2 \cdot 5 \pm 0 \cdot 5$
A/Port Chalmers/73	(H3 N2)	$2 \cdot 3$
A/Hannover/1/74	(H3 N2)	$4 \cdot 0$
A/Puerto Rico/74	(H3 N2)	$2 \cdot 2$

* 25 μg/ml amantadine in the egg piece system (Fazekas de St Groth & White, 1958).

Influenza inhibitory effects of Ribavirin. Ribavirin is a
synthetic nucleoside analogue, 1-β-D-ribofuranosyl-1,-2,4-triazole-3-
carboxamide (RTCA, Figure 3) which inhibits the replication of a
wide range of DNA and RNA containing viruses (Sidwell et al., 1972).
The compound also inhibits the replication of influenza virus in
mice (Sidwell et al., 1972) and ferrets (Potter, C.W. and Oxford,
J.S., unpublished). We have shown recently that the compound acts
at an early stage in the influenza virus infected cell, possibly by
inhibiting the production of essential nucleotides and hence RNA
synthesis. The compound as a reversible inhibitor has a dual interest in the analysis of the early steps in influenza virus RNA
replication and as a potential compound for the chemoprophylactic
control of influenza. The nucleoside analogue caused a very significant inhibition of the replication in egg pieces of a range
of influenza A strains (Table 2). In addition, influenza B/HK/8/73
virus was inhibited to a similar degree to the influenza A viruses.
Separate toxicity studies indicated that 0.4 mM concentrations of
RTCA had no effect on the uptake and incorporation of ^{75}Se
methionine or ^{3}H uridine into acid precipitable product after prior
incubation with the compound for 72 h. although the compound did
inhibit uptake of H^{3}-thymidine (R. Bucknall, I.C.I., personal communication) and there is some evidence of immunosuppressive activity
(C. W. Potter & J. S. Oxford, in preparation).

Virus	Inhibition $\log_{10}$ ID_{50}/ml
A/HK/1/68	$4·0\pm0·5$
A/PC/1/73	$3·5$
B/HK/8/73	$3·5$
A/FPV	$5·2$

* 0·04 mM-RTCA added at the time of virus infection. Egg piece technique of Fazekas de St Groth &
White (1958).

Inhibitors of influenza RNA-dependent RNA polymerase. As described above, inhibitors of virus RNA-dependent RNA polymerase
activity would have potential application as chemoprophylactic
agents against RNA-containing viruses. Ho & Walters (1971) initiated
studies using this approach and have described the inhibition of
cell-associated RNA-dependent RNA polymerase of influenza A/PR8
(HON1) virus by selenocystine. More recently we have described the
in vitro inhibition of influenza virion-associated RNA-dependent
RNA polymerase by selenocystamine dihydrochloride, bathophenanthroline disodium disulphonate and certain heterocyclic thiosemicarbazones. A property common to these compounds is the ability
to chelate soft, heavy, metal ions such as zinc and copper. Conversely, similar types of compounds in which the possibility of
chelation was diminished showed significantly less inhibitory
activity against influenza virus RNA-dependent RNA polymerase. This

and other data (Oxford & Perrin, 1974) suggested that the RNA polymerase of influenza was a zinc metalloenzyme. However the hypothesis requires the demonstration of zinc association with the enzyme polypeptide and this is not possible at present. In vivo studies are in progress using chelating agents encapsulated in liposome preparations.

References

Aoyagi, T. et al. Biochemica et Biophysica Research Communication, 57, 271 (1974).

Cooper, P.D. et al. Intervirology, 1, 1 (1973).

Dourmashkin, R.R. & Tyrrell, D.A.J. Journal of General Virology, 24, 129 (1974).

Dowdle, W.R. et al. Journal of Virology, 13, 269 (1974).

Downey, K.M. et al. Biochemica et Biophysica Research Communications, 56, 227 (1974).

Ho, P.P.K. & Walters, C.P. Annals of the New York Academy of Science, 173, 438 (1971).

Krug, R.M. & Etkind, P.R. Antimicrobial Agents and Chemotherapy, 334 (1973).

Kuo, C.H. & August, J.T. Nature (New Biology), 237, 105 (1970).

Oxford, J.S. & Perrin, D.D. Journal of General Virology, 23, 59 (1974)

Oxford, J.S. et al. Annals of the New York Academy of Sciences, 173, 300 (1970).

Palese, P. et al. Virology, 59, 490 (1974).

Pons, M.W. Virology, 47, 823 (1972).

Sidwell, R.W. et al. Science, 177, 705 (1972).

Skehel, J.J. Virology, 49, 23 (1972).

Subak-Sharpe, J.H. et al. Nature, 222, 341 (1969).

METALLOENZYMES: A NEW FOCUS FOR ANTIVIRAL DRUG DESIGN?

Douglas D. Perrin

Professorial Fellow, John Curtin School of Medical
Research, The Australian National University, P.O.Box
334, Canberra City, A.C.T., Australia, 2601

The very intimate relation that exists between a virus and its
host can be seen by considering the influenza virus and its "life"
cycle in Man. The core of this virion comprises a nucleoprotein
coat or capsid surrounding the viral RNA. It includes a virion
transcriptase enzyme which transcribes a copy of the single strand
RNA (complementary strand mRNA). Surrounding the core is the matrix protein, and this, in turn, is encased in a lipoprotein envelope which is bounded by an outer lipid membrane. The virion interacts with its environment by means of two types of spikes it carr-
ies on the envelope. The first of these contains haemagglutinin
which binds to sialic acid residues on cell membranes. The second
type of spike contains the enzyme neuraminidase which removes
neuraminic acid side chains from mucoproteins, a process which may
facilitate penetration of the virion into the cell or help in the
release of newly formed virus particles.

When the free virion comes into contact with the outer surface
of a cell it binds to sialic acid residues at receptor sites, prior
to entering the cell by pinocytosis (Fazekas 1948; Dourmashkin and
Tyrrell 1974). Inside the cell the virion is stripped of its
envelope, possibly by cytoplasmic proteases and lipases, and its
transcriptase enzyme is activated. The complementary strand mRNA
in the cytoplasm directs the host cell to synthesise viral structural proteins and enzymes. These are reassembled and new virus
particles are finally released by budding from the cell membrane.

This dependence of viral metabolism on host cell metabolism,
and the fact that the virus is protectively wrapped when it is
outside the cell, makes the possible avenues for chemotherapeutic

control of virus infection more limited than for diseases of bacterial origin. It is fortunate that many diseases of viral origin,
including smallpox, yellow fever and poliomyelitis, can be controlled adequately by the use of vaccines. However, in cases such as
influenza and the common cold, vaccines are of only limited use
because of variability in antigenicity or of multiplicity in the
number of serotypes.

It has been known for a long time that certain chemical substances possess antiviral activity and also form metal chelates,
although it has not been conclusively established that the two
properties are related. Thus, benzaldehyde thiosemicarbazone,
shown in 1950 (Hamre et al. 1950) to have some activity against
vaccinia virus, is also a chelating agent by virtue of its thiosemicarbazone moiety. Similarly, the thiosemicarbazones of
nicotinaldehyde, isonicotinaldehyde, 2-thenylaldehyde and
3-thenylaldehyde are chelating agents and have antiviral activity
(Thompson et al. 1953). Isatin thiosemicarbazone has three sites
through which it can coordinate to a metal ion: it also has greater
activity against vaccinia virus (Thompson et al. 1953). Derivatives of isatin thiosemicarbazone having even greater activity have
been synthesised (Bauer and Sadler 1960), and one of these,
methisazone (1-methylisatin 3-thiosemicarbazone) has been used
successfully in clinical trials as prophylaxis against smallpox
(Bauer et al. 1963). This was the first time that a drug had been
shown to be effective in the prevention of a virus disease in man.
Another metal-chelating agent, 4-bromo-3-methylisothiazole-5-
carboxaldehyde thiosemicarbazone, also afforded substantial protection against smallpox when it was administered in a controlled
prophylactic trial but was ineffective once the disease was
established (Rao et al. 1965).

Methisazone is active against other viruses, including tumour-
causing viruses (Levinson et al. 1971), adenovirus (Bauer and
Apostolov 1966; Apostolov 1967), and alastrim (do Valle et al.
1965), and is useful for treating complications following
vaccination (Bauer 1965).

It is likely that in all cases this antiviral activity is due
to the ability of the methisazone to form terdentate chelates with
essential heavy metal ions by bonding through a sulphur, a nitrogen
and either an oxygen or a nitrogen atom. A similar structure-
activity relation has been suggested (French and Blanz 1966) to
explain the anticancer effects of a number of related compounds.
The effect of methisazone on adenovirus is abolished if the sulphur
is replaced by oxygen (Bauer and Apostolov 1966). The antiviral
activity of methisazone and related thiosemicarbazones affects a
late stage of the pox virus cycle (Appleyard et al. 1965) by
interfering with viral mRNA translation (Woodson and Joklik 1965).

Similarly, methisazone has been found to reduce the reverse transcriptase activity and cytopathic effect of the RNA slow viruses
producing certain scrapie-like diseases of sheep in Iceland, and
hence may provide a chemotherapeutic method for their control
(Haase and Levinson 1973).

Recently, John Oxford and I (1974) found evidence that the
RNA-dependent RNA polymerase activity of influenza virus, which is
essential to the replication of influenza virus, is due to a zinc
metalloenzyme. With hindsight, this is not unexpected. Thus the
RNA polymerase of E.coli is a zinc metalloenzyme (Valenzuela et al.
1973) and so are the DNA polymerases of E.coli, sea urchin,
bacteriophage, and avian myeloblastosis virus (Poiesz et al.1974).
These results, taken in conjunction with inhibition studies using
1,10-phenanthroline (Valenzuela et al. 1973), suggest that many if
not all DNA and RNA polymerases and nucleotidyl transferases are
metalloenzymes. It is important to emphasise the clear distinction
between the heavy metal such as zinc that is an integral part of
the metalloenzyme and the magnesium or manganese ions that are
essential cofactors in enzymic activity (Chow and Simpson, 1971;
Skehel, 1971) and which are ordinarily present in large excess.

The 'flu virus RNA polymerase can be inhibited in vitro by a
number of chelating agents, including bathocuproine, bathophenanthroline and some heterocyclic thiosemicarbazones. The zinc ion
is not removed from the enzyme, and activity can be restored by
dialysing against distilled water.

The observation that one or more metalloenzymes are involved
in the synthesis of viral nucleic acid may explain the fact that
some antiviral agents appear to owe their activity to their metal-
chelating ability. In addition to direct involvement of a chelating agent in reversible metal-complex equilibria, two other types
of action can be envisaged. First of all, by chelating the metal
ion and hence greatly decreasing the level of free metal ion, it
may be possible to inhibit the formation of the metalloenzyme.
Secondly, involvement of the metalloenzyme in mixed-complex formation may block its activity. We suggest that this is what
happens with influenza RNA polymerase.

The hypothesis that influenza virus requires the action of one
or more zinc metalloenzymes for its replication raises the possibility of using chelating agents to control influenza by lowering
the free zinc ion concentration in cell cytoplasm and hence the
rate and extent of virus production. This would allow more time
for the mobilisation of the body's defence mechanisms. Alternatively, formation of a mixed-ligand complex by the metalloenzyme
with the chelating agent would competitively inhibit virus
synthesis.

In combating influenza, it is difficult to deliver a chelating agent to the desired site,˄the cytoplasm of cells in the respiratory tract. For example, the negatively charged CaEDTA complex and the EDTA anion cannot readily cross cell membranes to chelate any of the free zinc ions in the cytoplasm or to react with zinc bound in the RNA polymerase. Also, rapid excretion of EDTA by the kidney affords little opportunity to deplete the tissues of the zinc they contain (although removal of free zinc ion from blood plasma takes place as expected). Hence, results of in vitro testing of RNA polymerase inhibition, using buffered ATP, CTP, GTP and tritium-labelled UTP in a single-phase system, do not have direct application to whole-animal or human studies. In the enzyme test CaEDTA is an effective inhibitor but it has little effect in vivo. Similarly, bathophenanthroline disulphonate ion would not pass cell barriers and would be excreted rapidly. Bathophenanthroline, itself, would be more effective if it was not so sparingly soluble. Methisazone and related compounds would also seem to have limited potential in treating influenza, the main advantage of such chelating agents being their persistence in the body. This arises from their slow systemic absorption and their low solubility so that the body tissues are continuously exposed to low concentrations of them. The rates of excretion will decrease with their liposolubility, so that no direct correlation is likely between antiviral activity and chelating ability as measured in aqueous solutions.

Metal ions such as zinc and copper are essential in traces to living organisms. Thus, zinc occurs in metalloenzymes such as carbonic anhydrase, alcohol dehydrogenase, glutamic dehydrogenase and lactic dehydrogenase; it is also associated with carboxypeptidase and alkaline phosphatase activity. Depletion of general body levels of zinc to an extent that RNA polymerase synthesis or activity is significantly affected may thus have serious biological disadvantages. This sets definite limits to the possible level of chelating agent that can be injected into an animal. For example, because of its effect on body zinc ion, a dose level of only 2mM calcium DTPA (diethylenetriaminepentaacetic acid)/kg is toxic (Auth 1973).

Systemic control of levels of free metal ions is, therefore, likely to be difficult to achieve and maintain, and there may be only a narrow region in which viral inhibition is possible without overt toxicity. In proposing any chelating agent for use in this way it is also necessary to establish that the suggested agent can compete effectively for metal ions against biological ligands, such as amino acids, that are also present. Provided the necessary stability constants are available, this can be tested by using the computer programme COMICS (Perrin and Sayce 1967) which enables the equilibrium concentrations of species in mixtures of metal ions and complexing agents to be computed, given total concentrations and relevant equilibrium constants (pK_a values and stability constants).

As currently programmed, COMICS can handle up to 500 equilibria. In principle there is no inherent difficulty in including mixed-ligand complexes in the model.

However, to combat influenza virus, systemic control of metal ions is not required. It is necessary only to protect cells of the respiratory tract. This makes the use of liposome-encapsulated chelating agents an attractive possibility.

Liposomes are finely dispersed phospholipid spherules (Sessa and Weissman 1968) which can be formed by shaking a mixture of lecithin and cholesterol in an aqueous solution. If the solution contains a chelating agent some of this is trapped in the interior of the liposome whereas the outside is made up of lipid materials so that such a liposome looks like a fat droplet and, in the body, is treated as such. It can be taken up into a cell by pinocytosis or it can be engulfed by phagocytes. Once inside the cell, the liposome is broken down and the chelating agent is liberated. In getting the active agent through the cell wall a liposome functions rather like the Trojan horse of Greek antiquity.

With this approach a number of difficulties disappear. Liposome-encapsulation may make it possible to selectively deliver a particular chelating agent to an appropriate target area. Results from in vitro testing become applicable and it now becomes an advantage to use ionized ligands that are retained inside the target cells.

The choice of chelating agents is reasonably wide so long as they are not inherently toxic or exert undesirable long-term effects. CaEDTA (or better, CaDTPA) is chemically stable, would not leak out of the cell or disturb calcium metabolism, and it chelates zinc and copper by selectively displacing bound calcium ions. At a concentration of 1mM CaEDTA, in a solution 1mM in free calcium ion, at pH 7.4, free zinc ion concentration would be depressed to 1 millionth of what it would be in the absence of CaEDTA. CaDTPA would lower it by a further factor of one hundred. The induced zinc deficiency in the cytoplasm of the particular cell would persist until sufficient zinc ion had been transported across the call membrane from the blood plasma. In vitro tests suggest that sodium bathophenanthroline disulphonate would also be effective, and this agent is also likely to be long-persisting. By comparison, heterocyclic thiosemicarbazones would be less suitable, firstly because they could not be prepared in high enough concentrations inside the liposomes and secondly because absence of charge would favour their rapid diffusion from the active site.

Currently we are investigating this approach to see if influenza can be prevented (Oxford and Perrin 1975). Liposome-encapsulated chelating agents, prepared as described by Rahman et

al.(1974), are administered by aerosol so as to reach the respiratory tract. Ideally, all cells that are invaded by an influenza
virus should also have taken up one or more liposomes. This may be
less difficult than expected to achieve because Dourmashkin and
Tyrrell's (1974) work suggests that added ferritin (and hence,
presumably, a liposome) is taken up synergistically by cells
invaded by influenza virus.

Appleyard, G., Hume, V.B.M., and Westwood, J.C.N. (1965)
    Ann. N.Y. Acad.Sci. 130, 92.
Apostolov, K. (1967) Proc. 5th Inter.Congr.Chemotherapy, Vienna.
    4, 319.
Auth, U. (1973) Strahlentherapie, 146, 490.
Bauer, D.J. (1965) Ann. N.Y. Acad. Sci. 130, 110.
Bauer, D.J., and Apostolov, K. (1966) Science, 154, 796.
Bauer, D.J., and Sadler, P.W. (1960) Brit. J. Pharmacol. Chemother.
    15, 101.
Bauer, D.J, St. Vincent, C., Kempe, C., and Downie, A. (1963)
    Lancet 2, 494.
Chow, NL., and Simpson, R.W. (1971) Proc. Nat. Acad. Sci. U.S.A.
    68, 752.
Dourmashkin, R.R., and Tyrrell, D.A.J. (1974) J. Gen. Virol.24, 129.
do Valle, L.A.R., de Melo, P.R., de Salles Gomes, L.F., and
    Proenca, L.M. (1965) Lancet, 2, 976.
Fazekas, S. (1948) Nature, 162, 294.
French, F.A., and Blanz, E.J. (1966) J. Med. Chem. 9, 585.
Haase, A.T., and Levinson, W. (1973) Biochem. Biophys. Res. Comm.,
    51, 875.
Hamre, D., Bernstein, J., and Donovick, R. (1950)
    Proc. Soc. Exp. Biol. Med., 73, 275.
Levinson, W., Woodson, B., and Jackson, J. (1971) Nature, 232, 116.
Oxford, J.S., and Perrin, D.D. (1974) J. Gen. Virol., 23, 59.
Oxford, J.S., and Perrin, D.D. (1975) Unpublished results.
Perrin, D.D., and Sayce, I.G. (1967) Talanta, 14, 833.
Poiesz, B.J., Battula, N., and Loeb, L.A. (1974) Biochem. Biophys.
    Res. Comm. 56, 959 and refs therein.
Rahman, Y.E., Rosenthal, M.W., Cerny, E.A., and Moretti, E.S.
    (1974) J. Lab. Clin. Med. 83, 640.
Rao, A.R., McFadzean, J.A., and Squires, S. (1965)
    Ann. N.Y. Acad. Sci. 130, 118.
Sessa, G., and Weissmann, G. (1968) J. Lipid Res. 9, 310.
Skehel, J.J. (1971) Virology, 45, 793.
Thompson, R.L., Minton, S.A., Officer, J.E., and Hitchings, G.H.
    (1953) J. Immunol. 70, 229.
Valenzuela, P., Morris, R.W., Farao, A., Levinson, W., and Rutter,
    W.L. (1973) Biochem. Biophys. Res. Comm. 53, 1036.
Woodson, B., and Joklik, W. (1965) Proc. Nat. Acad. Sci. U.S.A.
    54, 946.

INHIBITION OF INFLUENZA VIRUS REPLICATION BY 2-DEOXY-2,3-DEHYDRO-N-TRIFLUOROACETYLNEURAMINIC ACID (FANA)

Jerome L. Schulman and Peter Palese

Department of Microbiology
Mount Sinai School of Medicine
of the City University of New York

Myxoviruses and paramyxoviruses are unique among animal viruses by virtue of their possession of a virus-coded enzyme (neuraminidase) which is capable of liberating free N-acetyl-neuraminic acid (NANA) from a variety of sialoprotein and sialolipid substrates. Although the precise role of neuraminidase in myxovirus replication had not been defined, numerous attempts were made over a period of more than 3 decades to inhibit influenza virus replication by the use of neuraminidase inhibitors. A variety of compounds have been shown to inhibit neuraminidase activity in vitro including polyanions such as congo red and trypan red, dextran sulfate etc., sulfhydryl reagents, concanavalin A, oxamic acid derivatives, and benzimidazole derivatives but neuraminidase inhibition by these compounds is either non-specific or requires very high concentrations of inhibitor.

Dihydro and tetrahydroisoquinoline derivatives were observed to inhibit neuraminidase activity in vitro and were found to be active against influenza virus infections in mice and humans. However, subsequent experiments revealed that these compounds did not inhibit neuraminidase but interfered with the thiobarbituric acid assay of neuraminidase activity. In the light of these findings it is likely that the protective effects observed in vivo with isoquinoline derivatives are not related to neuraminidase inhibition.

More recently, Meindl and Tuppy synthesized a series of derivatives of deoxyneuraminic acid and found them to have potent inhibitory activity against bacterial and viral neuraminidases. These synthetic analogs of N-acetylneuraminic acid differ from the latter in containing a double bond between carbon atoms 2 and

215

3. Additional derivatives were obtained by substitution of the N-acetyl group. A total of 18 derivatives were tested in vitro against bacterial and viral neuraminidases and the most active was found to be 2-deoxy-2,3-dehydro-N-trifluoroacetylneuraminic acid (FANA).

Kinetic studies indicate that FANA is a competitive inhibitor with a KI of 7.9×10^{-7}M for influenza A/Mel/35 (HON1) virus neuraminidase and the affinity of viral neuraminidases for small as well as large molecular weight substrates is approximately 1000 fold lower than their affinity for FANA. The capacity of FANA to inhibit elution of virus from red cells was tested by mixing varying concentrations with virus and red cells and allowing agglutination to occur at 4°. The tubes then were placed at 37° and aliquots of supernatant fluid were removed at intervals to measure the titers of eluted virus. Depending on the test virus employed, FANA inhibited virus elution, when present in concentrations ranging from $10^{-4}-10^{-6}$M. In the course of these experiments, it was observed that FANA had no effect on hemagglutination by influenza viruses, but did inhibit hemagglutination by some (but not all) parainfluenza viruses.

FANA was also shown to inhibit influenza WSN virus replication in MDBK cell culture. This inhibition was most readily demonstrated in multicycle replication where concentrations from $10^{-3}-10^{-6}$M reduced virus yields obtained after 72 hrs. However, concentrations as high at 10^{-3}M had no effect on virus yields obtained during single cycle replication (except with one temperature sensitive mutant of WSN virus which will be discussed later). Apparently, even at concentrations of inhibitor which reduce neuraminidase activity by more than 90%, only slight reductions in virus yields are produced in a single growth cycle. During multicycle replication these reductions are magnified during each subsequent cycle of replication. The inhibitory effects of FANA were also observed in plaque size reduction assay with a variety of influenza A viruses grown in clone 1-5C-4 cells. In this system, FANA is incorporated in the agar overlay added after infection of the monolayer, and inhibition is assessed by a reduction in the size but not the number of plaques observed. after 4-5 days. In the course of these experiments we observed marked differences in susceptibility among different strains of virus. Plaque size reduction with NWS (HON1) or WSN (HON1) viruses was observed at concentrations of FANA as low as 10^{-6}M whereas 100 fold higher concentrations of inhibitor were required to produce an equivalent effect with X-7 (HON2) virus -- a recombinant strain which derives its hemagglutinin from NWS and its neuraminidase from A/RI/5/57 (H2N2) virus. Systematic examination of several wild type viruses and antigenic recombinant viruses derived from them revealed that viral susceptibility to FANA is determined by the kind of neuraminidase contained in the virus.

Regardless of the source of their hemagglutinins, viruses which derive their neuraminidase from NWS virus are inhibited at concentrations of FANA of 10^{-6}M. Conversely, virus containing N2 neuraminidase (derived from either H2N2 or H3N2 strains) are not inhibited at concentrations lower than 10^{-4}M. Viruses with N1 neuraminidase derived from A/PR$_8$/34 (H0N1) were intermediate in their sensitivity. Kinetic studies in vitro with X7 and NWS viruses using fetuin as a substrate demonstrated that the affinity of NWS neuraminidase for FANA was 6 fold greater than that of X-7 neuraminidase. Similar studies using a synthetic low molecular weight substrate revealed no differences. The fact that viruses with the same hemagglutinin but different neuraminidases vary in their response to FANA is one indication that the antiviral effect of FANA is specifically mediated by its neuraminidase inhibiting activity. Additional evidence derives from the observation that FANA has no effect on the replication of other enveloped viruses such as measles and vesicular stomatitis virus which do not possess neuraminidase. Furthermore, even at concentrations of 10^{-3}M, FANA had no effect when it was present during the period of attachment and penetration but was removed 4 hrs after infection of the monolayer.

Preliminary experiments have been conducted to determine whether FANA could inhibit influenza virus replication in intact animals. Mice were infected with influenza A/NWS (H0N1) virus and were injected subcutaneously every 12 hrs with .5 ml of FANA in a concentration of 4×10^{-3}M. This dose was calculated to achieve an extracellular fluid concentration of 10^{-4}M. Pulmonary virus titers 48 and 72 hrs after infection and lung lesions 7 days after infection in FANA treated mice were not reduced when compared to those observed in control animals. However, attempts to demonstrate FANA in the sera of mice 12 hrs after injection failed to detect FANA despite the fact that assay procedures were employed which are capable of detecting concentrations of FANA as low as 5×10^{-6}M. From these results it seems that FANA is metabolized or excreted very rapidly in the intact animal and that to achieve an effect in vivo more frequent administration of higher concentrations of inhibitor are probably required. In another experiment, FANA was administered intranasally under ether anesthesia again at 12 hr intervals following infection for 3 days. Again no differences in virus titers or lung lesions between FANA treated and control animals were observed.

Despite these failures to modify influenza virus infection in intact animals with a highly potent inhibitor of neuraminidase we believe that such an approach is promising. By further modification of the compound it may be possible to concentrate it within cells or to slow its metabolism or excretion. In

addition newer methods of synthesis may make it convenient to
deliver larger doses of inhibitor at more frequent intervals.

The experiments conducted in cell culture confirm that
neuraminidase activity is essential for optimal replication of
influenza virus, but they do not define the function of neuraminidase in virus replication. From a variety of experiments,
it seems clear that neuraminidase is not required for virus
attachment, penetration or for early events in the replicative
cycle. More recently, it has been proposed that neuraminidase
is required to permit virus maturation at the cell surface or
for release of the mature particles from the cell membrane.
Recent experiments by Palese et al. with a temperature sensitive
mutant of WSN virus containing a defect in its neuraminidase have
revealed that at the nonpermissive temperature virus particles
are shed which still contain neuraminic acid in their envelopes.
Presumably as a consequence of attachment of one particle to
another by hemagglutinin molecules and neuraminic acid receptors
the particles which are shed are found in large aggregates.
Similar observations have been made when the mutant is grown at
permissive temperature in the presence of FANA. Thus at least
one function of neuraminidase may be to strip neuraminic acid
off of budding virus particles thereby preventing aggregation.

VIRUS SPECIFIED ENZYMES IN HERPES SIMPLEX VIRUS INFECTED CELLS

J. H. Subak-Sharpe and J. Hay

M.R.C. Virology Unit, Institute of Virology

University of Glasgow, Scotland

The genome of Herpes simplex virus (HSV) is a molecule of double-stranded DNA with molecular weight of about 100×10^6 and consequently the polypeptide-specifying potential of herpesviruses is considerable. Although over fifty polypeptides - induced following herpes virus infection of cells in tissue culture - have been recognised, the function of most of them is still unclear, but in a few cases induced enzyme activities have been identified and studied. The present discussion is concerned chiefly with the possible role of these enzymes in antiviral chemotherapy, and in this context only herpesvirus-induced (and coded) DNA polymerase and pyrimidine deoxynucleoside kinase activities can be related to current knowledge of antiviral reagents. However, the several other enzymes implicated as herpesvirus induced-DNA exonuclease (Morrison and Keir, 1968) ribonucleotide reductase (Cohen, 1972), dTMP kinase (Nohara and Kaplan, 1963), ATPase (Randall et al., 1972), dCMP deaminase (Keir, 1968) and protein kinase (Rubenstein et al., 1972) - may well include potential target molecules for chemotherapy.

In HSV infected cells, a new DNA polymerase activity can be detected which is quite distinct in biochemical, immunological and genetical properties from any of the DNA polymerase activities of the uninfected cell. The most striking biochemical difference is the stimulated activity of the viral enzyme in high monovalent cation concentrations, which enables the assay in vitro of virus-specific enzyme essentially free of inter-

ference from cell activities (Keir et al., 1966a; Keir et al.,
1966b).   The HSV type 1 DNA polymerase has been extensively
purified (Weissbach et al., 1973) and may be associated oper-
ationally with a virus-induced exonuclease activity.   The native
molecular weight of the enzyme has been estimated to be 150-
200,000 daltons and recent estimates of its polypeptide molecular weight suggest, that this may be a single molecular.   The
DNA polymerase has been shown to be a DNA binding protein
(Bayliss et al., 1975).   Other members of the herpesvirus
group are known to induce a salt-stimulated DNA polymerase
activity after infection e.g. Pseudorabies virus (Hay and Moss,
unpublished observations); Marek's disease virus (Boezi et al.,
1974).   This may be a characteristic feature of the group.

       Using HSV specific antiserum it has been demonstrated
with HSV infected cells of different species that the DNA polymerase is not only virus induced but virus specified (Keir et al.,
1966b).

       Genetic studies with herpes simplex virus types 1 and 2
have shown that over 50% of randomly-selected temperature-
sensitive mutants are defective in viral DNA synthesis (Halliburton and Timbury, 1973; Brown et al., 1973; Schaffer et al.,
1973).   Two of these mutants, ts 6 from HSV type 2 and ts H
from HSV type 1, appear to be in the structural gene for DNA
polymerase, which constitutes direct evidence for the essential
nature of viral DNA polymerase for herpes virus growth and
DNA synthesis (Hay et al., 1975; Crombie, 1975).   In addition, mutants in three separate cistrons of HSV type 2: ts 1,
9 and 11; and in two cistrons - ts K and J - of HSV type 1 possess lesions which affect DNA polymerase synthesis, but not
its function: these must constitute failure of essential control
mechanisms normally operating during virus replication.

       In terms of DNA polymerase induction and viral DNA
synthesis complementation and recombination have been demonstrated between two mutants of HSV type 2: ts 6 and ts 9.
Although the complementation is surprisingly inefficient, a correlation between DNA polymerase activity and DNA synthesis
can be seen (Timbury and Hay, 1975).

       Phosphonoacetic acid (PPAA), a potent anti-herpesvirus
agent in animals (Overby et al., 1974) has been shown in vitro
to be a specific inhibitor of the salt-stimulated viral DNA poly-

merase (Mao et al., 1975).   If its antiviral action is also mediated in vivo through specific interaction with the HSV DNA
polymerase, one might be able to isolate mutants of HSV which
are resistant to the action of PPAA and which may possess
altered DNA polymerase activity.   We have now isolated mutants from HSV type 1 and 2 which are resistant to 100 μg/ml
PPAA.   The viral DNA polymerase activity induced by these
mutants shows considerable resistance to PPAA in vitro relative to either wild-type, which is further strong support for
the hypothesis that PPAA acts through the viral enzyme.   In
addition, these results confirm the essential as well as the
virus-coded nature of the induced DNA polymerase and suggest
uses of the system not only for possible chemotherapeutic exp-
loitation, but also as a marker in genetic studies.

          One of the earliest features of the herpes virus growth
cycle is the appearance of thymidine kinase activity (Kit and
Dubbs, 1963).   This enzyme is unique in that it possesses both
deoxycytidine and thymidine kinase activity and has been classified as a HSV specified pyrimidine deoxynucleoside kinase
(dPyK) (Hay et al., 1971; Jamieson et al., 1974).   Until recently regarded as a dispensible virus function, the enzyme has
now been shown to be essential for virus growth in "resting"
cells in culture, a situation considered more closely analogous
to the whole animal system (Jamieson and Subak-Sharpe, 1974).
Major biochemical and immunological differences have been
demonstrated between dPyK and the cell's enzymes which exist
as separate thymidine-(TK) and deoxycytidine-kinases (dCK).
One of these biochemical properties, the in vitro pH optimum,
is used to emphasise assay conditions for viral enzyme (Jamieson
and Subak-Sharpe, 1974).   dPyK has not been successfully purified, probably owing to the formation of aggregates, but the
activity seems to have a denatured molecular weight of 43,000
daltons and exist as a dimer (or higher order structure) in the
infected cell with no host polypeptides required for activity
(Honess and Watson, 1974).   The enzyme dPyK has provided
a useful selective marker in transfection experiments, using
thymidine kinaseless LM cells and selecting for the ability to
utilise dT as sole thymidylate source (Munyon et al., 1971);
but examination of cells generally transformed with HSV has
failed to reveal the consistent appearance of viral enzyme (recognised by its characteristic heat sensitivity, RF value etc.) in
detectable amounts (Jamieson and Hay, unpublished observations).

A virus expressing thymidine and deoxycytidine kinase activity should be susceptible to inhibition by BUdR and araC, and the proof that these two activities were herpes virus coded has come from such experiments: mutants resistant to each analogue were readily obtained. When it became clear that in every case a mutant selected against one drug had simultaneously gained resistance to both, the classification of the enzyme as a virus-specified dPyK was made and has subsequently been verified biochemically (Jamieson and Subak-Sharpe, 1974). IUdR and araC have been used as anti-herpes therapeutic agents, the latter chiefly against eye infections where the blood supply is poor and little transfer to adjacent tissue can take place, but both these pyrimidine nucleoside analogues have only limited usefulness as clinical agents as they affect DNA synthesis and other pathways in the uninfected cells.

BUdR, IUdR and araC are converted intracellularly into antiherpes agents by the lethal synthesis of their phosphorylated nucleotides mediated by both pre-existing host-enzymes (TK or dCK) and the virus-programmed enzyme (dPyK). Any similar inhibitor recognised only by the HSV enzyme and not by host enzymes would have much greater therapeutic potential. The search for such compounds seems now to have succeeded. Prusoff and his collaborators (Cheng et al., 1975) have described 5' amino, 2'-5' dideoxyiodouridine which specifically inhibits HSV replication. It appears to block viral DNA synthesis, and may exert specificity by acting as a substrate for the viral dPyK but not for the various kinase activities in uninfected cells. A similar viral dPyK specificity seems to exist for bromodeoxy-cytidine, which has been used to halt the growth of HSV type 1 (Cooper, 1973).

The role of HSV dPyK may not simply be to 'scavenge' for deoxypyrimidines inside the infected cell. The large alterations in the pool sizes of deoxynucleotides - particularly of TTP - in HSV infected cells have been suggested to be due to the action of kinases (Jamieson and Bjursell, unpublished observations, 1975). Such action would constitute an additional controlling influence of the enzyme on nucleotide metabolism and consequently on viral DNA synthesis and replication.

Virus-coded dPyK activity can be shown to function in infected cells, in that dCMP can be formed in vivo even in dCK⁻ cells, but there, paradoxically, conversion of this dCMP to dCTP

cannot be detected.   Further, radioactively-labelled deoxycytidine cannot be incorporated into DNA in infected TK⁻, dCK⁻
cells which contain only the viral dPyK activity although infectious HSV is produced there.   (If araC is added virus production
is blocked).   However, it can be shown that infected cell extracts
form dCTP from deoxycytidine in vitro.   It seems clear that at
the level of the nucleoside monophosphate kinase, the deoxycytidine triphosphate synthesising system no longer functions in
HSV infected cells.   This raises the question of the inhibitory
activity of araC, which is presumed to act as araCTP, after
phosphorylation by the deoxycytidine phosphorylating mechanism.
The above evidence suggests that araCTP cannot be formed in
infected cells by the deoxycytidine phosphorylating mechanism
(Jamieson, 1974), and the finding that the HSV DNA polymerase
in vitro is not inhibited by araCTP (Muller et al., 1974) would
be compatible with this: it would be interesting to find what
action araCMP or araCDP have on HSV DNA polymerase activity.

        A new herpesvirus-specified RNA polymerase has so far
not been detected, but the possibility that the host enzyme following infection becomes virus-modified has not been fully excluded.
Therefore, specific attack on virus multiplication at the level of
RNA synthesis could still prove a possible chemotherapeutic
approach.

        Agents used in antiviral chemotherapy have most often
been found by trial and error and their action retrospectively
described in terms of inhibition of particular virus functions. As
more knowledge becomes available on the nature of virus-induced
functions, it should prove increasingly possible to design potential
antiviral compounds with specific and exclusive effects on virus
infected cells.   Viral gene products like the HSV DNA polymerase, or the several genetically detected HSV control genes which
act specifically on viral functions (like DNA synthesis or polypeptide cascades) could ultimately prove more useful as substrates for chemotherapy than virus gene products of more general
metabolic action (e.g. dPyK).   As genetic and biochemical analysis identifies more of the relevant genes in the large HSV genome, this should reveal additional promising points for chemotherapeutic attack.

        In general, currently used antiviral agents are active
against viruses in the lytic growth phase.   However, in cells
transformed by virus in tumour cells produced by virus in vivo and in

tumours produced by inoculation of virus transformed cells viral
antigens can be detected which appear to be essential expression
of the oncogenic viral agent.   Thus, a role for specific chemotherapy against the production of such viral antigens as well as
against cells manifesting them may exist.   This approach may
be able to avoid the problems inherent in the use of compounds
effective against all growing cells, and with intrinsic unwanted
side effects on normal tissues.

The very real problem of long term latency encountered
with herpes viruses could also prove tractable to this type of
approach once the genetic and biochemical regulation of the latent
herpes virus genome in nerve cells begins to be understood.

Bayliss, G., Marsden, H. and Hay, J. (1975).   Virology, in
        press.
Boezi, J. A., Lee, L. F., Blakesley, R. W., Keenig, M. and
        Towle, H. C. (1974).   J. Virol. 14, 1209.
Brown, S. M., Ritchie, D. A. and Subak-Sharpe, J. H. (1973).
        J. Gen. Virol. 18, 329.
Cheng, Y. C., Goz, B., Neenan, J. P., Ward, D. C. and
        Prusoff, W. H. (1975).   J. Virol. 15, 1284.
Cohen, G. (1972).   J. Virol. 9, 408.
Cooper, G. M. (1973).   Proc. Nat. Acad. Sci. (Wash.) 70, 3788.
Crombie, I. K. (1975).   Ph.D. Thesis, University of Glasgow.
Halliburton, I. W. and Timbury, M. C. (1973).   Virology 54, 60.
Hay, J., Moss, H. M., Jamieson, A. T. and Timbury,M. C.
        (1975).   J. Gen. Virol. Submitted for publication.
Hay, J., Perera, P.A. J., Morrison, J. M., Gentry, G. A.
        and Subak-Sharpe, J. H. (1971).   Ciba Foundation Symp-
        osium 'Strategy of the Viral Genome' p. 355.
Honess, R. W. and Watson, D. H. (1974).   J. Gen. Virol. 24,
        215.
Jamieson, A. T., Gentry, G. A. and Subak-Sharpe, J. H. (1974).
        J. Gen. Virol. 24, 465.
Jamieson, A. T. and Subak-Sharpe, J. H. (1974).   J. Gen.
        Virol. 24, 481.
Keir, H. M. (1968).   XVIII Symposium Gen. Microbiol. 67.
Keir, H. M., Hay, J., Morrison, J. M. and Subak-Sharpe,
        J. H. (1966a).   Nature 210, 369.
Keir, H. M., Subak-Sharpe, J. H., Shedden, W. I. H., Watson,
        D. H. and Wildy, P. (1966b).   Virology 30, 104.
Kit, S. and Dubbs, D. R. (1963).   Biochem. Biophys. Res.
        Commun. 11, 51.

Mao, J. C-H., Robishaw, E. and Overby, L. R. (1975). J. Virol.
        15, 1281.
Morrison, J. M. and Keir, H. M. (1968).   J. Gen. Virol. 3, 337.
Muller, W. E. G., Falke, D. and Zahne, R. K. (1973). Arch
        ges Virusforsch. 42, 278.
Munyon, W., Kraiselburd, E., Davis, D. and Mann, J. (1971).
        J. Virol. 7, 813.
Nohara, H. and Kaplan, A. S. (1963).   Biochem. Biophys. Res.
        Commun. 12, 189.
Overby, L. R., Robishaw, E. E., Schleicher, J. B., Reuter, A.,
        Skipkowitz, N. L. and Mao, J. C-H. (1974). Antimicrob.
        Agents Chemother. 6, 360.
Randall, C., Rogers, H., Downer, D. and Gentry, G. A. (1972).
        J. Virol. 9, 216.
Rubenstein, A. S., Gravell, M. and Darlington, R. (1972.).
        Virology 50, 287.
Timbury, M. C. and Hay, J. (1975).   In "Herpesvirus and
        Oncogenesis".   World Health Organisation.
Weissbach, A., Hong, S., Aucker, J. and Muller, R. (1973).
        J. Biol. Chem. 248, 6270.

STUDIES WITH IBT RESISTANT AND IBT-DEPENDENT MUTANTS OF VACCINIA VIRUS TO CLARIFY THE MECHANISM OF THE ANTIPOX ACTIVITY

Ehud Katz, Eva Margalith, Bela Winer, Haya Felix and
Natan Goldblum
Chanock Centre for Virology, Hebrew University-Hadassah
Medical School
Jerusalem, Israel

SUMMARY

The macromolecular events of vaccinia virus growth which are inhibted by isatin thiosemicarbazone (IBT) were followed. It was found that the maturation of the virus was blocked, although viral DNA, "early" poly-peptides and most of the "late" viral polypeptides were synthesized in the presence of the drug. A similar maturational block occurred with the IBT-dependent mutant when growing in the absence of IBT.

Eight thiosemicarbazone-containing compounds which inhibited the growth of the wild-type strain and to which the IBT-resistant mutant showed resistance, supported the gorwth of the IBT-dependent mutant. This indicates that there is a correlation between the abilities of the compound to inhibit the wild-type growth and to enhance the growth of the IBT-dependent mutant. Two compounds which did not follow this rule and inhibited the growth of all three virus strains were found to inhibit virus growth by a mechanism different from that of IBT, which resulted in failure of the virus to synthesize its DNA. Their antiviral action is not attributed to the thiosemicarbazone component of the molecule but to the chemical structure attached.

INTRODUCTION

The antiviral effect of thiosemicarbazones was first demonstrated by Hamre et al. (1950, 1951) who showed that the compound para-aminobenz-aldehyde-3-thiosemicarbazone and several of its derivatives inhibited the lethal effect of vaccinia virus in chick embryos and in mice. These studies were extended by Minton (Minton et al., 1953) and by Tompson (Tompson et al., 1951, 1953a,b), who showed that the benzene, thiophene, pyridine, quinoline and isatin derivatives of thiosemicarbazides also protected mice against vaccinia-induced encephalitis.

In 1955 Bauer (Bauer, 1955) began a study on the effect of IBT and other thiosemicarbazone derivatives on vaccinia infection as well as on other members of the poxviruses group (Bauer and Sadler, 1959, 1961; Bauer,1963). Following the demonstration of the antipox activity of N-methyl derivatives of IBT in mice (Bauer and Sadler, 1960; Bauer et al., 1962), a clinical trial with the N-methyl derivative of IBT, clinically known as methisazone or Marboran, was initiated in Asia, Africa and South America.

The objectives of our study were to elucidate the mechanism by which IBT exerts its antiviral activity on vaccinia virus and to learn more about the component of the drug molecule which determines the antiviral activity. A drug-resistant mutant (IBT^R) and a drug-dependent mutant (IBT^D) which we recently isolated were very helpful in this research.

MATERIALS AND METHODS

Isolation and Characterisation of IBT-resistant and IBT-dependent Mutants of Vaccinia Virus

The two vaccinia mutants IBT^R and IBT^D were isolated from chick fibroblasts infected with wild-type (wt) virus after treatment with the mutagenic agent, iododeoxyuridine, in the presence of IBT (Katz et al., 1973d). It was found that the wild-type strain is inhibited more than 99% by IBT concentrations larger than 20 µM, while concentrations of 10 µM and lower allowed its partial growth. Full growth rate of the IBT^D mutant was obtained even with a concentration of 3µM of IBT. The IBT^R mutant was able to grow equally well in the absence and presence of IBT concentrations up to 40 µM (the highest concentration used by us, which did not cause visible toxic effects to the host cell). The reversion from dependence on IBT was examined following infection of HeLa cells with the IBT^D mutant in the absence of IBT. The revertants (2% of the progeny virus) were found to be sensitive or resistant to IBT, thus exhibiting the wt or the IBT^R characters (Katz et al., 1973d).

Several physical and biochemical characteristics of the three virus strains were compared. Using sedimentation of virus particles in sucrose gradient we could not detect differences between the two mutants, as compared with the wild-type strain (Katz et al., 1973c). Autoradiography of ^{35}S-methionine-labelled virus particles, following polyacrylamide gel electrophoresis in the presence of sodium dodecyl sulphate, did not reveal significant qualitative differences in the molecular weights of the main structural polypeptides of the IBT^R and IBT^D mutants, except for some quantitative differences of several viral polypeptides (Katz, et al., 1973c). The two mutants were neutralized by antiserum which was obtained from rabbits immunized with the wild-type strain (Felix and Katz, to be published).

Since the multiplication of the wild-type strain is inhibited in the presence of IBT, and the growth of the IBT^D mutant depends on a constant supply of IBT in the culture media, we studied whether the viruses can interact during their co-cultivation. It was found that it is possible to rescue the we strain in the presence of IBT, during mixed infection with either IBT^R or IBT^D, and to rescue IBT^D in the absence of IBT, by mixed infection with wt or IBT^R (Katz et al., 1973c). These findings suggest that there are common events in the multiplication of these three strains and that they are capable of sharing an event or a factor(s) involved in their multiplication.

The Mechanism of the Inhibition of Vaccinia Virus by IBT

The mechanism by which IBT exerts its antipox activity is not yet clear. Studies which were done in wt-infected tissue cultures revealed that IBT does not affect early events which occur during the multiplication cycle of the virus: uncoating is normal, "early" enzymes are synthesized (Woodson and Joklik, 1965) a number of "early" structural viral proteins are made (Appleyard et al., 1965) and viral DNA replicates (Easterbrook, 1961; Woodson and Joklik, 1965). The rate of transcription of mRNA is not affected and the formed mRNA combines with ribosomes to form polyribosomes; however, polyribosomes which are formed by "late" mRNA are rapidly broken down (Woodson and Joklik, 1965). On the basis of this finding, Woodson and Joklik (1965) suggested that a deficiency of late viral protein is the target for the inhibition of poxviruses by IBT.

New techniques, like the separation of radioactively labelled polypeptides by polyacrylamide gel electrophoresis which were developed during the last few years, enabled us now to follow the synthesis of viral polypeptides in the presence of IBT. Host protein synthesis is progressively inhibited after virus infection, thus permitting the specific labelling of viral polypeptides (Holowczak and Joklik, 1967; Moss and Salzman, 1968; Moss, 1968; Salzman and Sebring, 1967; Shatkin, 1963). In order to distinguish between specific and non-specific effects of IBT on the synthesis of viral polypeptides, we used in these experiments a control of polypeptides synthesized in the presence of the drug by the IBT-resistant mutant of vaccinia virus. We could show that both "early" and "late" viral polypeptides were formed in the presence of IBT by the wild-type strain (Katz et al., 1973b).

A major vaccinia-virus structural polypeptide is formed from a higher molecular-weight precursor. This process appears to be a late step associated with virus maturation and is completely prevented by rifampicin (Katz and Moss, 1970a, b). We followed the formation of this structural polypeptide and found that, although the precursor polypeptide is formed in the presence of IBT, only partial cleavage of it occurs in the presence of IBT (Katz et al., 1973b). We cannot conclude whether the partial inhibition of this cleavage is the target of IBT or a secondary effect due to the failure of virus maturation, which occurs in the presence of the drug.

The Need for IBT of the IBT-dependent Mutant

The need for IBT of the IBT-dependent mutant raised the question as to whether IBT is required for the growth of this mutant at the same stage of virus development which is the target of the inhibition of the growth of the wild-type strain by IBT. We followed virus macromolecule synthesis in IBT^D-infected cells in the presence of IBT. It was found that, although virus DNA is synthesized under these conditions, it fails to acquire resistance to deoxyribonuclease. When "early" and "late" viral structural and non-structural polypeptides were examined by polyacrylamide gel electrophoresis, it was found that their synthesis was not affected by the absence of IBT. However, the formation of vaccinia virus core polypeptide from its polypeptide precursor was greatly inhibited under these conditions (Katz et al., 1973a). Electron microscopy studies of cells infected with the wt strain in the presence of IBT and of IBT^D-infected cells in the absence of IBT could not reveal differences between the structures of the two developing virus strains, the morphogenesis of which stopped as a result of the non-permissive growth conditions (Katz et al., 1973c).

The Effect of IBT-related Compounds on the Wild-type Strain and on the Two Mutants, IBT^R and IBT^D

Many reports on the antiviral effect of thiosemicarbazone-containing compounds against pox viruses appeared in the scientific literature during the last 25 years. However, the mechanism of inhibition of virus growth by these compounds was not clarified and was not compared with that of IBT. We thought that the growth capability of the three strains of vaccinia virus, the wild-type and the two mutants, IBT^R and IBT^D, in the presence of these drugs, can indicate whether the tested drugs behave similarly to IBT and therefore might have a similar mechanism of antiviral activity. The ten tested compounds, which inhibit the growth of the wild-type strain, can be divided into two groups (Table 1). Compounds of the first group act similarly to IBT; support the growth of the IBT^D mutant and the IBT^R mutant can grow in their presence. The chemical structure of all these compounds is composed of a combination of a thiosemicarbazone chain and another part containing an aromatic closed ring. The thiosemicarbazone side chain in all these compounds has the structure – C_1N NHCSNH$_2$, while the structure of the attached chemical component is quite different from one another. The antiviral activity of compounds of the first group against wild type strains of poxviruses was previously reported; of compounds 1, 2 and 3 by Bauer (1965); of compound 5 by Winkelman and Rolly (1971); of compound 6 by Tsunoda et al., (1971); and of compound 8 by Singh and Sugden, (1971).

The second group of compounds inhibit the growth of all the three virus strains: wild-type, IBT-resistant and IBT-dependent mutants. The two compounds which belong to this group are picolinaldehyde-5-dydroxythio-semicarbazone and 1-formylisoquinoline thiosemicarbazone. When examining the step of virus growth which is affected by these compounds, it was found that they completely inhibit vaccinia virus DNA synthesis. These findings are well correlated with previously reported observations indicating that these compounds are inhibitors of DNA synthesis during cell growth and also of herpes virus DNA synthesis (Brockman et al., 1970; DeConti et al., 1972). It is suggested that the thiosemicarbazone part of these two compounds does not play a primary role in their antiviral activity and that their involvement in nucleic acid metabolism is caused by the other part of the molecule.

In conclusion, by examining the growth of the three vaccinia virus strains: wild-type, IBT^R and IBT^D in the presence of thiosemicarbazone-related compounds, it is possible to suggest whether these compounds exhibit a similar mechanism of antipox activity as that of IBT. We could not find until now a thiosemicarbazone-containing compound which inhibits the growth of the wild-type strain and to which IBT^R show growth resistance, that fails to enhance the growth of the IBT-dependent mutant. It seems that for compounds of the thio-semicarbazone group, of which the thiosemicarbazone part of the molecule determines the antipox activity, the inhibition of the growth of the wild-type strain and the capability to support the growth of the IBT-dependent mutant are characteristics which are related one to the other. Additional IBT-related compounds which we will examine in the future will show whether there are compounds which behave differently.

Formation of plaques of vaccinia virus WR strain (wt) and of the two mutants
IBT^D and IBT^R in the presence of IBT-related compounds

Group	No	Compound	Conc (µM)	wt	IBT^D	IBT^R	Group	No.	Compound	Conc	wt	IBT^D	IBT^R
I	1	Isatin β thiosemicarbazone (IBT)	14	−	+	+	I	6		3.5	−	+	+
	2		14	−	+	+		7		28	−	+	+
	3		14	−	+	+		8		14	−	+	+
	4		112	−	+	+	II	1		14	−	−	−
	5		56	−	+	+		2		14	−	−	−

Monolayers of BSC1 cells were infected with end-point dilutions of stock
suspensions of the three virus strains and overlaid with Eagle's media containing 1% special Agar noble (Difco Laboratories, Detroit, Michigan), 5%
inactivated calf serum, and the tested compounds at the concentration
indicated.   Neutral red (0.0025%) was added 4 days following infection and
plaques were counted on the following day.   The compounds were kindly
obtained: group I-compound 1 from Mann Research Laboratories, New York,
N.Y.; Compounds 2 and 3 from D.J. Bauer, Wellcome Research Laboratories,
Kent, England; compound 4 from K. and K. laboratories Inc., Plain View,
New York; compound 5 from H. Rolly Farbwerke Hoechst AG, Frankfurt,
W. Germany; compound 6 from H. Isoyama, Meiji Seika Ltd., Tokyo, Japan;
compound 7 from S.J. Lucania, The Squibb Institute for Medical Research,
Princeton, N.J.; compound 8 from J.K. Sugden, Leicester Polytechnic,
Leicester, England; compound 1 of group II from H.B. Wood, National
Institutes of Health, Bethesda, Md.; and compound 2 from F.A. French, Mt.
Zion Hospital Medical Center, PaloAlto, California.

A part of this study was supported by a grant of the United States – Israel
Binational Science Foundation.

REFERENCES

Appleyard, G., Hume, V.B.M. and Estwood, J.C.N. (1965). Annual N.Y. Academy of Sciences, 130, 92.

Bauer, D. (1955). British Journal of Experimental Pathology, 36, 105.

Bauer, D. (1963). British Journal of Experimental Pathology, 44, 233.

Bauer, D., Dumbell, K., Fox-Hulme, P., and Sadler, P. (1962). Bulletin W.H.O., 26, 727.

Bauer, D. and Sadler, P. (1959). Nature (London) 184, 1496.

Bauer, D. and Sadler, P., (1960). Lancet, 1, 1110.

Bauer, D. and Sadler, P. (1961). Nature (London), 190, 1167.

Easterbrook, K.B. (1961). Virology, 17, 245.

Hamre, E., Bernstein, J. and Donovick, R. (1950). Proceedings of the Society of Experimental Biology and Medicine, 73, 275.

Hamre, D., Brownlee, L., and Donovick, R. (1951). Journal of Immunology, 67, 305.

Holowczek, J.A. and Joklik, W.K. (1967). Virology, 33, 726.

Katz, E., Margalith, E. and Winer, B. (1973a). Journal of General Virology, 21, 477.

Katz, E., Margalith, E., Winer, B. and Goldblum, N. (1973b). Antimicrobial Agents and Chemotherapy, 4, 44.

Katz, E., Margalith, E., Winer, B. and Lazar, A. (1973c). Journal of General Virology, 21, 469.

Katz, E. and Moss, B. (1970a). Journal of Virology, 6, 717

Katz, E. and Moss, B. (1970b). Proceedings of the National Academy of Sciences (USA), 66, 677.

Katz, E., Winder, B., Margalith, E. and Goldblum, N. (1973d). Journal of General Virology, 19, 161.

Minton, S., Officer, J. and Thompson, R. (1953). Journal of Immunology, 70, 222.

Moss, B. (1968). Journal of Virology, 2, 1028.

Moss, B. and Salzman, N.P. (1968). Journal of Virology, 2, 1016.

Rolly, H. and Winkelman, E. (1971). In: Advances of Antimicrobial and Antineoplastic Chemotherapy. Edited by M. Hejzlar, M. Semansky and S. Masak, p. 305.

Salzman, N.P. and Sebring, E.D. (1967). Journal of Virology, 1, 16.

Shatkin, A.J. (1963). Nature (London), 199, 357.

Singh, M. and Sugden, J.K. (1971). Pharmaceutica Acta Helvetiae, 46, 627.

Thompson, R., Davis, J., Russell, P. and Hitchings, G. (1953b). Proceedints of the Society of Experimental Biology and Medicine, 84, 496.

Thompson, R., Minton, S. Jr., Officer, J., and Hitchings, G. (1953a). Journal of Immunology, 70, 229.

Thompson, R., Price, M. and Minton, S. (1951). Proceedings of the
       Society of Experimental Biology and Medicine, 78, 11.
Tsunoda, A., Miyazaki, K., Aota, T., Matsumoto, S., Kumagai, K. and
       Ishada, N. (1971). Japanese Journal of Microbiology, 16, 61.
Woodson, B. and Joklik, W.K. (1965). Proceedings of the National
       Academy of Sciences (USA), 54, 946.

THE ROLE OF CELL-MEDIATED IMMUNITY IN THE THERAPEUTIC ACTION OF

ISOPRINOSINE OF VIRAL DISEASE PROCESSES

A.J. Glasky, G.E. Friebertshauer, J.W. Holker,
R.A. Settineri, & T. Ginsberg

Newport Pharmaceuticals Int'l., Inc.
Newport Beach, California, U.S.A.

Summary: Isoprinosine has been shown to enhance certain aspects
of the immune response in experiments employing sensitization of
mouse spleen lymphocytes with sheep erythrocytes in vivo and
mitogen-induced proliferation of human peripheral blood lymphocytes
in vitro. Clinical studies demonstrated utility for the treatment of
influenza, herpes simplex and measles virus infections in man.

Modification of the cell-mediated immune response represents a
new approach to the therapeutic cure of viral disease. Isoprinosine
(a 1:3 molar complex of inosine and N,N-dimethylamino-2-propanol
p-acetamidobenzoate) is an agent which affects the immune response
in a selective manner. It has been tested extensively for its
safety in animals and man as well as for its efficacy against a
variety of viral diseases.

Animal studies have demonstrated that the antiviral effect of
Isoprinosine in vivo is optimalized when the following interrelated
experimental conditions are taken into consideration: (1) adequacy of
drug dosage; (2) employment of a therapeutic dosing schedule with
initiation of dosing delayed to about 1 day after virus challenge;
(3) use of a non-overwhelming virus challenge approximating a natural
exposure; (4) continuous and frequent dosing throughout the course of
the infection and; (5) employment of the oral route of drug
administration to slow absorption, catabolism and excretion. Previous
reported experiments in animals (Gordon et al, 1974) have shown that
pretreatment of rats with Isoprinosine produced a structural modification of polyribosomes such that their ability to accept and
translate foreign messenger RNA is impaired. Further, a number of
studies (see Glasky et al, 1975) in animals and man indicated that the
immune response was a major component of the activity of Isoprinosine.

These observations lead us to study the effect of Isoprinosine on the sensitization and response of mouse spleen lymphocytes.

Mice were immunized using sheep erythrocytes as an antigenic stimulus and their spleens were removed after 4 days. The spleens were homogenized and assayed for the number of immunocompetent cells (Mishell and Dutton, 1967). In addition, several in vivo prophylactic treatments were employed during immunization.

Table 1 (first column) shows that non-immunized controls have few immunocompetent cells. Animals receiving saline treatment in vivo developed approximately 1500 immunocompetent cells per 10^6 spleen cells. Those animals treated with Isoprinosine both prophylactically and throughout the 4 days of the experiment showed a mild suppression in the number of immunocompetent cells but nowhere near the suppression seen with the potent immunosuppressive agent 6-mercaptopurine. If we added Isoprinosine to the in vitro assay of more or less sensitized spleen cells, we saw that therapeutic addition of Isoprinosine in vitro caused an increase in the number of immunocompetent cells in all immunized groups – even those suppressed in vivo by 6-mercaptopurine.

One of the standard laboratory techniques for assessing immunocompetence is the measurement of mitogen-induced proliferation of human peripheral blood lymphocytes (Park and Good, 1972). DNA synthesis was measured by H^3-thymidine uptake after exposure to the mitogen, phytothemaglutinin (PHA). Isoprinosine produces a consistent stimulation of the PHA-induced response over a broad dose range. The 50% stimulation observed at the optimal dose of Isoprinosine (50mcg./ ml.) compares favourably with the lesser degree of stimulation usually seen with other agents which are active in this system. This Isoprinosine response has been seen consitently in all subjects studied. In addition, it is important to consider that Isoprinosine has no direct effect on proliferation in the absence of PHA or other mitogens.

TABLE 1   EFFECT OF ISOPRINOSINE ON THE IMMUNE RESPONSE

Prophylactic Treatment in vivo		Therapeutic Treatment in vitro			
		No Drug	100 ug/ml	300 ug/ml	500 ug/ml
Non-Immunized Group	A	0	50	60	20
	B	10	30	60	0
Immunized+Saline	A	k845	2745	2550	2910
	B	1215	3150	2490	2610
Immunized+Isoprinosine (500 mg/kg b.i.d.)	A	1260			2040
	B	720			2085
Immunized-6-mercapto- purine Treated	A	240		1080	
	B	285		870	

We investigated the effects of Isoprinosine on RNA synthesis in human lymphocytes using H^3-uridine in the system described above. Figure 1 represents typical results obtained when a single dose of Isoprinosine is administered simultaneously with PHA. Shown is the dose response to PHA when the pulse is administered from either 0-2 hours or from 24-26 hours after mitogen and drug. The early pulse shows no stimulation of RNA synthesis but rather a weak high dose inhibition. The 24-26 hour pulse shows a stimulation of RNA synthesis that appears dose related at 2 mcg./ml. of PHA.

The expression of cell-mediated immunity involves three steps: (1) sensitization of lymphocytes; (2) proliferation of sensitized lymphocytes and; (3) production by sensitized lymphocytes of certain factors which act on the recovery process at the site of the viral infection. Based on these considerations and the experimental observations reported, we propose the following mechanism of action of Isoprinosine on the cell-mediated immune response. Isoprinosine suppresses the sensitization of the lymphocytes when administered prophylactically. However, once sensitization has occurred, Isoprinosine enhances both the proliferation of the sensitized lymphocytes as well as the response of these sensitized lymphocytes. The response phase is either direct cytolysis of virus-infected cells or the production of the lymphokines.

Following are a few representative examples of the clinical experience with Isoprinosine (also see Glasky et al, 1975).

In carefully monitored studies in normal healthy volunteers (Glasky et al, 1975), the administration of up to 6 grams of Isoprinosine per day for 4 weeks produced no serious adverse signs or symptoms. There was an occasional report of nausea at the higher doses. The increased uric acid seen was a reflection of the normal metabolism of the inosine portion of the drug and thus is the excretory product of the drug rather than a product of a toxicological reaction. No clinical sequelae of this were observed. There were no abnormalities in the other blood and urine chemistries. Hematologic, ophthalmologic and liver function tests were all normal as was the EKG. When doses up to 6 gm per day were given for periods of from 6 months to $4\frac{1}{2}$ years to several hundred patients, we observed the same pattern of safety evident in the acute studies.

In an open field trial (Ink et al, 1971) of Isoprinosine given therapeutically against influenza, it was observed that the duration of symptoms were decreased from approximately $5\frac{1}{2}$ days to $1\frac{1}{2}$ dyas duration. Similar results have been obtained in a recently completed double-blind study using therapeutic administration of Isoprinosine to normal volunteers artificially infected with Rhinovirus 21 (Waldam, 1975). In a double blind study (Sternberg and Macotella, 1972) of herpes simplex infections of the lips and body, 18 out of 21 Isoprinosine treated patients showed a rapid recovery while only 4 out of 12 controls responded. In another double blind study (Chang and Weinstein, 1973), statistically significant clinical improvement in primary herpes progenitalis was seen when Isoprinosine was administered.

A double-blind study (Waldman, 1975) in human volunteers artificially infected with measles virus by administering the measles vaccine showed that therapeutic administration of Isoprinosine significantly suppressed clinical symptomatology while having no inhibitory effect on the normal antibody response. The effect of Isoprinosine was studied on subacute sclerosing panencephalitis (SSPE), and extremely serious and fatal encephalitis caused by the measles virus (Mattson, 1974).

The first patient studied was a 10 year old female when first seen in August of 1970. She had measles at age two and received oral measles vaccine in May 1970. Two months later, she was noted to be emotionally labile and began to have periodic myoclonic jerks. EEG showed characteristic periodic slow wave complexes. Her clinical state deteriorated through mid 1971. A brain biopsy and CSF measles antibody titer performed in February 1971 provided a confirmation of the diagnosis of SSPE. The patient began receiving 5 grams of Isoprinosine per day in August of 1971 and has continued on drug since that time. No further deterioration has been seen; the patient has in fact improved. She now attends high school.

In conclusion, we have described an interesting new chemotherapeutic agent. Isoprinosine is an effective and safe drug for the therapeutic treatment of viral diseases. It acts by enhancing the immune response while suppressing disease symptomatology. Thus making it the first agent for the treatment of viral diseases that acts through a PRO-HOST mechanism.

REFERENCES

1.   Glasky, A.J., Pfadenhauer, E.H., Settineri, R.A. & Ginsberg, T. (1975), in Combined Immunodeficiency Disease and Adenosine Deaminase Deficiency, Academic Press, New York, p. 157.
2.   Gordon, P., Ronsen, B. & Brown, E.R. (1974). Antimicrob. Ag. Chemother., 5, 153.
3.   Ink, J., Andres, F.J., Antonini, G.M., Stepano, J.C., Scarpie Scarpiello, U., Vaninetti, C., Ink, R.L., Ink de Vila, H.N.H. & Goijam, I. (1971). La prensa med. arg. 58, 1875.
4.   Mishell, R.I. & Dutton, R.W. (1967) J. Exp. Med., 126, 423.
5.   Park, B.H. & Good, R.A. (1972) Proc. Nat. Acad. Sci U.S. 69 371.
6.   Sternberg, T.H. & Macotella Ruiz, E. (1972) Prensa Med. Mexico, 37, 159.
7.   Waldman, R.H. (1975), personal communication.

BONAPHTON - A NEW ANTIVIRAL CHEMOTHERAPEUTIC

DRUG

G.N. Pershin, N.S. Bogdanova, I.S. Nikolaeva,
A.N. Grinev, G.Ya. Uretskaya, N.V. Arkhangelskaya

All-Union Chemical Pharmaceutical Research Institute
Moscow, U.S.S.R.

Orthonaphthoquinone and many of its derivatives exert antiviral activity. Conditional estimation of antiviral action of
compounds studied is represented in Table 1.

The data on antiviral efficacy of orthonaphthoquinone
and its derivatives against virus of APR-8 strain influenza
are given in Table 2. From II compounds studied 9 are active.
The most effective is 7-hydroxyorthonaphthoquinone (+++++).
Compounds I, IV, V and X are highly active (++++). In the
experiments on chick embryos only four substances were active
(II, VI, VIII, X) and in the treatment of experimental influenzal
pneumonia of mice the only compound 6-bromorthonaphthoquinone,
named bonaphton (X), was active.

In contact with virus-containing suspension of mouse lung
0.05 mcg, 0.5 mcg and 5 mcg doses of bonaphton neutralize I LD_{100},
10 LD_{100}, and 100 LD_{100} of influenza virus, respectively
(activity ++++).

In the experiments on chick embryos bonaphton in a dose
of 7 mcg per embryo inhibits the development of 10 infective
doses of virus.

Bonaphton gives therapeutic effect against influenzal
pneumonia of mice infected with A2/Frunze and A2/Hong-Kong/68
viruses.

Maximum tolerated dose of bonaphton hasn't revealed curative
effect. Apparently, complex action of toxic effects of the drug
and influenzal virus takes place.

Table I

Estimation of antiviral action of compounds studied

Estimation	Doses of compounds (in mcg) neutralizing I LD$_{100}$ of influenza virus	Inhibition of growth of influenza virus in chick embryos at the infective doses (ID 80)
+	50 – 100	I
+ +	5 – 10	10
+ + +	0. 5 – 1.0	100
+ + + +	0.05 – 0.1	1000
+ + + + +	0.005 – 0.01	10000

Designations: LD – lethal dose
ID – infective dose

Table 2:   Antiviral action of o-naphtoquinone and its derivatives
           with respect to influenza APR-8 virus.

Nos. of compounds	Chemical formulae of compounds	Activity		
		Virucidal action in vitro	Virostatic action in ovo	Chemotherapeutic action in vivo
I		+ + + +	0	no
II		+ + + + +	+	no
III		+ +	0	no
IV		+ + +	0	no
V		+ + + +	0	no
VI		+ +	+ +	no
VII		0	0	not studied
VIII		+ + +	+ +	no
IX		+ +	0	no
X	Bonaphton	+ + + +	+ +	active
XI		0	0	no

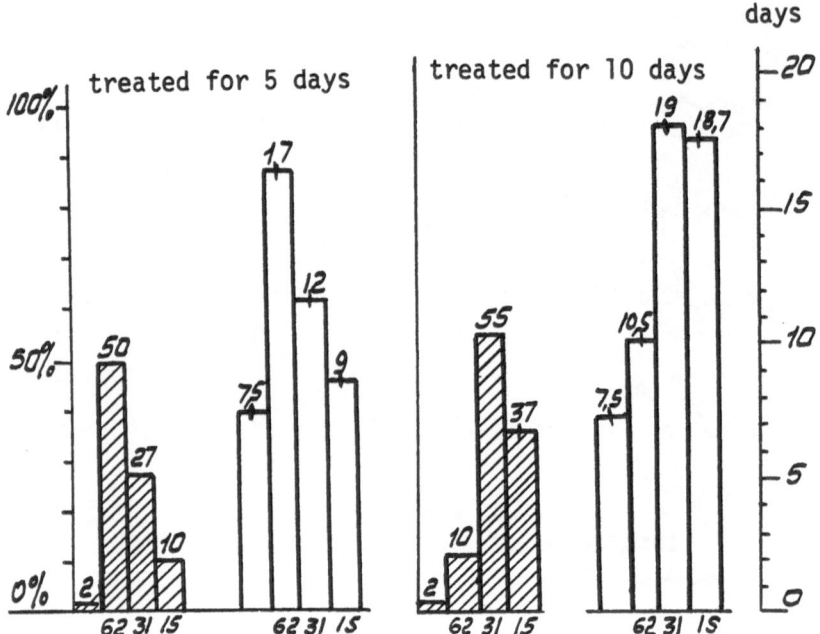

Fig. 3.   Effect of peroral bonaphton on survival and life span of
mice infected with $1 LD_{100}$ of influneza A_2/Frunze virus.
▨ - survival (%), ▭ - medium life span (days ± m), c – control
(non treated mice) 62;31;15 – bonaphton doses (mg/kg a day).

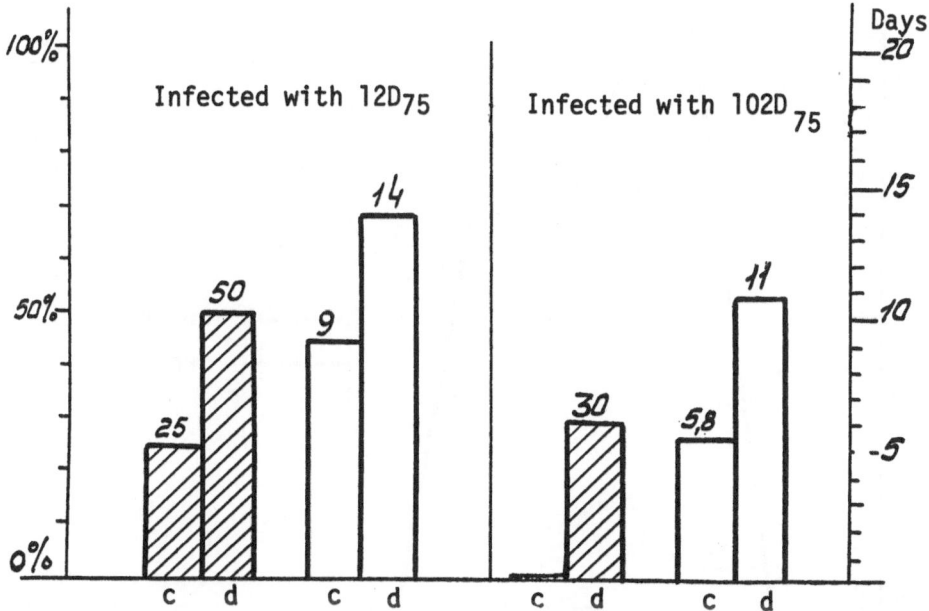

Fig. 4. Effect of peroral bonaphton (62 mg/kg a day for 5 days) on survival and life span of mice infected with influenza A_2/Hong Cong/68 virus. ▨survival (%), ☐-medium life span (days ± m), c - control (non treated mice), d - bonaphton 62 mg/kg a day.

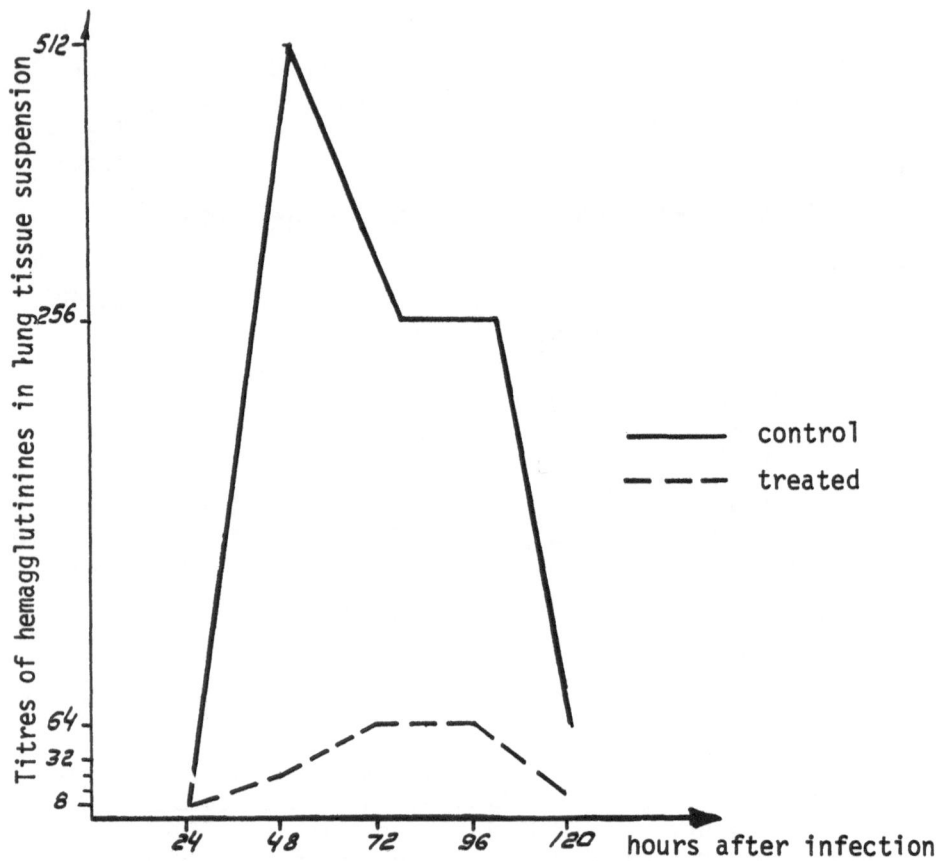

Fig. 5.   Effect of bonaphton (6.2 mg/kg/day) on accumulation
dynamics of influenza A_2/Hong Cong/68 virus in lung tissue of mice
infected with LO LD_{50} virus.

Bonaphton used during 5 days after infecting of mice with I LD_{100} of A2/Frunze influenza virus (daily dose of the drug being 62 mg/kg) gives survival of 50% of the animals. Administration of 31 mg/kg does of bonaphton prevents death of 25% of the animals while I5 mg/kg dose slightly prolongs living period of infected animals. (Fig. 3).

62 mg/kg dose of bonaphton used for 10 days is too high, not giving essential survival of infected mice but extending their living. 31 and 15 mg/kg doses exert pronounced chemotherapeutic effect promoting survival of 50% and 30% of animals infected with I LD_{100} of influenza virus (Fig. 3).

As well, marked therapeutic efficiency is observed in the treatment of mouse influenza provoked by A2/Hong-Kong/68 influenza virus (Fig. 4). Curative effect takes place only when the treatment begins before or simultaneously to inocculation. Administration of bonaphton even 3 hours after inocculation gives no precise chemotherapeutic effect.

Special investigations have demonstrated that accumulation of virus is inhibited in lung tissue under the action of effective doses of bonaphton. (Fig. 5).

Pathohistologic changes in lungs of the mice treated are considerably less pronounced comparatively to the controls.

Bonaphton inhibits the development of herpes simplex virus in cell culture. The addition of bonaphton to culture medium (cell culture Hep-2, medium N199) in a concentration I mcg/ml increases cytopathic dose of virus by 100 times. Local and oral administration of bonaphthon gives therapeutic effect in experimental herpetic keratitis of rabbits (detailed data will be presented in a separate report).

Preliminary clinical studies indicate perorally bonaphton to be active as a remedy for the prophylaxis of influenza as well as for medication of herpetic diseases.

CHEMOTHERAPEUTICAL ACTIVITY OF BONAPHTON IN

HERPETIC KERATITIS IN RABBITS

N.S. Bogdanova, I.S. Nikolayeva, S.N. Kutchak,
G.N. Pershin

All-Union Chemical Pharmaceutical Research Institute
Moscow, U.S.S.R.

The virus of Herpes simplex type 1, was taken for experiment. Keratitis was induced in rabbits by applying the virus to the scarified cornea. Bonaphton treatment was started 48-72 hours after the infection, with the clinical picture of keratitis well developed, and continued till complete recovery.

0.25%, 0.1% and 0.05% ointments on a vaseline base were applied only topically to one group of rabbits. The second group received bonaphton only per os, while the third one underwent combined treatment (per os + topical application). Two groups of rabbits were taken for control, one of them getting 0.1% kerecide solution, and the other -- placebo. The preparations's effectiveness was estimated by comparing the gravity of the clinical course of keratitis and the pathomorphological picture of the eyes of the treated and control groups of rabbits.

It was established that the administration of bonaphton for the treatment only orally in a 200mg/kg dose (i.e. 2.5 times less than the maximum tolerance does) without topical treatment caused a manifested therapeutic effect, comparable to the curative effect produced by an 0.1% solution of 5-iodine-2' desoxyuridine, administered topically. Recovery took 10-18 days, an average of 13 ± 0.9 ($p > 0.002$) days from the beginning of treatment. In the control group of animals self-recovery took place within 21-40 days, an average of 24.0 ± 3.1 days (Fig. 1). A good therapeutic effect was also observed with combined bonaphton treatment, i.e. per os and topically. With this method of administration, started on the 3rd day after infection, recovery took 13.0 ± 0.7 ($p < 0.001$) days on an

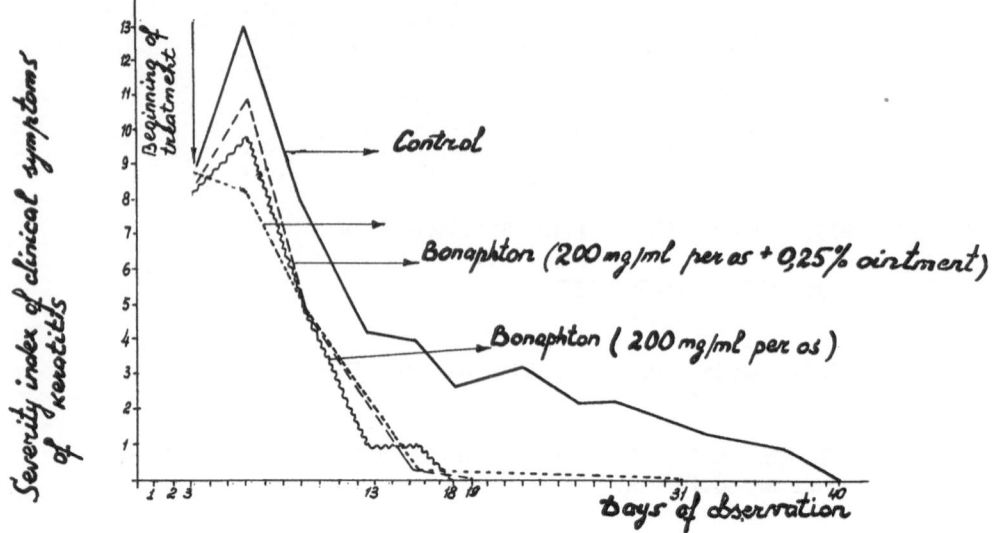

Fig. 1. Dynamics of clinical course of experimental keratitis in rabbits treated with Bonaphton

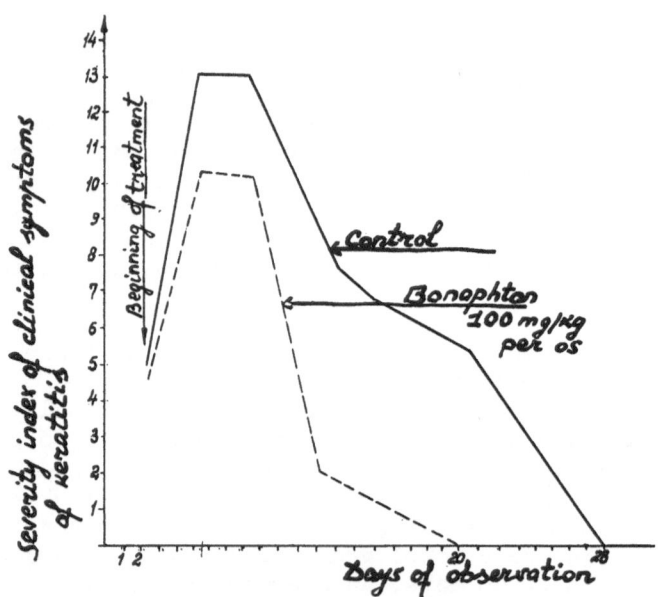

Fig. 2. Dynamics of clinical course of experimental keratitis in rabbits treated with Bonaphton

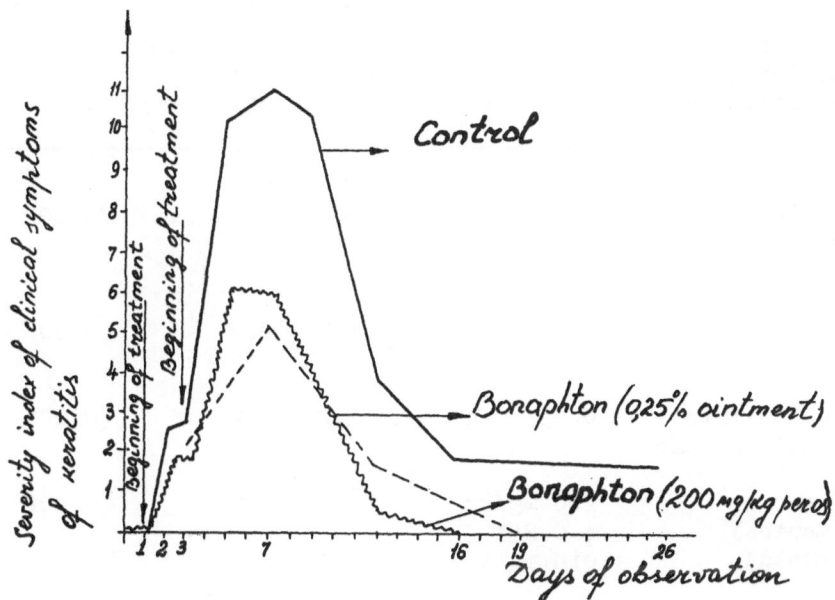

Fig. 3.   Dynamics of clinical course of experimental keratitis in
rabbits treated with Bonaphton.

TABLE 1

Effectiveness of Bonaphton Treatment of Experimentally Induced
Herpetic Keratitis in Rabbits with Different Methods of
Administration

Method of bonaphton administration	Dose of bonaphton	Average duration of keratitis treatment (days)	P
per os (72 hours after infection	200 mg/kg	13.0 ± 0.9	<0.002
per os (6 hours before infection)	200 mg/kg	11.7 ± 0.7	<0.001
topically into conjunctival sac	0.25% ointment	12.2 ± 1.2	<0.001
oral per os and topical (combined)	200 mg/kg + 0.25% ointment	13.0 ± 0.7	<0.001
kerecide	0.1% solution	13.2 ± 2.2	<0.01
Control		24.0 ± 3.1	

Note: Bonaphton was administered once a day, daily, for

14-16 days, topically bonaphton and kerecide were used

daily, four times a day for 14-16 days.

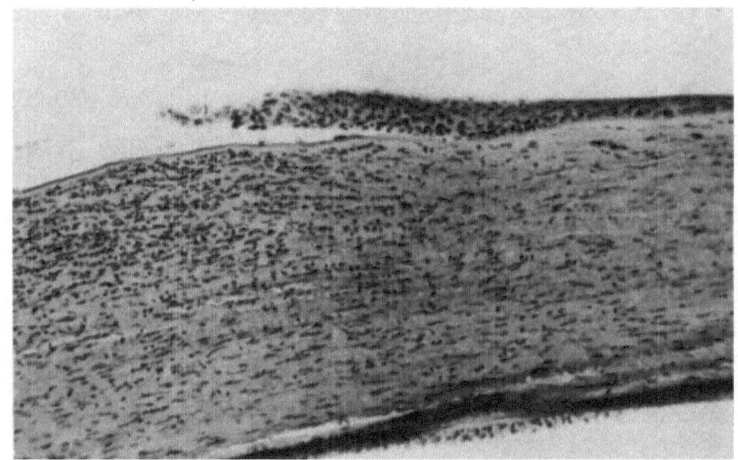

FIG. 4   Cornea of the eye of the untreated rabbit infected
          with herpes simplex virus. Epithelium is absent
          in site of cornea ulceration, substantia propria
          of cornea is oedematous and infiltered with leucocytes
          (II day after infection).
          Haematoxylin-eosin x22o

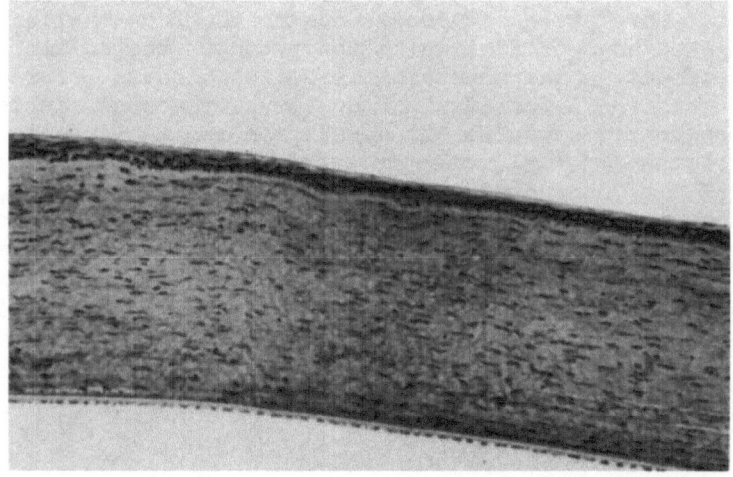

FIG. 5   Cornea of the eye of the rabbit infected with herpes
          simplex virus and treated with bonaphton (200 mg/kg/
          day per os). Ulcerated surface is epithelized, signs
          of inflammation in substantia propria of cornea
          disappeared (II day after infection).
          Haematoxylin-eosin x22o

average. In the untreated group recovery took 24.0 ± 3.1
(Fig. 1).

An authentic therapeutic effect, though less pronounced, was
produced by the oral administration of bonaphton in a 100 mg/kg
does (one fifth of the maximum tolerance dose). Keratitis took
an average of 14.8 ± 0.6 days to heal, while in the control
group of animals the infectious process lasted on an average
21 ± 5.3 days (Fig. 2).

A still more pronounced bonaphton action was observed at
its early (6 hours before infection) oral administration in
a 200 mg/kg dose. Healing took 11.7 ± 0.7 (p < 0.001) days
from the moment of infection. The gravity of the clincieal
course of keratitis in this group of rabbits was about half
that of the control group.

Bonaphton administration to rabbits with developed keratitis
in the form of 0.25%, 0.1% and 0.05% ointments only topically
produced a clearly manifested therapeutic effect (Fig. 3).

A comparison of average indices of the duration of keratitis
treatment with nonaphton, and using various methods of administration, shows that combined oral and topical treatment in the
most effective doses is not superior to its separate administration when treatment is started at the developed stage of
keratitis. This may be obviously due to the fact that even any
one of the methods of administration produces the maximum
possible effect. Bonaphton administration 6 hours before the
rabbit's eyes are infected with the virus of Herpes simplex and
then subsequently given for 10 days, promotes the speediest
recovery (Table 1). Microscopic examination of eye-ball of
teated rabbits, conducted on the 11th day after infection,
revealed recovery well under way irrespective of the way of
bonaphton administration (topical or oral), whereas an examination of the eyes of untreated animals at the same date revealed
a picutre of grave, acute ulcerous keratitis (Fig 4; Fig 5).

EFFECT OF RIBAVIRIN ON INFLUENZA VIRUS INFECTION IN FERRETS

Karen P. Schofield, C.W. Potter, J.P. Phair,
J.S. Oxford and R. Jennings
Academic Division of Pathology (Virology)
University of Sheffield Medical School
Sheffield S10 2RX, U.K.

SUMMARY

The effect of 1- -ribofuranosyl-2, 4-triazole-3-carboxamide
(ribavirin) on influence virus infection was studied in ferrets.
Ferrets were given 100 mg/kg of ribavirin intraperitoneally one
day before and 1 and 24 hrs following intranasal infection with
$10^{3.0}$ ferret infective doses of A/Port Chalmers/73 virus. Ribavirin caused a reduction in the febrile response, and the peak
temperature reaction occurred 24 hrs later than for control animals. Drug-treated ferrets produced both nasal wash antibody and
increased levels of protein, but the peak levels, similar to those
of control ferrets, occurred later than in untreated animals.
Titres of virus isolated from nasal washings were similar for the
two groups, but peak titres occurred later after infection in
treated ferrets.

The response of ferrets to influenza infection was also
examined in animals given ribavirin one day before, one hr before
and daily for five days after virus infection. These animals
showed no temperature response, no increase of nasal wash protein
and did not produce nasal antibody following virus infection. In
addition, drug-treated ferrets had markedly reduced titres of virus
in nasal washings, and did not produce serum antibody following
virus infection. The absence of an antibody response was probably
due to the immunosuppressive action of the compound.

The compound 1- -D Ribofuranosyl-1, 2, 4-triazole-3-carbox-
amide (Ribavirin) has been reported to inhibit the replication of a
number of DNA and RNA viruses (Sidwell et al, 1972- Witkowski et
al, 1972- Huffman et al, 1973); specifically, ribavirin was found

to inhibit influenza virus infection in vitro (Huffman et al, 1973; Todo, 1973; Oxford, 1975) and in vivo (Sidwell et al, 1972; Khare et al, 1973). In the present study, the effects of ribavirin on influenza virus A/Port Chalmers/73 infection of ferrets was examined, since influenza in these species closely approximates the disease in man)Smith et al, 1933; Haff et al, 1966; Potter et al, 1972) and this recommends the ferret for the investigation of influenza inhibiting compounds. Thus, ferrets infected with influenza viruses show a sharp febrile response, produce high titres of virus, produce nasal wash and serum antibody and show a marked increase in nasal wash protein (Smith et al, 1933; Francis and Stuart-Harris, 1938; Lui, 1955; Haff et al, 1966). Using these parameters, the effects of antiviral compounds on influenza virus infection can be measured qualitatively (Cochran et al, 1965; Squires, 1970; Potter et al, 1972; Haff and Pinto, 1973; Potter and Schofield, 1975).

METHODS AND MATERIALS

Virus and Virus Vaccines

Influenza virus A/Port Chalmers/73 (H3N2) was obtained from Dr. G.C. Schild, National Institute for Medical Research, Mill Hill, London. A virus pool was prepared in 10 day embryonated eggs, and the infectivity of the virus for ferrets was established by titration in normal animals. Using the temperature response, virus isolation and the serum antibody response as indices of infection, the 50% ferrets infective dose (FID_{50}) was calculated as $10^{3.0} EID_{50}$. Ferrets were lightly anaesthetised with ether and inoculated with $10^{3.0} FID_{50}$ of the A/Port Chalmers/73 virus; the virus was given dropwise intranasally in a 1.0 ml volume of PBS.

A formaldehyde, inactivated influenza virus A/England/42/72 (H3N2) vaccine, containing 16,000 international units (IU)/ml, was kindly supplied by Dr. I. Furminger, Evans Biologicals Ltd., Speke, Liverpool. The vaccine virus was dialysed against medium '199' for 24 hr at 4°C immediately prior to use in macrophage migration inhibition tests.

Ribavirin

Ribavirin was kindly supplied by Dr. R.W. Sidwell, ICN Nucleic Acid Research Institute, Irvine, California and by Lederle Labs., Gosport, Hants. and was stored at room temperature. The drug was weighed out fresh each day and dissolved in phosphate buffered saline, pH 7.2, at a concentration of 100 ug/ml. Ferrets were inoculated daily by the intraperitoneal route with 100 mg/kg during the period of treatment.

Experimental Design

Adult ferrets, aged 4-8 months and weighting 500-800g, were obtained from accredited dealers and housed in individual cages for seven days prior to experimentation. During this period, nasal washings were collected for protein estimation and temperatures taken to establish normal values. Ferrets were test bled and inoculated intraperitoneally with 100 mg/kg of ribavirin. The following day, the ferrets were given a second dose of ribavirin, and two hours later the animals and a group of control ferrets were infected with influenza virus A/Port Chalmers/73. In one group of drug-treated ferrets a third dose of ribavirin was inoculated 24 hr after virus infection, and in the second experiment ferrets were inoculated with ribavirin daily for five days after virus infection.

Following virus infection, ferret temperatures were taken twice daily for four days, and once daily for three days. Nasal washings were collected daily for six days after virus infection for virus isolation, and on alternate days from day 5-15 for protein and neutralising antibody studies. Blood samples were taken 10 and 21 days after virus infection to determine the serum antibody response to infection.

To determine the effect of ribavirin on the immune response to influenza virus vaccine, a group of guinea pigs were inoculated intraperitoneally with 100 mg/kg of ribavirin for 10 days. On the second day, the drug-treated animals and a group of untreated guinea pigs were inoculated intramuscularly with 400 IU of A/England/42/72 influenza virus vaccine in an equal volume (0.5 ml) of Freund's complete adjuvant (Difco Laboratories, Detroit, Michigan). Serum specimens were collected from all guinea pigs prior to and 10 days after immunisation, and tested for serum HI antibody. Some guinea pigs from each group were inoculated intraperitoneally with 10 ml of sterile paraffin oil 4 days after immunisation and killed six days later; the peritoneal macrophages were removed and tested for cell-mediated immunity to influenza virus vaccine by the macrophage migration inhibition test.

In a further study, a group of CBA mice were inoculated intraperitoneally with 100 mg/kg of ribavirin on day -1, 0, 1, 2, 3, 6 and 7; on day 0 the animals and a group of control mice each received 150 ug of purified, whole influenza virus X31 (H3N2) in FCA. The virus used in this experiment was purified in linear sucrose gradients and inactivated by exposure to UV light. The mice were bled prior to and eight days after immunisation, and the sera were tested for antibody by the single radial diffusion method.

Virus Isolation

Bovine serum albumin, at a final concentration of 2.0% (v/v) and antibiotics (250 units/ml of penicillin and 200 ug/ml of streptomycin) were added to nasal washings taken for six days after virus infection; the washings were collected in 10 ml of PBS as described previously (Potter et al, 1972), and stored at -80°C. The titre of virus in these specimens was determined by titration by the allantois-on-shell method (Fazekas de St.Groth et al, 1958), or by titration in whole, 10 day embryonated eggs inoculated by the allantoic route (Potter et al, 1972).

Serological Tests

1. Haemagglutination Inhibition (HI) Antibody Tests

Ferret and guinea pig serum specimens were tested for HI antibody by the microtitre technique (Sever, 1962). Before testing, the ferret sera were treated with five volumes of cholera filtrate (Burroughs Wellcome Ltd.) for 18 hrs at 37°C, and then heated for 1 hr at 56°C. Guinea pig sera were heat-inactivated and absorbed overnight at 4° with kaolin (Flow Laboratories, Irvine, Scotland), and 50% suspension of fowl erythrocytes to remove non-specific inhibitors, as described previously (Oxford and Potter, 1970).

2. Single Radial Diffusion (SRD) Tests

Post-infection ferret sera and post-immunisation mouse sera were analysed for antibodies to influenza virus haemagglutinin by SRD, as previously described (Schild et al, 1975). The haemagglutinin for these tests was obtained from purified X31 recombinant influenza virus by treatment with bromelain- the freed haemagglutinin was purified in sucrose gradients (Schild et al, 1975).

3. Neutralization Tests

Nasal washings collected for neutralizing antibody and protein determinations were shaken with glass beads, and centrifuged at 3,000 rpm for 10 mins. The supernatant fluid was then concentrated 10-fold by dialysis against 30% Carbowax. The concentrated nasal wash specimens were tested for neutralizing antibody by the allantois-on-shell (AOS) method (Fazekas de St.Groth et al, 1958) using standard methods.

4. Macrophage Migration Inhibition (MMI) Tests

The cell-mediated immune response of guinea pigs to immunisation with influenza virus vaccine was measured by the direct MMI test (George and Vaughan, 1962; David et al, 1964). Six days prior to test, the guinea pigs were inoculated intraperitoneally with 10 ml of sterile paraffin oil; this induced a peritoneal cell

exudate which was removed by washing the peritoneal cavity with a
total of 100 ml of medium "199". The cells were washed and packed
into capillaries, as described previously (Rees and Potter, 1973),
anchored in the wells of plastic migration chambers (Sterilin Ltd.)
and covered with medium "199" containing 20% foetal bovine serum
and either 40 IU or 4.0 IU of inactivated influenza virus vaccine.
The wells were sealed, and the tests incubated for 48 hr at $37^{\circ}C$
in an atmosphere of 4% CO_2 in air. After incubation, the areas of
macrophage migration were measured by planimetry, and the percent
inhibition of migration calculated from the formula:-

$$\% \text{ inhibition} = 100 - \frac{(\text{average migration with antigen(9-12) tests}}{\text{average migration with normal allantoic fluid (9-12 tests)}} \times 100)$$

In each experiment, the effects of virus vaccine on normal guinea
pig macrophages was examined, but on no occasion did vaccine cause
inhibition of migration.

RESULTS

Two separate studies were carried out to determine the effect
of ribavirin on influenza virus A/Port Chalmers/73 infection in
ferrets. In the first test the drug was given daily for three days
from 24 hr prior to virus infection, and in the second experiment
ribavirin was given daily for seven days from 24 hr before virus
infection. In both studies the response of ferrets to infection
was measured by five parameters; these were the temperature response, virus replication, serum and nasal wash antibody production
and increase in nasal wash protein.

1. Temperature Response

In the first study, all four control ferrets inoculated with
$10^{3.0}FID_{50}$ of A/Port Chalmers/73 virus showed a sharp febrile response to virus infection, which was maximal at 24-48 hr after
infection. Thus, for each animal the temperature rose $\geqslant 1^{\circ}C$ above
the mean, pre-infection level to a peak of $\geqslant 40.0^{\circ}C$ on two occasions; this was taken as indicating both a significant temperature and a significant rise in temperature (Potter et al, 1972).
In contrast, ferrets treated with three doses of ribavirin showed
a less marked temperature response. For three of the four ferrets
in this group the temperature did not increase to over $40^{\circ}C$ on two
occasions, and for three animals the temperature did not increase
to $1^{\circ}C$ above the mean, pre-infection temperature. Thus, by both
parameters, ribavirin modified the febrile response to influenza
virus infection. In addition, the peak temperature response in
ferrets treated with ribavirin was seen 3-5 days following virus
infection (Fig. 1).

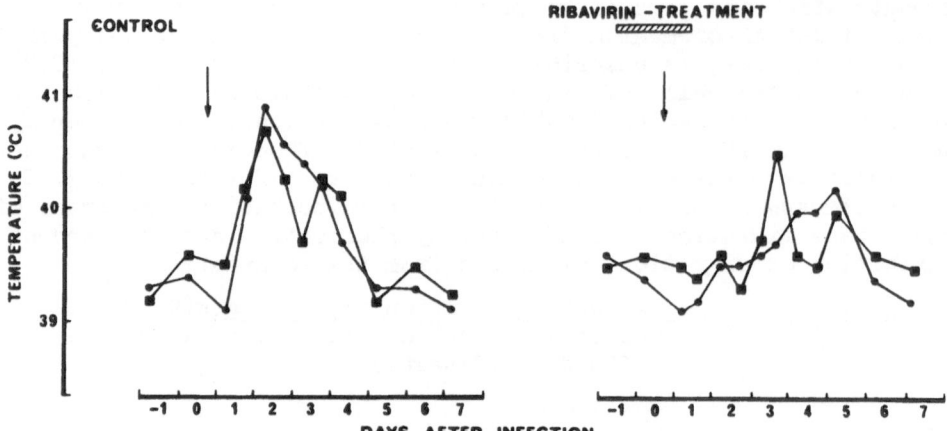

Fig. 2. Tmperature response of ferrets treated with Ribavirin
and infected with influenza virus A/Port Chalmers/73.

In the second study, the control ferrets again exhibited a
marked febrile response to infection with $10^{3.0}$ FID_{50} of A/Port
Chalmers/73 virus; the temperatures of two of the animals are
shown in Fig. 2. Both the criteria of a significant rise in
temperature and a significant peak temperature, maximal at 24-
48 hr after infection, were found in all four ferrets in this
group. In addition, a second peak of temperature was observed in

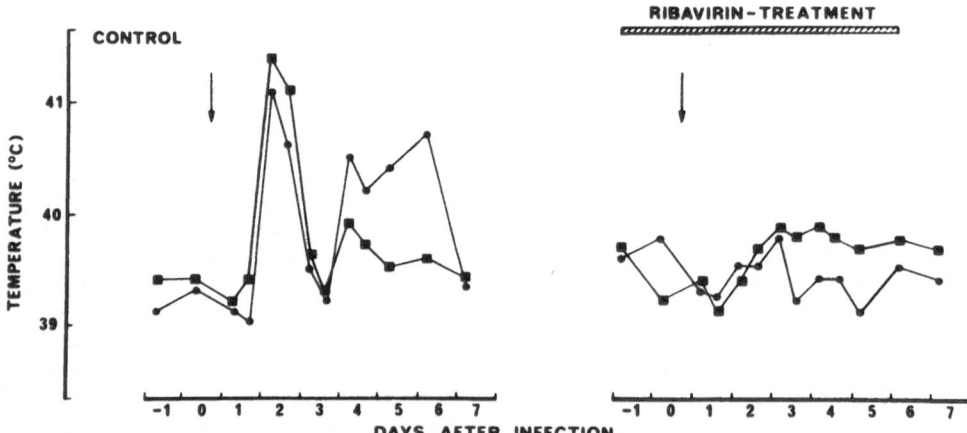

Fig. 1. Temperature response of ferrets treated with Ribavirin
and infected with influenza vir-us A/Port Chalmers/73

two of the control ferrets; this had been seen in previous experiments as an infrequent and random observation. In contrast to the
control ferrets, ferrets given seven daily doses of 100 mg/kg of
ribavirin intraperitoneally exhibited no febrile response to infection with A/Port Chalmers/73 virus. Thus, none of the ferrets in
this group developed either a significant temperature or a significant rise in temperature following virus infection (Fig.2).

2. Virus Isolations

Nasal washings were collected daily for six days following
virus infection, and were titrated for infective virus by the AOS
method. The results for the first experiment are shown in Fig.3.
For control ferrets, virus was detected 24 hrs after infection
and peak titres were found 2-3 days after infection; after this
time the titres of virus recovered progressively declined. In
contrast, virus was not recovered 24 hr after virus infection
from ferrets treated with three doses of ribavirin; however,
virus was recovered 48 hr post-infection and peak titres, higher
than those found in control ferrets, were found three days after
virus infection (Fig.3). From three days after infection, the
titre of virus recovered from drug-treated ferrets fell, but the
mean titre was consistently greater than that found in control
animals.

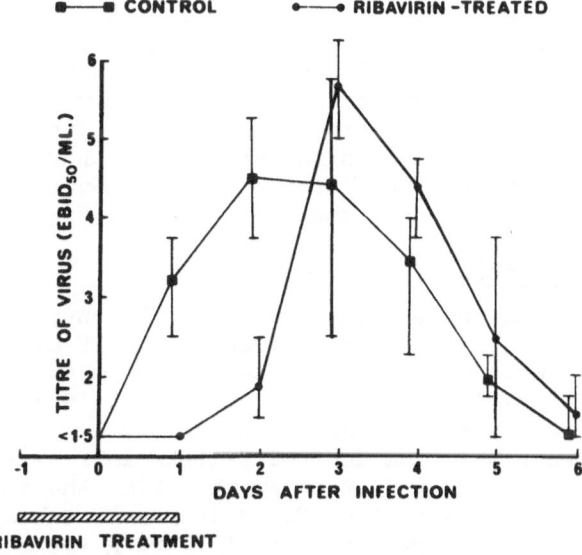

Fig. 3. Titre of virus in nasal washings of ferrets infected
with influenza virus A/Port Chalmers/73.

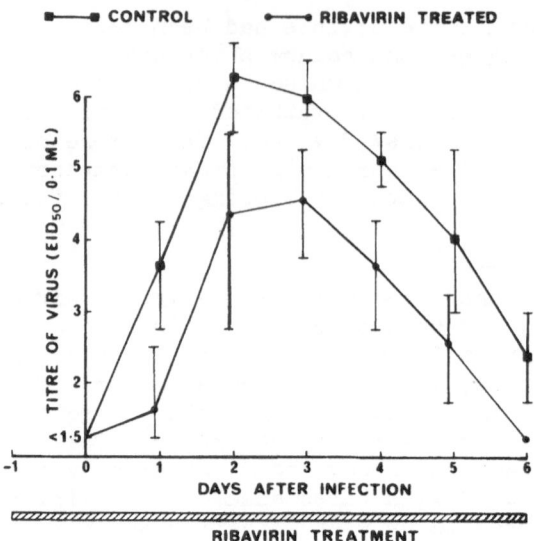

Fig. 4. Titre of virus in nasal washings of ferrets infected
with influenza virus A/Port Chalmers/73.

The characteristics of virus shedding shown by control
ferrets infected with A/Port Chalmers/73 virus in the second experiment were similar to that seen in the first study; in this
experiment the nasal washings were titrated in whole eggs, and
the titres of virus recovered were 10-100 fold greater than found
by titration on AOS. The results are shown in Fig.4. The titre
of virus recovered from nasal washings from control ferrets
infected with influenza virus increased to a maximum 2-3 days
following infection; after this time virus shedding declined.
Ferrets treated with ribavirin for seven days showed the same
result, but on each day the titre of virus recovered was 10-50
fold less than that found on control ferrets. (Fig.4).

3. Nasal Wash Protein

Nasal washings were collected from all control and ribavirin
treated ferrets on alternate days from days 5-15 after virus infection. The specimens were concentrated 10-fold, and the amount of
protein measured by the method of Lowry et al (1951). The results
are shown in Fig.5. In both experiments, the concentration of protein in nasal washings from control ferrets increased to a maximum
at 5-7 days after virus infection;at this time the concentration
was 2-4 times greater than that found in nasal washings collected
prior to infection. After day seven following virus infection the
concentration of protein declined, and by day 13-15 the concentration had returned to normal levels.

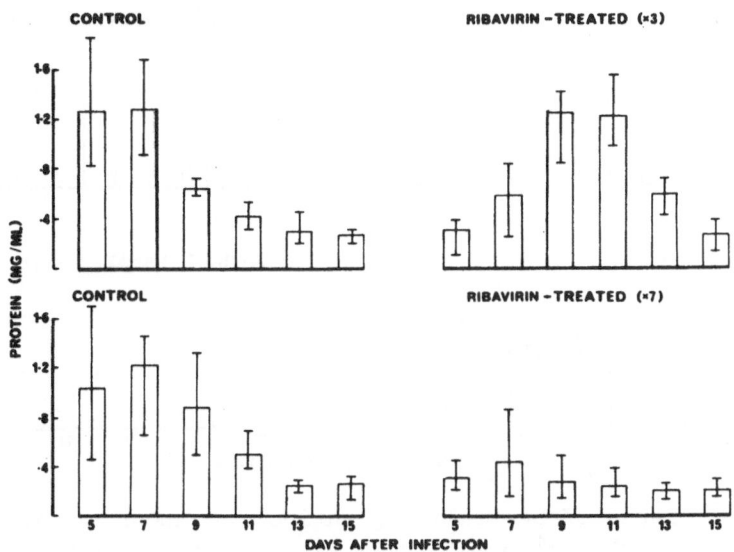

Fig. 5. Concentration of protein in nasal washings of ferrets infected with influenza virus A/Port Chalmers/73

For virus infected ferrets treated with three doses of riba-virin, the concentration of protein in nasal washings increased to a maximum level at 9-11 days after infection before declining; thus ribavirin delayed the appearance of peak concentrations of nasal wash protein (Fig.5). For ferrets treated with ribavirin for seven days, no increase in the concentration of protein in nasal washings was found in specimens collected 5-15 days after virus infection. A small increase in the protein level was found in washings taken seven days after infection; however, the inc-rease was relatively small, and not considered significant (Fig.5).

4. Nasal Wash Neutralizing Antibody

The titre of neutralizing antibody in concentrated nasal washings from control and ribavirin-treated ferrets is shown in Fig.6. For control ferrets in the first experiment, the maximum titre of neutralizing antibody was found on days 9 and 11 after virus infection when the mean antibody titres were 1:10 and 1:6, respectively. Similar results were obtained for the control fer-rets in the second experiment; thus, peak titres of neutralizing antibody were again found 9 and 11 days, post-infection, and the mean antibody titres were 1:14 and 1:8, respectively. In neither experiment was neutralizing antibody detected in nasal washings collected five days before or 13 days or more after virus infection. For ferrets treated with three doses of ribavirin, neutralizing antibody was detected in nasal washings collected on days 11 and 13

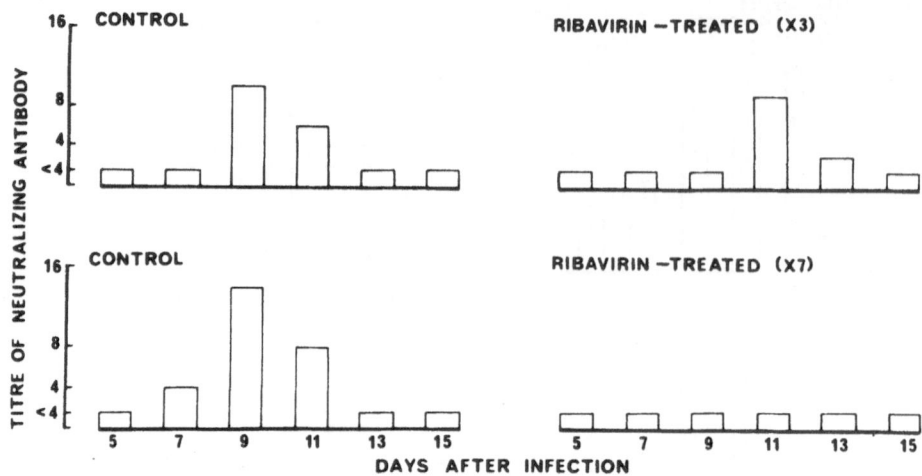

Fig. 6. Titres of neutralising antibody in nasal washings of
ferrets infected with influenza virus A/Port Chalmers/73

following infection (Fig.6); thus, no significant decrease in the
titre of nasal wash neutralizing antibody was observed in drug-
treated ferrets, but the production of antibody was delayed. No
detectable neutralizing antibody was found in nasal washings from
ferrets treated with seven doses of ribavirin (Fig.6).

5. Serum HI Antibody Response

        None of the ferrets had detectable serum HI antibody to
influenza virus A/Port Chalmers/73 prior to virus infection.
Serum specimens taken 10 days after virus infection of control
ferrets contained HI antibody at a titre of 1:250 (gmt) in one
experiment and at a titre of 1:233 (gmt) in the second experiment
(Table I).   These serum HI antibody titres increased in both experiments, and for serum specimens collected 21 days post-infection,
the HI antibody titres were 1:595 and 1:463.   For virus-infected
ferrets treated with three doses of ribavirin, the mean serum HI
antibody titre to A/Port Chalmers/73 virus at 10 days post-infection was 1:83; this titre was significantly less than that found
in control animals (Table I).   However, the HI antibody titre at
21 days was similar to that of control animals.   In the second
experiment, where seven doses of ribavirin were given, no detectable serum HI antibody was found at either 10 or 21 days after
virus infection.

Table 1.   Serum HI antibody response of ferrets treated with Ribavirin and infected with influenza virus A/Port Chalmers/73

EXP. 1

Ribavirin Treatment	Ferret No.	Serum HI antibody titre to A/Port Chalmers/73		
		pre - infection	post - infection (day 10)	post - infection mm(day 21)
100 mg per Kg/ day (X3)	611	<5	80	160
	612	<5	60	960
	613	<5 } <5	80 } 83*	640 } 466
	614	<5	120	480
NIL	607	<5	320	640
	608	<5	320	320
	609	<5 } <5	240 } 250	480 } 595
	610	<5	160	1280

EXP. 2

Ribavirin Treatment	Ferret No.	pre - infection	post - infection (day 10)	post - infection mm(day 21)
100 mg per Kg/ day (X7)	623	<5	<5	· <5
	624	<5	<5	<5
	626	<5 } <5	<5 } <5	<5 } <5
	630	<5	<5	<5
NIL	621	<5	240	480
	622	<5	240	960
	625	<5 } <5	320 } 233	320 } 463
	627	<5	160	320

* Geometric Mean Titre

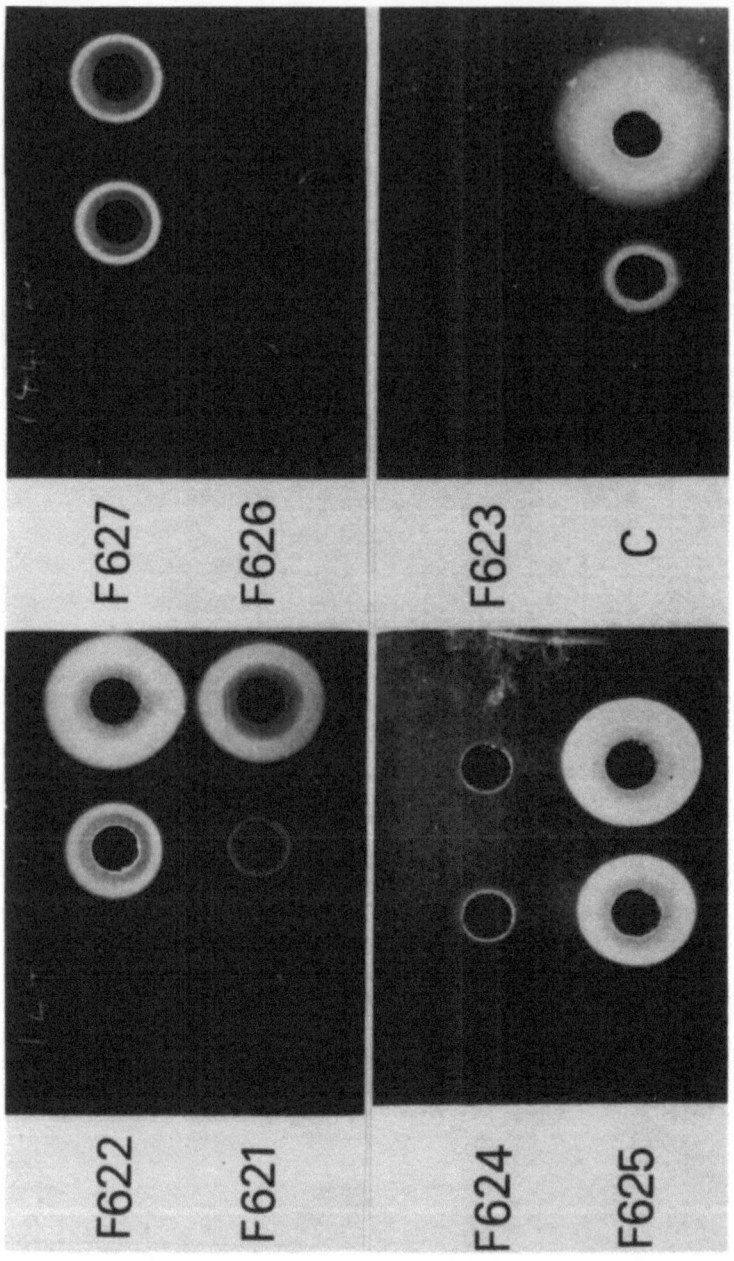

Figure 7. Single radial diffusion tests of sera from ferrets infected with influenza virus A/Port Chalmers/73. Three sera were tested from each ferret; the left hand well was inoculated with pre-infection sera, the centre well with sera collected 10 days after infection and the right hand well was inoculated with sera collected 21 days after infection. Sera from ferrets Nos. F623, F624 and F626 were from ferrets treated with riavirin. Sera from ferrets Nos. F621, F622, F625 and F627 were from untreated ferrets and show zones of reaction which indicate the presence of antibody. The wells of row C were inoculated with control sera.

The ferret sera collected prior to and 10 and 21 days following infection with influenza virus A/Port Chalmers/73 were
also examined for HI antibody by the SRD method. The results are
shown in Fig.7. For the four control ferrets, No.621, 622, 625
and 627, no antibody was found before infection, but antibody was
detected at 10 and 21 days after infection in all four animals.
In contrast, no antibody was found in any of the sera from the
three ferrets, No.623, 624 and 626, which had received seven doses
of ribavirin.

Effect of Ribavirin on the Immune Response of Guinea Pigs and Mice

In view of the above result, the effect of ribavirin on both
the cellular immune response and humoral antibody production was
examined further. A group of eight guinea pigs were immunised
with 400 IU of inactivated influenza virus A/England/42/72 vaccine in FCA; four animals were given ten daily doses of ribavirin
(100 mg/kg) from 24 hr prior to immunisation whilst the remainder
were untreated. Ten days after immunisation of the serum HI antibody response and the cellular immune response were measured.
The results are shown in Table II. Ribavirin treatment of guinea
pigs immunised with influenza virus vaccine prevented the development of serum HI antibody; however, the compound did not inhibit
the development of delayed hypersensitivity to influenza virus
antigens, as measured by the direct MMI test. Thus, the migration
of peritoneal macrophages from immunised guinea pigs was inhibited
by inoculation with 40 IU of inactivated influenza A/England/42/72
vaccine (Table II).

The antibody response of CBA mice to immunisation with purified influenza virus haemagglutinin was measured by SRD. The
results are shown in Fig.8. In the control mice, the mean area
of reaction was 25.9 mm^2, and for immunised mice treated with
fibavirin the mean area was 15.6 mm^2. These results indicated a
39.5% reduction of the antibody response for mice treated with
ribavirin. Sera collected from immunised mice four weeks after
the last treatment with ribavirin showed high concentrations of
antibody; at this time the antibody titres in control mice had
fallen, and were less than those in treated animals.

DISCUSSION

The results of the present study have shown that ribavirin
inhibited the response of ferrets to infection with influenza
virus A/Port Chalmers/73. Thus, three daily doses of 100 mg/kg
of ribavirin given intraperitoneally modified the temperature
response to influenza virus infection, and delayed the appearance
of peak titres of virus in nasal washings, nasal wash protein and
antibody and serum antibody. For influenza virus-infected ferrets
treated with seven daily doses of ribavirin, the effects of the

Table 2: Immune response of guinea pigs to inoculation with 400 IU of inactivated influenza virus A/England/42/72 vaccine in FCA.

Ribavirin Treatment	Animal No.	Serum HI antibody (gmt)		Area of Macrophage Migration		
		day -1	day 10	Test ± SD	Control ± SD	% Inhibition
100 mg/kg daily from day -1 to 10	1	<5	<5	NT	NT	NT
	2	<5) <5	<5) <5	0.25 ± 0.007	0.48 ± 0.041	54 *
	3	<5	<5	0.66 ± 0.017	1.25 ± 0.107	47 *
	4	<5	<5	NT	NT	NT
Nil	5	<5	512	0.75 ± 0.051	1.79 ± 0.220	58 *
	6	<5) <5	128) 124	1.33 ± 0.067	2.91 ± 0.572	54 *
	7	<5	32	0.47 ± 0.060	0.73 ± 0.016	36 *
	8	<5	128	0.31 ± 0.005	0.40 ± 0.005	22 *

* Significant inhibition of macrophage migration ($P = <0.05$)

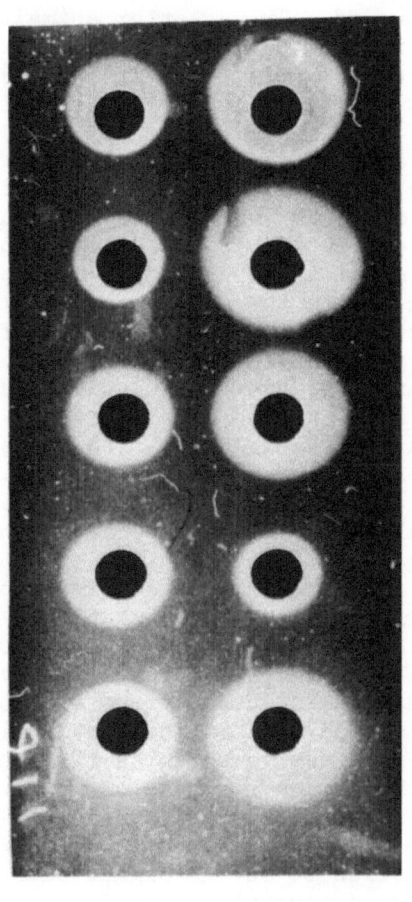

Mice immunised with :-

HA + Ribavirin

HA only

Figure 8. Single radial diffusion tests of sera from mice inoculated with 150 μg of haemagglutinin from influenza virus X31 in FCA. The top row are from mice treated with rivabirin, and the bottom row are from untreated mice. The reduced zone of reaction in the wells of the top row indicate lower titres of HI antibody.

compound were more pronounced. These latter animals showed no temperature response to infection, the titres of virus produced were reduced during the entire period of viral replication, and there was no significant increase in nasal wash protein.

Of particular interest was the observation that virus-infected ferrets treated with seven daily doses of ribavirin failed to develop either local or serum antibody to influenza virus, despite evidence of viral replication in the nasal mucosa. The absence of a detectable serum antibody response to the virus haemagglutinin may have been due to the chemoprophylactic effect of ribavirin which inhibited virus infection to a level that failed to stimulate antibody production; alternatively, ribavirin may have suppressed the immune response. To test the latter possibility, guinea pigs and mice treated with ribavirin were inoculated with inactivated influenza vaccine or purified virus haemagglutinin in FCA. Immunised guinea pigs treated with ribavirin failed to develop detectable levels of serum HI antibody; however, these animals did develop a cellular immune response to influenza virus antigens, as measured by the MMI test. Similar tests carried out in CNA mice showed that ribavirin significantly reduced the serum antibody response to purified virus haemagglutinin. These results indicate that ribavirin has a suppressive activity on the serum antibody response, and the absence of serum antibody in drug-treated ferrets infected with influenza virus A/Port Chalmers/73 was probably not due to the partial inhibition of virus replication, but to the immuno-suppressive activity of ribavirin. The effect of ribavirin on the immune response of mice was reversible. Thus, mice tested for serum antibody to virus haemagglutinin had reduced titres immediately after treatment, but four weeks later the antibody titres had risen to levels higher than those of control animals. Presumably, a persistence of depot antigen in FCA throughout the period of ribavirin treatment induced a serum antibody response when drug treatment was stopped. The absence of late serum antibody response in ferrets infected with influenza virus was probably due to the elimination of virus antigen during the period of treatment.

Ideally, a chemotherapeutic agent against influenza virus infection would allow a subclinical infection and the development of antibody to the virus, since the presence of serum HI antibody has been shown to correlate with immunity to infection in ferrets (Potter et al, 1973) and in man (Hobson et al, 1972). No attempt was made in the present study to determine if ribavirin-treated ferrets infected with influenza virus were susceptible to further infection with homologous virus infection; however, previous observations would suggest that such animals would not be immune. Further studies are now in progress to determine the effects of lower concentrations of ribavirin on influenza virus infection of ferrets and on the immune response to such infections, and the effect of administering the drug by different routes.

REFERENCES

Cochran, K.W., Maassab, H.E., Tsunoda, A. and Berlin, B.S. (1965)
Studies on the antiviral activity of amantadine hydrochloride.
Annals of the New York Academy of Science, 130, 432-440.

David, J.R., Al-Askari, S., Lawrence, H.S. and Thomas, L. (1964)
Delayed hypersensitivity in vitro. I. The specificity of
inhibition of cell migration by antigens. Journal of
Immunology, 93, 264-273.

Fazekas de St. Groth, S., Witchell, J. and Lafferty, K.J. (1958)
An improved assay for neutralization antibodies against
influenza viruses. Journal of Hygiene (Cambridge), 56,
415-426.

Francis, T. and Stuart-Harris, C.H. (1938) Studies on the nasal
histology of epidemic influenza virus infection in the ferret.
III. Histological and serological observations on ferrets
receiving repeated inoculations of epidemic influenza virus.
Journal of Experimental Medicine, 68, 813-830.

George, M. and Vaughan, J.H. (1962) In vitro cell migration as
a model for delayed hypersensitivity. Proceedings of the
Society of Experimental Biology (New York), 111, 514-521.

Haff, R.F., Schriver, P.W. and Stewart, R.C. (1966) Pathogenesis
of influenza in ferrets: nasal manifestation of disease.
British Journal of Experimental Pathology, 48, 435-444.

Haff, R.F. and Pinto, C.A. (1973) The nasal decongestant action
of aspirin in influenza infected ferrets. Life Sciences,
12, 9-14.

Hobson, D., Beare, A.S. and Ward-Gardner, A. (1972) Haemagglutinin-
inhibiting serum antibody titres as an index of response of
volunteers to intranasal infection with live, attenuated strains
of influenza virus. Proceedings of the Symposium on Life
Influenza Vaccines, Zagreb, 1971, pp.73-84. (Yugoslav Academy
of Sciences and Arts, Zagreb,1972).

Huffman, J.H., Sidwell, R.W. and Khare, G.P. (1973) In vitro effect
of 1- -D-Ribofuranosyl-1, 2,4-triazole-3-carboxamide (Virazole,
ICN 1229) on deoxyribonucleic acid and ribonucleic acid viruses.
Antimicrobial Agents and Chemotherapy, 3, 235-241.

Khare, G.P., Sidwell, R.W., Witkowski, J.T., Simon, L.N. and
Robins, R.K. (1973) Suppression by 1- -D-ribofuranosyl-1, 2,
4-triazole-3-carboxamide (Virazole, ICN 1229) of influenza
virus-induced infections in mice. Antimicrobial Agents and
Chemotherapy, 3, 517-522.

Lui, C. (1955) Studies on influenza infection in ferrets by
means of fluorescin-labelled antibody. I. The pathogenesis
and diagnosis of the disease. Journal of Experimental
Medicine, 101, 665-676.

Oxford, J.S. (1975) Specific inhibitors of influenza replication as potential chemoprophylactic agents. Journal of Antimicrobial Chemotherapy, 1, 7-23.

Oxford, J.S. and Potter, C.W. (1970). An immunologic marker technique for the Cendehill vaccine strain of rubella virus. Journal of Immunology, 105, 818-823.

Potter, C.W., Oxford, J.S., Shore, S.L., McLaren, C. and Stuart-Harris, C.H. (1972) Immunity to influenza in ferrets I. Response to live and killed virus. British Journal of Experimental Pathology, 53, 153-167.

Potter, C.W., Jennings, R. and McLaren, C. (1973) Immunity to influenza in ferrets. VI. Immunization with adjuvanted vaccines. Archi. fur die desamte Virusforschung, 42, 285-296.

Potter, C.W. and Schofield, K.P. (1975) The effect of amantadine on the response of ferrets to influenza virus infection. Ciba-Geigy Symposium - in press.

Rees, R.C. and Potter, C.W. (1973) Immune response to adenovirus 12-induced tumour antigens, as measured in vitro by the macrophage migration inhibition test. European Journal of Cancer, 9, 497-502.

Schild, G.C., Oxford, J.S. and Virilizier, J.L. (1975) The immune response to influenza. Methods of analysis for antibody and antigens. Proceedings of the Miles Symposium, London, 1975.

Sever, J.L. (1962) Application of a microtechnique to viral serological investigations. Journal of Immunology, 88, 320-329.

Sidwell, R.W., Huffman, J.H., Khare, G.P., Allen, L.B., Witkowski, J.T. and Robins, R.K. (1972) Broad-spectrum antiviral activity of Virazole: 1- -D-ribofuranosyl-1, 2, 4-triazole-3-carboxamide. Science, 177, 705-706.

Smith, W., Andrews, C.H. and Laidlaw, P.P. (1933) A virus obtained from influenza patients. Lancet, 2, 66-68.

Squires, S.L. (1970) The evaluation of compounds against influenza viruses. Annals of the New York Academy of Science, 173, 239-248.

Togo, Y. (1973) In vitro effect of virazole against influenza viruses. Antimicrobial Agents and Chemotherapy, 4, 641-642.

Witkowski, J.T., Robins, R.K., Sidwell, R.W. and Simon, L.N. (1972) The design, synthesis and broad spectrum antiviral activity of 1- -D-ribofuranosyl-1, 2, 4-triazole-3-carboxamide and related nucleosides. Journal of Medical Chemistry, 15, 1150-1154.

I.C.I. 73602 - A POTENT ANTI-RHINOVIRUS COMPOUND

D.L. Swallow, R.A. Bucknall, W.E. Stanier, Miss A.
Hutchinson and H. Gaskin
Imperial Chemical Industries Ltd., Pharmaceuticals
Division, Alderley Park, Macclesfield, Cheshire,
SK10 4TG, England

Guanidine has been known for a long time as a selective inhibitor of replication of small RNA viruses in tissue culture.[1] The biochemical basis for this activity was traced to an inhibition of the synthesis of viral RNA polymerase,[2] and thus was specific for viral replication, leaving cellular replication and function unaffected. The antiviral activity of guanidine cannot however be demonstrated _in vivo_, consequently much work has been carried out to try to find useful antiviral activity in derivatives of guanidine.

Two years ago we reported[3] the discovery of a substituted guanidine I.C.I. 65709 which had high activity against a number of RNA viruses particularly rhinoviruses.

I.C.I. 65709

1-p-chlorophenyl-3-(m-isobutylthioureidophenyl)-guanidine
hydrochloride

Subsequent development of this discovery led us to the structurally related compound I.C.I. 73602[4] which had a broader spectrum of activity against viruses causing "the common cold" i.e. rhinoviruses and coronaviruses.

I.C I. 73602

1-p-chlorophenyl-3-(m-isobutylguanidinophenyl)-urea hydrochloride

The method of testing for _in vitro_ antiviral activity has already been described,[5,6] but briefly consists in infecting human embryonic lung cells in 3 x 0.5 inch tubes with 100 TCD_{50} of test virus and then adding test compound at a range of concentrations. After incubation at 33° for 2 days the cells are inspected under a low-power microscope and the concentration of compound which causes 50% cytotoxic effect and that causing 50% inhibition of virus growth are determined. From these values a tissue culture "therapeutic ratio" can be calculated.

Table 1 shows the activity of I.C.I. 73602 against 15 strains of rhinovirus and one strain of coronavirus in human embryonic lung cells.

TABLE I

	Type	50% inhibition µg/ml	Therapeutic Ratio (based on 50% toxicity at 30µg/ml)
Rhinovirus	9	0.2	150
	1A, 2, 11, 19, 26, 36, 43	0.4	75
	1B, 4, 16	0.8	38
	5, 14, 17, 35	1.6	19
Coronavirus	229E	1.0	30

It can be seen that the compound has very considerable selectivity between effects on virus replication and effects on

cellular function. This was confirmed by studies on the synthesis
of cellular RNA, DNA and protein in human embryo lung cells.
Synthesis of these components was unaffected by concentrations of
compound up to 50 x greater than the antiviral levels. The most
stringent test of the effect of a drug on cellular function is to
grow cells in its presence. When human embryo lung cells are grown
in the presence of I.C.I. 73602 over 15 days the yield of viable
cells is completely unaffected by 1.0 μg/ml but is reduced by about
50% at 2.5 μg/ml. Thus antiviral activity at 0.2 μg/ml is indeed
selective.

The growth of rhinoviruses in fragments of human embryonic
trachea is also inhibited by I.C.I. 73602. A 50% reduction in
virus yield from a challenge of 100 TCD_{50} is produced by 2.5 μg/ml
while the 50% toxic dose, as judged by cessation of ciliary
activity, is about 20 μg/ml giving a therapeutic ratio of about 10.
In this type of experiment the drug is present throughout in the
culture medium which is renewed each day of the 4-5 day experiment.
To demonstrate further the effectiveness of the drug an intermittent
dosing schedule was devised in which the tracheal fragments were
treated for 5 seconds or 60 seconds each day for 4 days with I.C.I.
73602. The results of several tests are shown in Table II. Virus
yields are TCD_{50}/ml of culture fluid and as each experiment was
done on fragments from different tracheas, control virus yields from
fragments treated with isotonic saline for the same time, are given
for each test. It can be seen that the drug will produce effectively
complete inhibition of viral replication when dosed once per day for
1 minute at a concentration of 0.35 mg/ml.

Attempts to make rhinovirus cultures resistant to I.C.I. 73602
by repeated passage in sub-inhibitory concentrations of drug were not
successful. Thus the compound differs significantly from guanidine,
to which resistance begins to develop after only one passage.[7]

Preliminary mode of action studies,[8] by measuring virus yield
from tissue cultures 9-16 hr after infection and adding drug at
0-8 hr after infection, indicate that I.C.I. 73602 affects a late
stage in viral replication, possibly the assembly of virus RNA and
coat protein. Later biochemical studies[9] indicated that only 4%
of viral single stranded RNA found in infected cells was
encapsidated into mature virions when drug was present, confirming
our original finding. In addition however, it was found that RNA
dependent RNA polymerase activity was inhibited by the drug
although the synthesis of polymerase polypeptides appeared to be
unaffected.

I.C.I. 73602 is relatively non-toxic. It is well tolerated
when instilled into the nostrils of rats six times per day for 7
days at concentrations up to 400 μg/ml, and no abnormalities were
found on pathological examination of either these animals or in

TABLE II

Effect on rhinovirus yield from infected human embryonic tracheal
fragments when treated once per day with I.C.I. 73602

Concentration of I.C.I. 73602 at time of treatment	Period of daily exposure	Virus Yield TCD_{50}/ml on day				Total TCD_{50}
		1	2	3	4	
0.35 mg/ml	5 sec	250	160	63	5	478
0.35 mg/ml	60 sec	7	5	<2.5	<2.5	<17
Control	–	63	100	63	5	231
0.4 mg/ml	5 sec	160	100	4	5	305
1.36 mg/ml	5 sec	100	63	5	<5	<168
Control	–	400	25	8	5	438
0.8 mg/ml	5 sec	25	25	<5	<5	<50
Control	–	630	400	111	160	501
1.49 mg/ml	5 sec	40	10	5	–	55
Control	–	2500	630	630	–	3760

TABLE III

Activity of Substituted Guanidinoureas against Rhinoviruses

$$R_1 \text{—} \bigcirc \text{—NHCONH—} \bigcirc \text{—} \underset{NH}{\overset{NH.C.NHR_2}{C}}$$

R_1	R_2	Benzene Substitution	I.C.I. No.	Activity µg/ml	Toxicity µg/ml
p—Cl	H	m	94458	NA	25
	Me	m	81011	NA	>45
	^{n}Pr	m	81012	NA	45
	^{i}Pr	m	80656	1.8	9
	^{n}Bu	m	81013	NA	45
	^{i}Bu	m	73602	0.1	30
	^{s}Bu	m	81014	NA	45
	^{i}Am	m	81015	NA	45
	Ph	m	77868	0.04	5
	^{i}Pr	p	81262	1.8	45
	^{i}Bu	p	81263	5	45
p—Br	^{i}Bu	m	80497	1.0	30
	^{i}Bu	p	81679	NA	45
p—OMe	^{i}Bu	m	80459	NA	45
p—OEt	^{i}Bu	m	76961	1.5	30

NA indicates a ratio between toxicity and activity of < 5

another series dosed 100 mg/kg daily intraperitoneally for 14 days.
When dosed orally or intranasally there is little or no systemic
absorption.

An investigation of structure-activity relationships in this
type of compound served only to demonstrate that activity was
unpredictable as can be seen in Table III. Activity was most
frequently present when R_2 = ^{i}Bu, but even closely related R_1
eg. OMe and OEt gave inactive and active analogues respectively.
All compounds in which the central aromatic substitution was
ortho were inactive. Reversal of the relative positions of the urea
and guanidine moieties in the molecule led to compounds in which
activity appeared even less frequently.

In I.C.I. 73602 we have an anti-rhinovirus compound which has
very high activity in two types of _in vitro_ test system, is
relatively non-toxic to laboratory animals and studies in the only
satisfactory _in vivo_ system, homo sapiens, are in progress.

References

1. I. Tamm, and H.J. Eggers, Science, 1963, 142, 24.

2. D. Baltimore, H.J. Eggers, R.M. Franklin and I. Tamm,
    Proc.Nat.Acad.Sci., 1963, 49, 843.

3. R.A. Bucknall, D.L. Swallow, H. Moores, J. Harrad, Nature,
    1973, 246, 144.

4. U.K. Patent No. 1,311,432.

5. R.A. Bucknall, J.gen.Virol, 1967, 1, 55.

6. R.A. Bucknall in "Advances in Pharmacology and Chemotherapy",
    Academic Press, New York, p. 295, 1973.

7. N. Ledinko, Virology, 1968, 35, 584.

8. R.A. Bucknall (unpublished results).

9. S. Koliais and N. Dimmock (unpublished results).

ASSESSMENT OF SOME ANTIRHINOVIRUS COMPOUNDS IN TISSUE CULTURE AND AGAINST EXPERIMENTAL CHALLENGE IN VOLUNTEERS

Sylvia E. Reed and D. A. J. Tyrrell

Medical Research Council Common Cold Unit

Harvard Hospital, Salisbury, Wilts. SP2 8BW, U.K.

Four unrelated antirhinovirus compounds were compared by a standard method in vitro and three of these were assessed for antiviral effect in volunteers.

The compounds were the triazinoindole SKF 40491 (1), a substituted oxadiazole Glaxo R9–338, an imidazo-thiazole RP 19326 (Rhone-Poulenc), and ICI 73,602, a guanidine derivative related to ICI 65,709 (2). A method found applicable to assessment of all of these compounds in vitro involved titration of the yield of virus obtained from HeLa cells (3) or human embryo lung fibroblasts (HEL) which had been treated with the test compound incorporated in maintenance medium, and then inoculated with one of four rhinoviruses, RV3, 4, 9 or 31 at low input multiplicity. Cultures were harvested when the cytopathic effect in untreated controls involved about 75% of the cells (2 to 4 days). Yields of virus from treated and untreated cultures were titrated by a plaque-counting method in HeLa cells.

SKF 40491 had good activity against the four viruses in both types of cell, usually achieving a reduction of virus yield of between $10^{2.6}$ and 10^{6} PFU at a concentration of 4 µg/ml in comparison with the untreated control. GL R9–338 and RP 19326 were again active in both cell types but had variable effect against the different rhinovirus serotypes. Both gave a reduction of over $10^{2.0}$ PFU against RV9 in HeLa cells at 4 µg/ml. ICI 73,602 was active only in HEL cells, but inhibited a range of serotypes at 0.5 µg/ml.

Placebo-controlled double-blind studies were carried out in volunteers in isolation (4). The subjects were given intranasal

medication from one day before until three or four days after
challenge with 20 – 50 TCD_{50} of a sensitive serotype of rhinovirus.
Results were evaluated by daily scoring of symptoms, by titration
in HeLa cells of virus shed in nasal secretions, and by evaluation
of serum antibody responses to the challenge viruses. SKF 40491,
given 10 times daily in a total daily dose of 1 mg caused a slight
but not significant reduction virus shedding of RV3 by the treated
volunteers, and although the compound was not significantly
irritant in the absence of a virus challenge, it appeared to
enhance the severity of the symptoms. GL R9–338 and RP 19326 were
used respectively 5 times daily (15 mg/day total) and 13 times
daily (6.8 mg/day total). Both of these compounds caused a
significant reduction of shedding of RV9, and the serological
responses were also somewhat less in the treated groups.
Treatment with RP 19326 was also associated with diminished
symptoms in the treated group, but had the disadvantage that the
formulation used (and its placebo) had mildly irritant properties
when given intranasally. An investigation of some of the virus
strains re-isolated from volunteers by the yield-reduction method
in vitro suggested that resistance to GL R9–338 and RP 19326 may
possibly develop.

    In these studies in volunteers, reduction in virus shedding
was therefore more easily achieved than significant improvement
in symptoms of rhinovirus infection. The compound which
apparently had the most marked antiviral effect in vitro at least
at the higher of the concentration tested, 4 µg/ml, i.e. SKF 40491,
did not achieve a useful effect in man when used as described.
In considering antiviral compounds for intranasal use, factors
such as the total daily dose which can be administered, the
duration of the inhibitory effect which develops on contact
between the compound and the nasal epithelial cells, the frequency
of dosage and, not least, the possible irritancy of the medication may all be of considerable importance in determining the
result.

REFERENCES

1. Haff, R. F., Flagg, W. B., Gallo, J. J., Hoover, J. R. E.,
    Miller, J. A., Pinto, C. A. and Pagano, J. F. (1972). The
    in vitro antiviral activity of a triazinoindole (SK & F
    40491). Proc. Soc. Exp. Biol. Med. 141, 475 – 478.
2. Bucknall, R. A., Swallow, D. L., Moores, H. and Harrad, J.
    (1973). A novel substituted guanidine with high activity
    in vitro against rhinoviruses. Nature 246, 144 – 145.
3. Stott, E. J. and Tyrrell, D. A. J. (1968). Some improved
    techniques for study of rhinoviruses using HeLa cells.
    Archiv. fur ges. Virusforsch. 23, 236 – 244.
4. Tyrrell, D. A. J. (1963). The use of volunteers. Amer.
    Rev. Resp. Dis. 88, 128 – 134.

THE POTENTIAL OF NUCLEOSIDES AS ANTIVIRAL AGENTS

R.W. Sidwell, L.B. Allen, J.H. Huffman, J.T. Witkowski,
P.D. Cook, R.L. Tolman, G.R. Revankar, L.N. Simon and
R.K. Robins
ICN Pharmaceuticals Inc., Nucleic Acid Research
Institute, 2727 Campus Drive, Irvine, Ca.92664, U.S.A.

The world has seen a marked increase in the biochemistry of nucleosides, especially beginning in the early 1950's when we could consider the era of modern biology was introduced by the classical work of Watson and Crick (1953). This interest has been further stimulated by the discovery of a number of nucleoside anti-biotics (Suhadolnik, 1970). As we view antiviral chemotherapy, the nucleosides again have played a most significant role, perhaps beginning with Igor Tamm's demonstration in 1956 that 1-β-$\underline{D}$-ribo-furanosyl-5,6-dichlorobenzimidazole (Fig.1) was an in vitro inhibitor of both DNA and RNA viruses (Tamm, 1956). The 1961 report by Herrmann that the halogenated pyrimidine nucleosides 5-iodo-2'-deoxyuridine (IDU, Fig.2) and 5-bromo-2'-deoxyuridine inhibited the replication of DNA viruses in vitro (Herrmann,1961) was another key milestone, since IDU particularly was later found efficacious in treating herpetic keratitis in animals (Kaufman et al, 1962) and finally in man (Kaufman, 1962; Kaufman et al, 1962). We have since seen the advent of a multitude of nucleosides having great antiviral potential. 1-β-$\underline{D}$-arabinosyl-cytosine(ara-C, Fig.3) (Renis and Johnson, 1962),and 9-β-$\underline{D}$-arabinosyl-adenine (ara-A, Fig.4) (De Garilhe and De Rudder, 1964) are perhaps the most well known, both of which have progressed to the point of clinical investigation (Ch'ieu et al, 1973).

Where do we stand today as we consider nucleosides as anti-viral agents? To answer this question, we will take a rather biased approach in this review as research predominantly from our Institute will be presented.

In 1969 ICN Pharmaceuticals Nucleic Acid Research Institute
was established in California, with a major initial goal to pursue
nucleoside chemistry as a potential source of additional significant antiviral agents.

It was recognised the way may be difficult, for as those
familiar with the chemistry of this class of compounds know, nucleosides are not among the easier molecules to synthesise.

We were pleasantly surprised, then, when Joseph T. Witkowski
of our Institute submitted a triazole nucleoside (Witkowski et al,
1972) which we found in our earliest antiviral studies to have
marked activity against both DNA and RNA viruses (Sidwell et al,
1972). That compound, 1-β-D-ribofuranosyl-1,2,4-triazole-3-
carboxamide (ribavirin, Fig.5), has since been proven efficacious
in a wide variety of in vivo animal virus systems, and is currently
under widespread clinical investigation.

At this point, we should define how our initial in vitro antiviral studies are run, since the data derived from this method will
be used throughout the remainder of this presentation. We use
inhibition of virus-induced cytopathogenic effect (CPE), seen
after 72 hr incubation with varying dilutions of test compound, as
an initial criterion for evaluation. The drug is added within 15
min. after the virus to the established cell monolayer. Disposable
plastic microplates are used as described in detail previously
(Sidwell and Huffman, 1971). This CPE inhibition is determined
microscopically, and a numerical value originally termed the Virus
Rating (VR) by Ehrlich et al (1965) but modified somewhat by our
group (Sidwell and Huffman, 1971) is used as an expression of antiviral efficacy. Table 1 illustrates the overall method of this
evaluation. In our experience, a VR of 0.5 or greater usually
indicates definite anti-viral activity,but the higher the number,
the greater the therapeutic index of the drug.

In a previous symposium the antiviral activity of ribavirin,
as well as the structure-activity studies run with this class of
compounds, was documented in detail (Sidwell et al, 1971). It
was seen that the structural features of ribavirin which are necessary for antiviral activity are relatively specific. Substitution
of thio and imino groups on the 3-position maintained a degree of
HSV/1 activity (Fig.6). We have found that the triazole-3-carbo-
xamide base, the 5'-phosphate, the 2' and/or 3'-'hosphate, the
3',5'-cyclic phosphates, and the 2'3'-cyclic phosphates maintain
the potent and broad spectrum antiviral activity of the parent
nucleoside (Fig.7), whereas other modifications of the heterocycle,
the carbohydrate moiety, the ribosyl moiety and most substitutions
on the heterocycle all reduced or eliminated the original antiviral
activity.

TABLE 1

Determination of In Vitro Virus Rating

Drug conc. (µg/ml)	Visible tox.	72 Hr viral CPE*		Gross C-T		Toxicity adjust.	Net C-T	
Treated (T):								
1000	+++	Toxic		-		-	-	
320	++	0	0	4	4	2	2	2
100	+	0	0	4	4	2	2	2
32	+	1	1	3	3	2	1.5	1.5
10	-	1	1	3	3	None	3	3
3.2	-	2	2	2	2	None	2	2
1.0	-	3	3	1	1	None	1	1
0.32	-	4	4	0	0	None	0	0
0.1	-	4	4	0	0	None	0	0
Control (C):								
0		4	4					
Total $(C-T)_{net}$: 23								
$$VR = \frac{\Sigma(C-T)_{net}}{10\,n^{**}} = \frac{23}{10 \times 2} = 1.15$$								

* CPE: 0 = No cytopathic effect; 4 = complete cell destruction.

** n = number of cups used per drug concentration

1.   1-β-D-Ribofuranosyl-5,6-dichlorobenzimidazole

2.   5-Iodo-2'-deoxyuridine (IDU)   3. 1-β-D-Arabinofuranosylcytosine (ara-C)

5. 1-β-D-Ribofuranosyl-1,2,4-triazol
   3-carboxamide (ribavirin)

4. 9-β-D-Arabinofuranosyladenine (ara-A)

TABLE 2

REVERSAL OF RIBAVIRIN INHIBITION OF TYPE 1 HERPES SIMPLEX
VIRUS CYTOPATHOGENIC EFFECT BY GUANOSINE, XANTHOSINE, AND
INOSINE[a]

Ribavirin Conc.(µg/ml)	% CPE/% CYTOTOXICITY			
	Ribavirin only	Ribavirin+ Guanosine[b]	Ribavirin+ Xanthosine[b]	Ribavirin+ Inosine[b]
1000	0/50	0/50	0/50	0/75
320	0/50	13/50	13/50	0/50
100	0/50	38/50	50/50	0/50
32	19/25	68/25	71/25	13/50
10	50/0	88/0	75/0	71/0
3.2	88/0	88/0	94/0	100/0
1.0	88/0	94/0	94/0	94/0
0	94/0	94/0	94/0	94/0

[a] No reversal seen using orotodine, adenosine, deoxyadenosine,
cytidine, uridine, thymidine, AICAR, AICAR-5'-PO$_4$.

[b] 200 µg/ml added concomitantly with ribavirin.

We can make some educated guesses of the mechanism of ribavirin's antiviral activity, based on some limited studies completed to date. The drug does not induce interferon (Allen et al,
1973), inactivate viruses extracellularly (Huffman et al, 1973),
nor prevent attachment or penetration of viruses into the host cell
(Sidwell et al, 1975). A marked inhibition of nucleic acid synthesis associated with almost total stopping of production of
infectious virus particles which is exerted by ribavirin suggests
the inhibition of virus replication occurs at an early step in the
virus infective process (Streeter et al, 1972).

Reversal studies such as that seen in Table 2 indicate the
antiviral effect of drug is reversed by guanosine, xanthosine,
and to a lesser extent by inosine (Streeter et al, 1973). It is
pertinent to note in the table that the visible cytotoxicity of the
drug was not influenced by these metabolites, which suggests the
cytotoxicity and antiviral activity are not a result of the same
biochemical mechanism of the drug. These antiviral reversal studies
point to a step in the GMP biosynthetic pathway inhibited by

ribavirin, probably acting as an analog of guanosine or a guanosine precursor. Our later enzyme studies have shown that ribavirin acts as the 5'-monophosphate, inhibiting GMP synthesis at the step involving the conversion of IMP to XMP. Specifically, IMP dehydrogenase is markedly inhibited (Streeter et al, 1973). X-ray crystallographic studies indicate also that ribavirin in the crystalline state has a structure similar to guanosine (Prusiner and Sundaralingan, 1973).

One might, therefore, ask "would other guanosine analogs exert a similar antiviral effect?" We have intensively studied this possibility, finding that 3-deazaguanine, and the ring-opened base, 4(5)-cyanomethylimidazole-5(4)-carboxamide have activity resembling ribavirin (Cook et al, 1975). We may speculate that this latter compound is being cyclized in the cell to 3-deazaguanine, but preliminary studies have not indicated this to occur. The pertinent nucleoside and nucleotide of each were also active antivirals, particularly against HSV/1 (Figs. 8 and 9). 3-deazaguanine has recently been shown to have notable anticancer activity (Khwaja et al, 1975), as well as the antiviral activity seen in our studies.

Another nucleoside on which considerable work has been completed to correlate structure with antiviral activity has been adenine arabinoside. This purine nucleoside has striking anti-DNA virus activity, with positive antiviral effects seen also in clinical investigations recently initiated (Pavan-Langston et al, 1975). Approximately 100 analogs of ara-A have been synthetized and tested for antiviral efficacy. For brevity, we will only consider the structural modifications which resulted in positive anti-DNA virus activity.

Looking first at alterations in the 2-position of the base moiety (Fig.10), only chloro and methoxy groups could be substituted, and in each case, the activity was somewhat weakened, especially in animal studies (Miyai et al, 1964). Addition of monophosphate or methylphosphate to the 5'-position appeared to strengthen ara-A's activity (Sidwell et al, 1973- Revankar et al, 1975). It is interesting that ribosylation on the 3-position did not lessen the antiviral activity, and the α derivatives also retained some antiviral effect (Revankar et al, 1975). Substitutions in the N^1-position of ara-AMP did not improve its antiviral efficacy, although antiviral activity was still demonstrable following several alterations in that position (Fig. 11).

Early investigations with ara-A revealed that it apparently was metabolized to ara-hypoxanthine, ara-Hx, (Brink and LePage, 1964), which also had reasonable antiviral activity (Miller et al, 1969). Pavan-Langston et al (1973) have reported ara-A deaminates to ara-Hx in the eye, although they also have shown ara-Hx to be approximately 5 times less potent than ara-A when used against the established herpes simplex keratoconjunctivitis (Pavan-Langston et al, 1974). Investigations by Plunkett and Cohen (1975) indicate that the majority of ara-A is metabolized by the cell to ara-Hx, which would suggest that ara-Hx may indeed be the active material in the cell, although LePage (1970) has seen some deamination of ara-Hx to ara-A in murine tumor cells. We have synthetized the 5'-monophosphate of ara-Hx, ara-HxMP, as well as numerous derivatives of that molecule (Revankar et al, 1975). Fig.12 compares the efficacy of ara-Hx and ara-HxMP, as well as the 5'-methyl phosphate of ara-Hx. It is noted that ara-Hx loses its activity when ribosylated at the 3-position.

The 3',5'-cyclic phosphate derivatives of both ara-A (Sidwell et al, 1973; Mian et al, 1974) and ara-Hx (Revankar et al, 1975) also retained the initial strong efficacy (Fig.12). Ara-HxMP has proven experimentally to be a very significant antiviral drug, inhibiting the DNA viruses in vitro to a similar extent as ara-A (Huffman et al, 1974) as summarised in Table 3, and in certain

TABLE 3

IN VITRO ANTIVIRAL ACTIVITY OF 9-β-D-
ARABINOFURANOSYLHYPOXANTHINE-5'-MONOPHOSPHATE
(ARA-HxMP)

Virus	Cell Line Used	Maximum Virus Rating	Minimum Inhibitory Concentration (μg/ml)
AV/3	KB	0.0	0.0
HSV/1	KB	1.2	0.32
HSV/1	BHK	1.6	3.2
HSV/1	HEp-2	1.0	3.2
HSV/1	CE	1.1	1.0
HSV/1	HeLa	0.5	32.0
HSV/2	KB	1.1	1.0
HSV/2	Vero	0.6	100
PRV	RK-13	0.3	32
MCMV	ME	0.9	10
VV	KB	1.1	1.0
VV	RK-13	0.7	32
VV	HeLa	0.8	10
MV	RK-13	1.0	3.2

animal systems exerted a stronger antiviral effect than ara-A and
ara-Hx, particularly when used topically (Sidwell et al, 1975).
Of considerable importance was the finding that equimolar quantities of ara-HxMP are notably less cytotoxic than either ara-A
or ara-AMP (Huffman et al, 1974), a finding also seen by Plunkett
and Cohen (1975a).

        We have been attracted to the nucleosides because of a number
of rather unique features. They penetrate cells readily by a
facilitated transport mechanism (Pickard et al, 1973), making them
uniquely suited to combat intracellular infections. Many of the
nucleosides are converted to the nucleotide within the cell, and
it has been generally thought that they exert carcinostatic, and,
presumably, antiviral effects after conversions in the cell to
the corresponding mono-, di- or tri-phosphates. It is becoming
clear, however, that in many instances the biological effect may
be due to specific binding of the nucleoside itself, such as may
be the case with ara-Hx. Evidence is now also accumulating to
indicate the 3',5'-cyclic nucleotides do cross cell membranes.
This has been shown specifically for cyclic ara-AMP as reported
by LePage and Hersh (1972). This molecule, once in the cell, is
then converted to the 5'-nucleotide. We are intrigued by the
cyclic nucleotides since they could bypass the necessity of cells
to be in growth cycle with high kinase levels in order for them
to be susceptible to effects of the drug (LePage and Hersh, 1972).
Plunkett and Cohen have recently shown data indicating ara-AMP
also slowly penetrates cells in its intact form (1975a). Both the
cyclic phosphate and monophosphate derivatives of the compounds we
have studied usually markedly improved the solubility of the compound, a definite advantage since formulation, ability to admini-
ster intravenously, and possibly to more early penetrate cell
interfaces are enhanced. In addition, the nucleotide often blocks
the inactivating deamination of the nucleoside. Ara-AMP, for
example, has definitely been found not to be deaminated (Plunkett
and Cohen, 1975a), and LePage and his co-workers (1972) have demonstrated a marked prolongation of human plasma levels of ara-AMP
due to this lack of deamination, suggesting such nucleotides may
be useful as sustained release forms for the nucleosides. Ara-AMP
and the cyclic phosphate, however, also produce a sustained cytotoxic effect against L cells (Plunkett and Cohen, 1975a). The use
of inhibitors of the enzymes breaking down active nucleosides has
also been considered. Adenosine deaminase inhibitors are very
effective in prolonging the efficacy of ara-A, but also increase
the compound's toxicity (Plunkett and Cohen, 1975a), so from a
therapeutic index viewpoint, no advantage is seen.

        As we consider ara-A and its many derivatives, it would be
well to consider the possible metabolism of these compounds, seen
in Fig. 13. Ara-A may be acting, as originally speculated (York
and LePage, 1966; Furth and Cohen, 1967) as its mono-, di- or

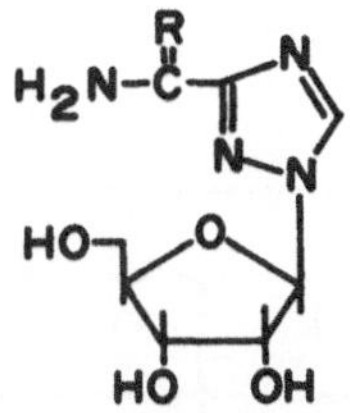

R	Virus Rating			
	HSV/1	VV	PIV/3	RV/13
O	0.7-1.3	0.7-1.3	0.5-1.1	0.5-1.2
S	0.5-1.0	0.3	0.0	0.2
NH·HCl	0.5-1.0	0.3	0.4-0.8	0.4-0.6

Fig. 6. Antiviral activity of substitutions on the 3-position of ribavirin.

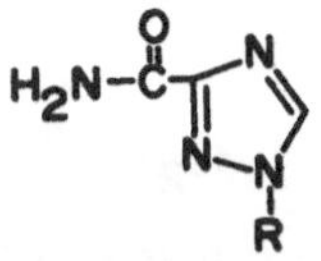

R	Virus Rating			
	HSV/1	VV	PIV/3	RV/13
H	0.6-1.1	0.8	0.6-0.9	0.0-0.3
β-D-Ribofuranosyl-5'-PO₄	0.7-1.3	0.7-1.3	0.5-1.1	0.5-1.2
β-D-Ribofuranosyl-3',5'-cyclic PO₄	0.7-0.8		0.0-0.3	0.2-0.6
β-D-Ribofuranosyl-2',3'-cyclic PO₄	0.8-1.2	0.6-0.7	1.0-1.1	0.2-0.6
β-D-Ribofuranosyl-2' and/or 3' PO₄	0.6-0.9		0.8-1.2	0.7

Fig. 7. Antiviral activity of substitutions on the 1-position of ribavirin.

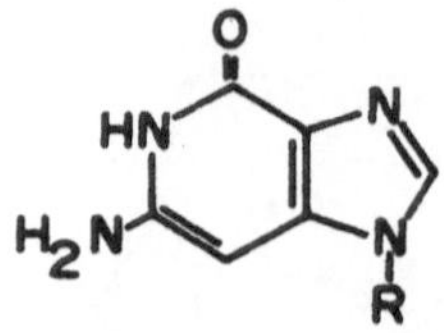

R	Virus Rating			
	HSV/1	VV	PIV/3	RV/13
H	1.0-1.4	1.1-1.3	1.1-1.4	0.7-1.2
β-D-Ribofuranosyl	0.8 1.1	0.7-1.1	0.7-1.1	0.4-0.8
β-D-Ribofuranosyl 5'-PO_4	1.0-1.1	1.0	0.7-1.0	0.8-1.0

Fig. 8. Antiviral activity of 3-deazaguanine, and its corresponding nucleoside and nucleotide.

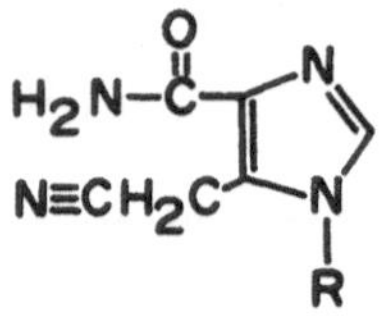

R	Virus Rating			
	HSV/1	VV	PIV/3	RV/13
H	0.7-0.8		0.8	0.4-0.8
β-D-Ribofuranosyl	0.6-0.7	0.4	0.4	0.2
β-D-Ribofuranosyl 5'-PO_4	0.6-1.0	0.3	0.0	0.0

Fig. 9. Antiviral activity of 4(5)-cyanomethylimidazole-5(4)-carboxamide and its corresponding nucleoside and nucleotide.

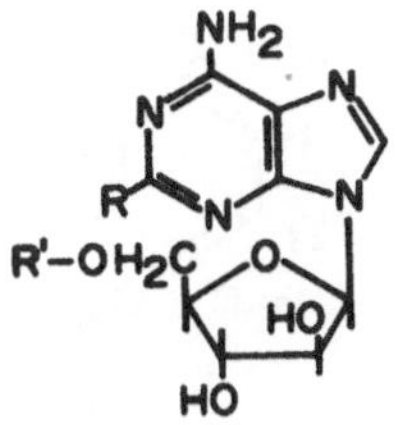

Fig. 10. Antiviral activity of substitutions on the 2 and 5'-positions of ara-A.

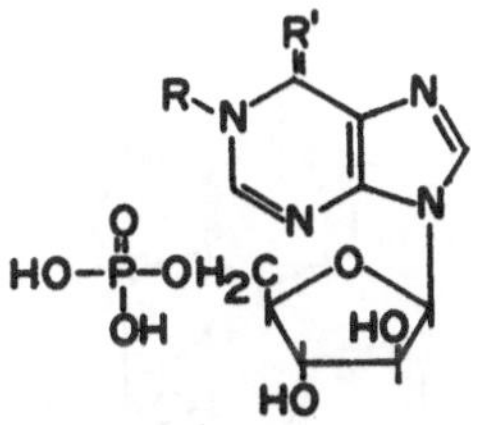

R	R'	Virus Rating	
		HSV/1	VV
H	H	0.6-1.1	0.5-0.9
H	H (α)	0.6	0.5
H	H (3-β-$\underline{D}$)	0.7-1.2	0.6
Cl	H	0.9	0.8-0.9
OCH3	H	0.4	0.4
H	PO$_3$H$_2$	0.8-1.2	0.6-1.1
H	PO$_3$H$_2$ (α)	0.1-0.6	0.3-0.6
H	PO$_3$H$_2$(3-β-$\underline{D}$)	0.7-1.1	0.2
H	PO$_3$H$_2$·CH$_3$	0.8-1.2	0.8
Cl	PO$_3$H$_2$	0.5-0.6	

R	R'	Virus Rating	
		HSV/1	VV
OH	O	0.1-0.7	0.1-0.4
OCH$_2$C$_6$H$_5$	O	0.1-0.2	0.0-0.2
CH$_3$	O	0.0	0.0
(CH$_2$)$_3$CH$_3$	NH	0.4-0.5	0.2-0.4
CH$_2$C$_6$H$_5$	NH	0.2	0.1
OCH$_3$	NH	0.3-0.5	0.4
O(CH$_2$)$_3$CH$_3$	NH	0.3	0.3
OCH$_2$C$_6$H$_5$	NH	0.4-0.7	0.3

Fig. 11. Antiviral activity of substitutions on the N^1-position of ara-AMP and ara-HxMP.

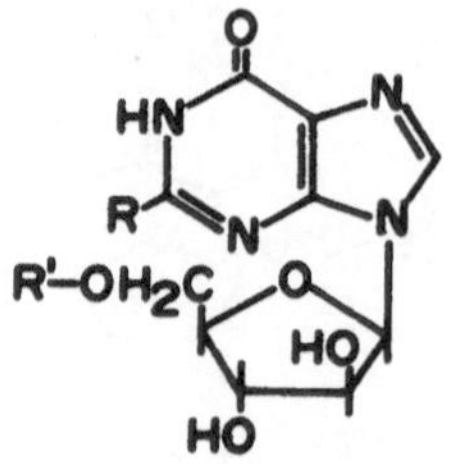

R	R'	Virus Rating	
		HSV/1	VV
H	H	0.6-1.1	0.6-0.9
H	H (3-β-$\underline{D}$)	0.1	0.0
NH_2	H	0.4-0.7	0.1-0.2
H	PO_3H_2	0.6-1.2	0.7-1.1
H	$PO_3H_2 \cdot CH_3$	0.4-0.7	0.4

Fig. 12. Antiviral activity of substitutions on the 2 and 5'-positions of ara-Hx.

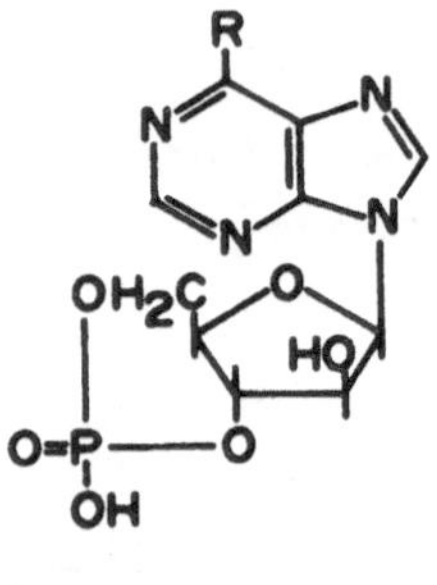

R	Virus Rating	
	HSV/1	VV
NH_2	0.8-1.3	0.7-1.2
OH	0.7-1.1	0.7

Fig. 13. Antiviral activity of the 3',5'-cyclic nucleotides of ara-A and ara-Hx.

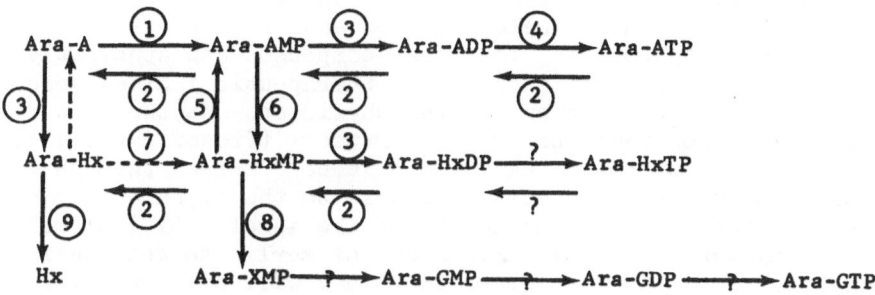

Legend

——————➤ Good activity (in vitro)
– – – –➤ Little or no activity
———?—➤ No available data

Enzyme

① Nucleoside kinase   ⑥ Adenylate deaminase
② Nucleotidase   ⑦ Nucleoside kinase
③ Nucleoside monophosphate kinase   ⑧ IMP dehydrogenase
④ Nucleoside diphosphate kinase   ⑨ Purine nucleoside
⑤ Adenylosuccinate lysase   phosphorylase

Fig. 14. Possible metabolic pathways of ara-A, ara-AMP, ara-Hx
and ara-HxMP.

triphosphate, but more evidence is accumulating to indicate the compound is being deaminated to its hypoxanthine form, ara-Hx. This compound, again, may be acting as the nucleoside, may be phosphorylated to ara-HxMP, or, more probably, is broken down to the inactive hypoxanthine. Ara-HxMP may also undergo several routes of alteration, although early metabolic data Jon Miller of our Institute (personal communication) has accumulated in rats suggests this drug may be absorbed orally and excreted in the urine as the intact molecule, suggesting it may be exerting the good antiviral effect we have seen as itself.

To summarize this brief review, we can again ask the question, "What is the potential of nucleosides as antiviral agents?" Our answer has to be optimistic, for these compounds can apparently exert a specific antiviral action with therapeutic indices acceptable to, we hope, the most practicing physician. At the last meeting of this congress, Dr. William Prusoff (Prusoff et al, 1974) posed the problem of how we can find Ariadne's thread through the labrynth of potential syntheses available to the organic chemist in order to reach the nucleoside having the ideal antiviral efficacy. It may take wizardry reminiscent of Merlin to get the final answer, but I hope the work presented today will bring us close to that ideal.

REFERENCES

Allen, L.B., Huffman, J.H. and Sidwell, R.W. (1973) Antimicrob. Ag.Chemother., 3, 534.

Brink, J.J. and LePage, G.A. (1964) Cancer Res., 24, 1042.

Ch'ien, L.T., Schabel, F.M.Jr., and Alford, C.A.Jr. (1973) In W.A. Carter (ed) Selective Inhibitors of Viral Functions, p.227, CRC Press.

Cook, P.D., Rousseau, R.J., Mian, A.M., Meyer, R.B.Jr., Dea.P., Ivanovics, G., Streeter, D.G., Witkowski, J.T., Stout, M.G., Simon, L.N., Sidwell, R.W. and Robins, R.K. (1975) J.Amer. Chem.Soc., 97, 2916.

DeGarilhe, P.and DeRudder, J. (1964) C.R. Acad.Sci., 259, 2725.

Ehrlich, J., Sloan, B.J., Miller, F.A. and Machamer, H.E. (1965) Ann.N.Y.Acad.Sci., 130, 5.

Furth, J.J. and Cohen, S.S. (1967) Cancer Res., 27, 1528.

Herrmann, E.C.Jr. (1961) Proc.Soc.Exp.Biol.Med., 107, 142.

Huffman, J.H.,Allen, L.B., Tolman, R.L., Revankar, G.R., Simon, L.N., Robins, R.K. and Sidwell, R.W. (1974) 14th Intersci.Conf. Antimicrob.Ag.Chemother. Abstr.233.

Huffman, J.H., Sidwell, R.W., Khare, G.P., Witkowski, J.T., Allen, L.B. and Robins, R.K. (1973) Antimicrob.Ag.Chemother., 3, 235.

Kaufman, H.E. (1962) Proc.Soc.Exp.Biol.Med., 109, 251.

Kaufman, H.E., Maloney, E.D. and Nesburn, A.B. (1962) Invest. Opthalmol. 1, 686.

Kaufman, H.E., Martola, E. and Dohlman, C. (1962) Arch-Ophthalmol. 68, 235.

Khwaja, T.A., Kigwana, L., Meyer, R.B. and Robins, R.K. (1975) Proc.Amer.Assoc.Cancer Res., 16, 162.

LaPage, G.A. (1970) Canad.J.Biochem., 48, 75.

LaPage, G.A., Lin, Y.T., Orth, R.E. and Gottleid, J.A. (1972) Cancer Res., 32, 2441.

LaPage, G.A. and Hersh, E.M. (1972) Biochem.Biophys.Res.Commun., 46, 1918.

Mian, A.M., Harris, R., Sidwell, R.W., Robins, R.K. and Khwaja, T.A. (1974) J.Med.Chem., 17, 259.

Miller, F.A., Dixon, G.J., Ehrlich, J., Sloan, B.J. and McLean, I.W. Jr. (1969) Antimicrob.Ag.Chemother.-1968. p.136.

Miyai, K., Allen, L.B., Huffman, J.H., Sidwell, R.W. and Tolman, R.L. (1974) J.Med.Chem., 17, 242.

Pavan-Langston, D., Buchanan, R.A. and Alford, C.A. (eds) (1975) Adenine Arabinoside: An Antiviral Agent.

Pavan-Langston, D., Dohlman, C.H., Geary, P.A. and Sulzewski, D. (1973) Trans.Amer.Acad.Ophthalmol.Otolaryngol., 77, 455.

Pavan-Langston, D., Langston, R.H.S. and Geary, P.A. (1974) Arch. Opthalmol., 92, 417.

Pickard, M.A., Brown, R.A., Paul, B. and Paterson, A.R.P. (1973) Canad.J.Biochem., 51, 666.

Plunkett, W. and Cohen, S. (1975) Cancer Res., 35, 415.

Plunkett, W. and Cohen, S. (1975a) Cancer Res., 35, 1547.

Prusiner, R. and Sundaralingam, M.A. (1973) Nature New Biol., 244, 116.

Prusoff, W.H., Cheng, Y-C. and Neenan, J. (1974) Prog. in Chemother. 2, 881 (Proc. 8th Internat.Congr.Chemother., Hellenic Soc. Chemother., Publishers).

Renis, H.E. and Johnson, H.G. (1962) Bacterial Proc., p.140.

Revankar, G.R., Huffman, J.H., Allen, L.B., Sidwell, R.W., Robins, R.K. and Tolman, R.L. (1975) J.Med.Chem., 18, 721.

Sidwell, R.W., Allen, L.B., Huffman, J.H., Khwaja, T.A., Tolman,R.L. and Robins, R.K. (1973) Chemotherapy, 19, 325.

Sidwell, R.W., Allen, L.B., Huffman, J.H., Revankar, G.P., Robins, R.K. and Tolman, R.L. (1975) Antimicrob.Ag.Chemother. (in press)

Sidwell, R.W. and Huffman, J.H. (1971) Appl.Microbiol., 22, 797.

Sidwell, R.W., Huffman, J.H., Khare, G.P., Allen, L.B. Witkowski, J.T. and Robins, R.K. (1972) Science, 177, 705.

Sidwell, R.W., Khare, G.P., Allen, L.B., Huffman, J.H., Witkowski, J.T., Simon, L.N. and Robins, R.K. (1975) Chemotherapy, 21, 205.

Sidwell, R.W., Simon, L.N., Witkowski, J.T. and Robins, R.K. (1974) Prog. in Chemother., 2, 889 (Proc. 8th Internat. Congr. Che-other., Hellenic Soc.Chemotherapy Publishers)

Streeter, D.G., Khare, G.P., Sidwell, R.W. and Simon, L.N. (1972) Fed.Proc., 31,576.

Streeter, D.G., Witkowski, J.T., Khare, G.P., Sidwell, R.W., Bauer, R.J., Robins, R.K. and Simon, L.N. (1973) Proc. Nat.Acad.Sci.(USA), 70, 1174.

Suhadolnik, R.J. (1970) Nucleoside Antibiotics. Wiley – Interscience.

Tamm, I. (1956) Yale J.Biol.Med., 29,33.

Watson, J.D. and Crick, F.H.C. (1953) Nature 171, 737, 964.

Witkowski, J.T., Robins, R.K., Sidwell, R.W. and Simon, L.N. (1972) J.Med.Chem., 15, 1150.

York, J.L. and LePage, G.A. (1966) Canad.J.Biochem., 44, 19.

BICHLORINATED PYRIMIDINES AS POSSIBLE ANTIVIRAL AGENTS

P. LA COLLA, M.A. MARCIALIS, O. FLORE, A. FIRINU, A.
GARZIA & B. LODDO

Institute of Microbiology II, University of Cagliari,
Istituto Chemioterapico Italiano, Lodi

Cagliari and Lodi, Italy

Summary

Several dichloropyrimidines have been found able to inhibit the
growth of Polio 1, Coxsackie B_1, Vaccinia and HSV, but not of NDV
and VSV. The antiviral effect of the most active of them, 2-amino-
4,6-dichloropyrimidine (Py 11) is very probably due to impairment of
structural virus proteins.

It has been reported that 2-amino-4,6-dichloropyrimidine(Py 11)
inhibits the growth of Poliovirus 1. The degree of this inhibition
is much more pronounced in amino-acid free media than in complete
media, because of the antagonism exerted on Py 11 by glutamine and
cysteine (or cystine) (Marcialis et al. 1973). The successive demonstration that mercaptoethanolamine (or mercaptoethanol) reverses
this antagonism has given the opportunity to reveal that Py 11
inhibits, in complete media, the growth of polio, vaccinia and herpes
simplex virus (Marcialis et al. 1974). Data referred to here show
that several bichlorinated pyrimidines are endowed with antiviral
activity similar to that of Py 11. Details on the mode of action of
Py 11 are also given.

Materials and Methods

Chloropyrimidines were synthesized by Istituto Chemioterapico Italiano (ICI) Lodi. 3,5-dichlorosalicylic acid, 3,6-dichloropyridazine, 2,4 dichlorobenzoic acid and 2-mercaptoethanol by Eastman. Actinomycin D (AMD, Merck), 5-fluoro-2-deoxyuridine (FUdR, Merck), Cycloheximide (Calbiochem) and Guanidine-HCl (Eastman Kodak) were also used. ^{3}H thymidine (26 Ci/mMol), ^{3}H Uridine (24 Ci/mMol), ^{3}H leucine (15 Ci/mMol) were furnished by Amersham.

Virus strains (NIH), were: Poliovirus 1 Brunenders, Coxsackie B$_1$ virus, Newcastle disease virus (NDV), Vesicular stomatitis virus (VSV), Vaccinia virus and Herpes simplex 1 virus (HSV).

Experiments were carried out on HEp-2 cells (American type culture collection, Rockville), grown in Eagle's MEM (Hank's base, pH 7.3) supplemented with 7% calf serum. Eagle's MEM, Eagle's MEM with 1/5 of the normal leucine supplement, Eagle's MEM deprived of the whole aminoacid supplement (AFE), all with Earle's base, pH 7.3, supplemented with 2% calf serum, were used in different experiments.

The maximum non-cytotoxic doses of the drugs were determined in cell cultures incubated in Eagle's MEM at 37°C for 48 hours. Cell damages were checked both by direct observation at low magnification and by spectrophotometric measure of the amount of neutral red incorporated (Marcialis et al. 1972).

Two thirds of the maximum non cytotoxic doses were used in screening tests for antiviral activity. Cell monolayers (10^6 cells/sample) were infected at 20°C for 1 hour with 10 infectious units (I.U.) /cell, washed 3 times in Hank's BSS and incubated at 37°C in Eagle's MEM. Drugs were added at the end of the infection. 24 hours later the whole cultures were frozen-thawed 3 times, and deprived of cell debris at 3,000 rpm for 3 min. Infectious units produced by Polio, Coxsackie B$_1$, and VSV were titrated by the agar-plaque method (Dulbecco and Vogt 1954), while the end point titration (6 stationary tubes per decimal dilution) was used for Vaccinia, HSV and NDV.

With the same procedures the inhibitory action of Py 11 on the growth of Polio and Vaccinia virus, was investigated; the sole exception was that virus inputs were 100 and 30 I.U./cell, respectively and that Poliovirus yield was measured 10 hours postinfection.

AFE medium supplemented with AMD 2 µg/ml was used for Poliovirus . Cell protein inhibition was evaluated by 10 min pulses of ^{3}H leucine (0.5 µCi/ml) within 2.5 hours postinfection. Cytopathic effect was determined by intracellular incorporation of neutral red from 6 to 8 hours postinfection. The overall synthesis of viral RNA and proteins was determined by cumulative pulses of ^{3}H uridine and ^{3}H leucine, respectively (0.5 µCi/ml of each from 2.7 up to 4 hours postinfection). The assembly of viral proteins in procapsids and complete virus particles was determined by sucrose gradient centri-fugation (Jacobson and Baltimore, 1968) of extracts, obtained from cells labeled with ^{3}H leucine (2 µCi/ml) from 2.5 up to 4 hours postinfection. The same procedure was adopted to evaluate the assembly of ^{3}H uridine labeled viral RNA into complete virus.

TABLE 1

EFFECT OF CHLOROPYRIMIDINES AND OTHER CHLORINATED CYCLIC COMPOUNDS
ON THE GROWTH OF POLIO AND VACCINIA VIRUSES

Compounds in Eagle's MEM	MTD$^{(o)}$ ug/ml A = B	INHIBITORY EFFECT$^{(oo)}$ ON POLIO A B	VACCINIA A B
2,4-dimethoxy-6-chloro	200	0 0	0 0
2-amino-4-hydroxy-6-chloro	800	0 0	0 0
2-amino-4-ethanol-6-chloro	100	0 0	0 0
2-chloro-4,6-dimethyl	800	0 0	0 0
2,4-dichloro	12	1.2 2.1	1.0 2.0
4,6-dichloro	12	1.2 2.2	1.0 2.1
2-amino-4,6-dichloro	100	2.1 3.8	1.6 2.9
2-formamido-4,6-dichloro	25	1.6 2.9	1.2 2.4
2-acetamido-4,6-dichloro	25	1.4 2.7	1.2 2.4
3,5-dichlorosalicylic acid	50	0 0	0 0
3,6-dichloropyridazine	30	0 0	0 0
2,4-dichlorobenzoic acid	250	0 0	0 1.8

(°) Maximum tolerated dose (µg/ml) by uninfected cells
(°°) Inhibition of virus growth in logs given by 2/3 of the MTD
0 = less than 0.3 logs of inhibition
A and B = without and with 3 µg/ml of mercaptoethanol

Eagle's MEM containing 1/5 of the normal leucine supplement was used for studies on Vaccinia virus. Early cell damages were estimated as for polio. Cytopathic effect was roughly checked by microscopic observation of the cultures. The organization of Vaccinia particles was evaluated by sucrose gradient centrifugation (Joklik, 1962) of extracts from cells labeled with ^{3}H thymidine (2 μCi/ml) from 3 up to 7 hours postinfection, chased with 20 μg/ml of thymidine and harvested 24 hours postinfection.

Results

Data in table 1 show that the inhibitory effect of Py 11 on the growth of Polio and Vaccinia viruses, as well as the potentiation of that effect by mercaptoethanol, is shared by all the dichloro-pyrimidines tested. The monochloropyrimidines are inactive on both viruses, while among the non-pyrimidine molecules one is active, and on Vaccinia virus only.

TABLE 2					
ANTIVIRAL SPECTRUM OF DICHLOROPYRIMIDINES					
Pyrimidines in Eagle's MEM from time 0	MTD (°) ug/ml	MINIMAL DOSE (ug/ml) (°°) GIVING 95% INHIBITION ON THE GROWTH OF			
		POLIO COXS.B$_1$	VACC.	HSV	NDV VSV
2,4-dichloro	12	4	4	8	0(°°°)
4,6-dichloro	12	4	4	4	0
2-amino-4,6-dichloro	100	10	20	20	0
2-formamido-4,6-dichloro	25	8	8	16	0
2-acetamido-4,6-dichloro	25	8	8	16	0
(°) Maximum tolerated dose by uninfected cells (°°) In the presence of mercaptoethanol 3 μg/ml (°°°) No inhibition at 2/3 of the maximum tolerated doses					

Data in table 2 show that dichloropyrimidines also inhibit the growth of HSV, while they are ineffective on NDV and VSV. As far as the structure-activity relationship is concerned, the few molecules under study only allow to conclude that the 2,4 and 4,6 chlorine atom positions in the pyrimidine ring are both compatible with anti-viral action, and that the free amino group in 2 position decreases the cytotoxicity, thereby enhancing the rather low chemotherapeutic index of Py 11.

TABLE 3	
EFFECTS OF Py 11 ON POLIOVIRUS SYNTHESIS	
Py 11 30$^{(o)}$ in AFE	IN % OF CONTROLS
Py 11 added at 1 hour post infection (p.i.)	
Synthesis of virus proteins and RNA	85 and 80
Production of early and late cell damages	100
Organization of procapsids and complete particles	2
Production of infectious units (I.U.)	0.1
Py 11 added at 2.5 hours p.i.	
Production of infectious units	80
Py 11 added at 1 hour and removed at 4 hours p.i.	
I.U. produced in: AFE (A)	0.5
I.U. produced in: AFE + Glutamine 20$^{(o)}$ and Cysteine 20(B)	
I.U. produced in: AFE + Glutamine 20 + Cysteine and	80
Cyclohemide 20$^{(o)}$ (C)	0.2
Assembly into virus particles in B) of proteins previously made in the presence of Py 11	10
Py 11 added at 3.5 hours p.i., after 2.5 incubation in AFE and 1 hour in guanidine HCl 100$^{(o)}$	
Assembly into virus particles of virus RNA made in the presence of Py 11, by proteins previously made in the presence of guanidine	90
I.U. produced	77
(o) µg/ml Details of technique are in "Materials and Methods"	

The main features of the inhibitory action of Py 11 on Poliovirus growth are reported in table 3. The drug decreases the overall synthesis of viral RNA and proteins by about 20% while   not
affecting virus-induced cell damages; on the other hand Py 11 completely prevents the organization of both procapsids and mature
virus particles. This effect is apparently reversible; in fact upon
removal of Py 11 from the cultures and addition of both glutamine
and cysteine noteworthy amonts of infectious virus are produced.
This recovery, however, calls for new protein synthesis, and this
is in full agreement with the experimental evidence that very few
structural proteins, made under Py 11 treatment are incorporated
in newly made virus progeny. In addition, Py 11 has no effect   on
the assembly of viral RNA into complete and infectious virus,
provided that virus proteins, previously made in Py 11-free medium,
are available. Finally, to produce complete inhibition of Poliovirus growth, Py 11 must be added to the cultures within 2.5 hours

TABLE 4			
EFFECTS OF Py 11 ON VACCINIA VIRUS SYNTHESIS			
Py 11 66$^{(\circ)}$ + Mercaptoethanol (Met) 3$^{(\circ)}$ in the medium	CELL DAMAGES	IN % OF CONTROLS COMPLETE VIRUS	INFECTIOUS UNITS
Py 11 + Met added at 0 hours p.i.	10	5	0.4
Py 11 + Met added at 7 hours p.i. FUdR 5$^{(\circ)}$ added at 7 hours p.i.	80 100	5 81	0.6 75
Py 11 + Met added at 0 hours p.i. and replaced, at 9 hours, by MEM	90	65	70
Py 11 + Met added at 0 hours p.i. and replaced, at 9 hours, by FUdR 5	60	5	5
($\circ$) µg/ml Details of technique are in "Materials and Methods"			

postinfection. Treatment starting at 3 hours postinfection or later
on, when virus organization is already on the way, are far   less
effective.

Data of preliminary experiments on the mode of action of Py 11
on vaccinia virus growth are reported in table 4. These data show
that Py 11 prevents the production of complete infectious virus
even if added to the cultures at a time when, as shown by the lack
of effect of FUdR, virus DNA has already been made. The idea these
data give of a selective effect of Py 11 on late stages of vaccinia
virus development is tempered by two facts: I) when allowed to act
since the initial steps of infection, Py 11 also prevents the
appearance of virus induced cell damages; II) the recovery of virus
growth, occurring upon removal of Py 11 from the cultures, is
impaired by the presence of FUdR in the rescue medium, in spite of
the fact that FUdR is added after a Py 11 treatment that largely
exceeds the time needed for DNA synthesis in the controls.

Comments and conclusions

Among the chlorinated compounds tested for antiviral action,
dichloropyrimidines have proven to share with Py 11 both the
spectrum of activity (Polio 1, Coxsackie B_1, Vaccinia and Herpes
simplex virus are inhibited, while Newcastle disease and Vesicular
stomatitis viruses are not) and the enhancement of their antiviral
effect produced by mercaptoethanol. As for the monochloropyrimidines
the have been found inactive, in screening experiments, on both
the strains used (Vaccinia and polio viruses) while among the
bichlorinated cyclic compounds one is active, but on Vaccinia virus
only. In spite of the limited number of molecules examined, these
data support the idea that dichloropyrimidines may represent a new,
promising, group of antiviral agents.

In the Poliovirus system Py 11 prevents the assembly of particles at the procapsid stage, proveded that the drug is added to
the cultures early after infection, when, the synthesis of virus
proteins is on its initial steps. While poliovirus RNA, made in
the presence of Py 11 is assembled into complete infectious particles, very few of the structural proteins, synthesized in the
presence of the drug, become part of mature virus, when, upon
removal of the drug, infectious units are produced.

In the case of Vaccinia virus Py 11 prevents the production
of complete and infectious particles even if added to the cultures
very late in the virus cycle, when viral DNA has already been
synthesized and late proteins are being made.

Considered together, these data suggest that Py 11 acts on structural virus proteins, impairing their functions in   virus maturation. Whether Py 11 acts on virus proteins during the translation process or later on is, at present, only mather of speculation. In consideration of these findings, however, the fact that Py 11 is active on the growth of unrelated virus strains,endowed with cubic or mixed symmetry, while is ineffective on two viruses having helicoidal symmetry may not seem coincidental.

This work has been supported by a grant of Consiglio Nazionale del le Ricerche, Roma (Italy).

References

Dulbecco, R. and Vogt, M. (1954), Journal Experimental Medicine, 99, 167.

Jacobson, M. and Baltimore, D. (1968), Journal Molecular Biology, 33, 369.

Joklik, W.K. (1962), Biochimica et Biophysica Acta, 61, 290.

Marcialis,M.A., La Colla, P. and Loddo, B. (1972),Experimentia 2^,1117

Marcialis, M.A., Schivo, M.L., Atzeni, A., Garzia, A. and Loddo, B. (1973), Experientia, 29, 1559.

Marcialis,M.A., Flore, O., Firinu, A., La Colla, P., Garzia, A. and Loddo, B. (1974), Experientia, 30, 1972.

Experimental Chemotherapy of Arbovirus Infections

A.N. Fomina, A.K. Schubladze

The D.I. Ivanovsky Institute of virology,USSR
Acad. Med. Sci., Moscow
USSR, Moscow, Gamaleja st. 16

In a previous article we had presented evidence that
rimautadine HCl and combination of rimautadine with
interferon are capable of inhibiting the multiplication of arboviruses in tissue culture.
Therefore experiments were designed to study the prophylactic effect of rimautadine and of the combination of rimautadine with interferon in mice infected
with WEE and Semliki forest viruses.
White mice 3 weeks old were used in all experiments.
One group was treated with rimautadine HCl and another

Table I

Prophylactic Activity of Rimantadine HCl in mice infected with WEE and Semliki forest viruses

Viruses	Infection level (LD_{50})	Dose[a] (kg/kg)	Survivors[d] (%)	Increase in % Survival
WEE[b]	10	12.5	35.5	26.0
	5	12.5	51.0	41.5
SFV[c]	10	12.5	81.6	46.6

a. Animals were treated by i.p. injection 4 hr before
   infection.
b. Route of infection was i.p.
c. Route of infection was s.c.
d. Per cent surviving animals 2 weeks
   after challenge.

Table II
Activity of Rimantadine HCl and Interferon
against WEE virus

Infection level (LD_{50})	Drug[a] dose (mg/kg)	Interferon units[b]	Survivors (%)	Increase in % survival
IO	12.5	250	61.3	52.2
	12.5	0	35.5	26.4
	0	250	30.0	21.9
	0	0	9.1	-

a. Animals were treated by i.p. injection 4hr before
   infection.
b. Animals were treated by s.c. injection 24 and 2hr
   before infection.
c. Route of infection was i.p.

group was treated with rimautadine and interferon.
Mice were injected in traperitonially with rimautadine
4 hours before challenge with viruses.
The results as one can see in table I demonstrate the
protective effect in rimautadine - treated mice.
In table II the effect of combined treatment in mice
with rimautadine and interferon is shown.
This treatment resulted in an increase in per cent survival of arbovirus - infected animals.
Therefore experiments were designed to study the effect of rimautadine on virus accumulation in blood
serum and CNS, interferon production and antibody
response in mice infected with WEE virus.
WEE rivus titers in mice treated with rimautadine are

Table III
Effect of Rimantadine HCl on Virus Titer
in mice, infected with WEE virus

Infection level (LD_{50})[a]	Time after infection (hr)	Virus titer ($LGLD_{50}$)			
		Blood serum		CNS	
		Treated	Control	Treated	Control
IO	6	0	1.0	0	1.0
	24	1.5	2.75	2.5	5.0
	48	1.0	4.5	4.0	7.5
	72	0.5	1.75	1.5	7.5
	96	0	1.5	0.5	8.0

Animals were treated with Rimantadine HCl
4 hr before infection.
a. Route of infection i.p.

Table IV

Effect of Rimantadine HCl upon Interferon
production induced in mice by WEE virus

Infection level $(LD_{50})^a$	Time after in-fection (hr)	Interferon units (ml)			
		Blood serum		CNS	
		Treated	Control	Treated	Control
10	6	0	40	–	–
	24	160	320	80	320
	48	320	640	640	1280
	72	80	320	640	640
	96	80	40	160	640

Animals were treated with Rimantadine HCl
4 hr before infection.
a. Route of infection i.p.

shown in table III. Rimautadine treatment result was
associated with reduction of virus blood serum and
CNS.
However, rimautadine in this dosage schedule did not
significantly affect interferon production, as it is
shown in table IV.
As one can see from the data presented in table V the
recovery of the animals accurred concomitantly with
the appearance of humoral neutralizing antibodies.
Mice were treated with one dose of rimautadine, infected with virus and surviving animals bled 14 days
after infection for serum antibody determination.
The results demonstrate a certain correlation between
antibody production, infection levels and survival of
mice treated with drug.

Table V

Antibody Response to WEE Virus challenge
in mice treated with Rimantadine HCl

Infection level $(LD_{50})^{(a)}$	Dose mg/kg$^{(b)}$	Antibody titer $(IGLD_{50})^{(c)}$	Survivors (%)
5	12.5	1.25	41.5
10	12.5	1.75	36.8
100	12.5	2.75	16.7

a. Route of infection was i.p.
b. Animals were treated by i.p. injection
   4 hr before infection.
c. Animals bled 14 days after infection.

Since the antibody production increased with the infection dose one may suggest that rimautadine in the amount used in this experiment did not induce the immuno-depressive effect.
The data presented in this report suggest that the prophylactic antiviral effect of rimautadine in experimental arbovirus infection in white mice is due to its inhibitory action upon the reproduction of the virus in animals without any immuno-depressive effect.

THE USE OF LUNG WEIGHT CHANGES FOR EVALUATING THE ACTIVITY OF

DRUGS AGAINST INFLUENZA INFECTIONS IN THE MOUSE

M.F. Beeson and M.R. Boyd

Beecham Pharmaceuticals, Research Division

Brockham Park, Betchworth, Surrey RH3 7AJ, England

SUMMARY

The use of lung weight measurements in mice is described as a screening procedure for measuring the activity of drugs against an A_2 influenza. A sub-lethal virus challenge is given by aerosol and six doses of the drug administered subcutaneously. Lung weight is maximal after eight days and is paralleled by a decrease in body weight. Lung weight is statistically related to lung score. The technique has been used to demonstrate the activity of reference compounds.

INTRODUCTION

Several parameters have been used by ourselves and others to follow influenzal infections in the mouse, one of the most relevant being the quantitation of the virus content of the lung some days after infection, but such methods are time consuming. At high virus challenge levels the survival rate of infected animals can be used to study the protective effects of drugs (1), while greater precision is afforded by computing instead the mean survival time for each group of mice (2). At lower challenge levels rales (lung sounds) can be used (3). To permit the use of non-lethal challenge levels other parameters are necessary, the most widely used probably being a lung lesion score based on the superficial appearance of the lungs (1). Another terminal parameter which has been used is lung compliance (4). Continuous monitoring of infection is possible by measuring oxygen consumption (4), water intake (5) or body weight loss. We have developed our screen around the increase in lung weight which accompanies the pneumonic changes at low challenge levels. The use of this parameter was first proposed by Gordon and Brown (6).

METHODS AND RESULTS

The experiments described were mostly performed on groups of ten male Charles River CD-1 mice weighting about 20 gm at the start of the experiment.

Primary stocks of a mouse-adapted strain of the A/HK/1/68 (H_3N_2) virus, supplied by Dr. Oxford (N.I.M.R., Mill Hill) were passaged in eggs to provide a working stock which was stored at -70°C. Working dilutions were made in 1:1 nutrient broth:phosphate buffered saline. Virus was nebulized in an airflow of 15 l/min. into a chamber of volume 120 litres. Infection by the aerosol route was considered to be more convenient and reproducible than intra-nasal administration of virus suspension to anaesthetised mice.

Each experiment contained uninfected controls, infected controls and also a group both infected and dosed with a standard drug. Drugs were given subcutaneously twice daily for three days, the first dose being given three hours before infection and the second three hours after infection. Infection was with $1/30$ x LD_{50} of virus administered over 30 minutes. At termination animals were killed with an intraperitoneal injection of barbiturate. Body weights were recorded, the lung excised and then weighed.

Figure 1 shows the time course of this increase in lung weight. Peak lung weight occurred after about eight days. A good response was obtained with a challenge level of $1/100$ x LD_{50}. Challenges of $1/10$ x LD_{50} and higher can be complicated by deaths and so the challenge level was standardised at $1/30$ x LD_{50}. Experiments were terminated on day 8 (day of infection being day 0).

Body weight changes were recorded over the dosing period and used as an indication of drug toxicity. Group weights were determined both before infection and on the morning following the last drug treatment. Using a standard growth rate curve (prepared using accumulated data from infected but untreated mice), those drug treated groups with significantly low body weight increases after dosing could be identified. These groups were rejected and the treatment repeated at a lower dose level.

Between days 3 and 8 following infection, the body weight fell significantly below that in uninfected mice. Figure 2 shows that an infection level of $1/3$ x LD_{50} had a progressively deleterious effect on growth from day 2 onwards. A less marked influence on growth was evident at infection levels of $1/10$ and $1/30$ LD_{50} although these changes were reversible. This reversal occurred earlier at the lower challenge levels. The body weight change between days 3 and 8 was therefore used to confirm the lung weight changes. Improvements in lung weight which were not paralleled by improvements in body weight were regarded as suspect and probably

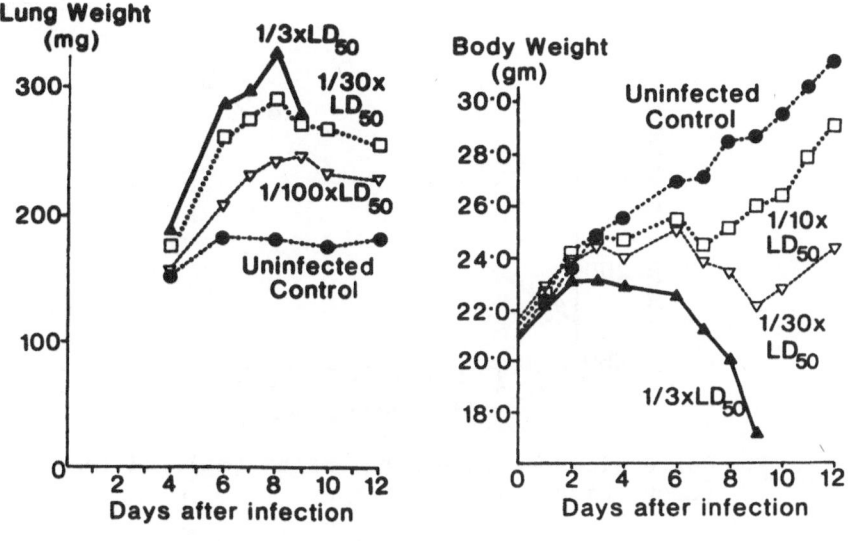

Figure 1   ### Figure 2

Lung weight and body weight changes in mice infected with A_2 influenza (group size = 10).

due to drug toxicity. The individual body weights on day 8 were used as a further measure of the success of the treatment. Results were routinely analysed by a method of least significant differences. Drugs were rated by their ability to return towards normal the virus-induced increase in lung weight. A statistical correlation can be demonstrated between lung weight and lung score, a parameter frequently used to quantitate virus infection levels (Figure 3).

The results of dose/response titrations with some standard drugs are represented graphically in Figure 4. Table 1 shows how the efficacy of six 30 mg/kg doses of spiroamantadine given s.c. over three days falls off when the first dose is delayed until 45 hours after administration of the virus. Accumulated values for the three control groups (uninfected control, infected control and positive control) from 32 screens are given in Table 2.

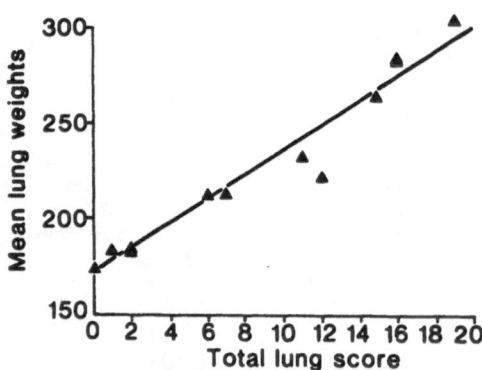

<u>Figure 3</u>   Correlation between lung weight (mg) and lung score
(Group Size = 10)

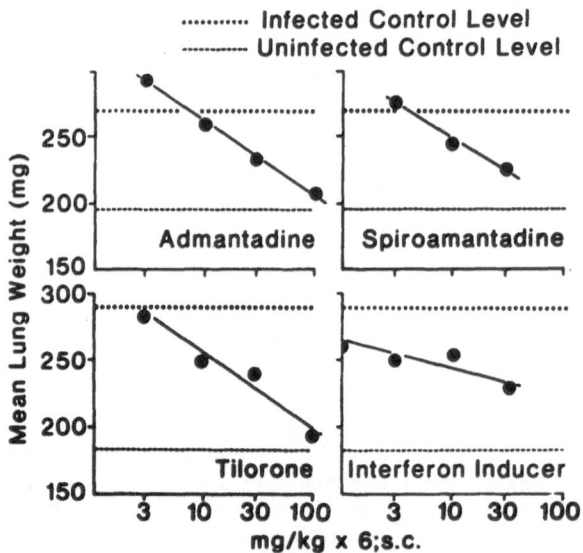

<u>Figure 4</u>   Effects of treatment of mice with six doses of standard
antiviral drugs (s.c., two times per day; first dose at -3 hours).
"Interferon inducer" = N,N-dioctadecyl-N',N'-bis (2-hydroxyethyl)
propanediamine.

Table 1   Influence of timing of first dose upon efficacy of
spiroamantadine (30 mg/kg, s.c., 6 doses, 2 per day) against A_2
influenza in mice (Group Size = 20).

Time of first dose relative to time of infection (Hours)	Percent return to uninfected levels	
	Lung Weight	Terminal Body Weight
+ 3	56	56
+ 21	55	38
+ 45	24	27
+ 69	20	31

DISCUSSION

These results show that the screening procedure described can
detect the activity of standard drugs against an A_2 influenza virus
in mice and that dose/responses can be demonstrated. The dosage
schedule routinely used (30 mg/kg s.c., -3 hours, +3 hours, 2 x day
+1, 2 x day +2) was not necessarily optimal for the drugs studied.

The procedure has no requirement for specialised equipment or
skills other than the infection apparatus and expertise at rapidly
and reproducibly removing lungs. It is sensitive to non-lethal
challenge levels below the level of sensitivity of comparable
techniques, and is readily subjected to statistical methods. It
was almost always possible in each screen to demonstrate a significant reduction in infection following the use of spiroamantadine so
that any other drugs having a beneficial effect of this magnitude
would also be selected statistically. We would normally follow up
any result better than a defined percentage improvement level as
long as body weight data supported possible antiviral activity.

Table 2   Control lung weight values (results from 32 groups of
          ten mice each)

	Mean (mg)	95% Confidence Limits
Uninfected control	186	181 - 191
Positive control (see text)	219	210 - 227
Infected control	289	278 - 301

Percent improvement due to spiroamantadine : 70%
Increase in lung weight induced by virus : 103 mg

REFERENCES

1.   Horsfall, F.L., J. exp. Med., 70, 209-222 (1939).

2.   Grunert, R.R., McGahen, J.W. and Davies, W.L.,
     Virology, 26, 262-269 (1965).

3.   Kaji, M. and Tani, H., Proc. 5th Int. Cong. Chemother. 2,
     19-22 (1967).

4.   Korotzer, T.I., Weiss, H.S. and Somerson, N.L.,
     Fedn. Proc. 33, 2400 (1973).

5.   McGahan, J.W. and Hoffmann, C.E., Proc. Soc. exp. Biol. Med.
     129, 678-681 (1968).

6.   Gordon, P. and Brown, E.R., Canad. J. Microbiol. 18,
     1463-1470 (1972).

IN VIVO TOPICAL ACTIVITY OF THE INTERFERON INDUCER BRL 5907 AND

RIBAVIRIN IN FERRETS INFECTED WITH INFLUENZA VIRUS

M.R. Boyd and M.F. Beeson

Beecham Pharmaceuticals, Research Division

Brockham Park, Betchworth, Surrey RH3 7AJ, England

Many workers have shown that influenza infection in ferrets provides a highly relevant model for the infection in man (1) (2). The virus is readily transmitted from infected to non-infected animals and the progress of the disease can be monitored by body temperature, virus isolation and antibody assay. In this paper, we present data to show that the course of experimental infection in ferrets is favourably altered by treatment with the double-stranded RNA interferon inducer BRL 5907 and by the virus inhibitor Ribavirin. We also hope to show that measurement of nasal airway resistance in ferrets provides a useful additional method for evaluating anti-viral compounds.

BRL 5907

The double-stranded RNA, BRL 5907, used in this study was pre-pared and highly purified in our laboratories from a strain of Penicillium crysogenum containing virus-like particles (3). We present data in Figure 1 showing that treatment of ferrets infected with influenza with an aerosol of BRL 5907 will effectively reduce and delay the febrile response resulting from the infection. We have previously shown (Boyd, M.R., unpublished) that an altered response of this magnitude would result from a reduction of greater than 2 $\log_{10}$ in the virus challenge.

Further data, shown in Table 1, indicates that virus isolation from the respiratory tract is markedly reduced after treatment with aerosolised BRL 5907. The difference between the treated and un-treated groups in this experiment was statistically significant (p <0.05). Nevertheless, antibody assays carried out on pre- and

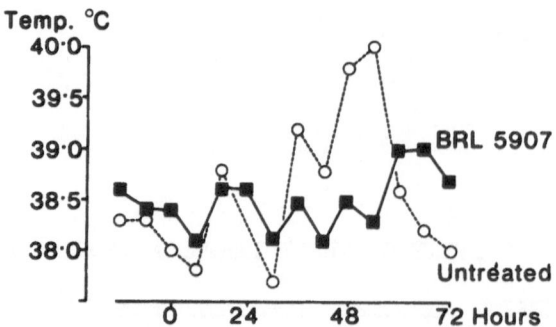

<u>Figure 1</u>   Effect of treatment with an aerosol of BRL 5907 on rectal temperature in ferrets infected with 300 EID$_{50}$ A/Hong Kong/68 (H3N2). (Each point represents the mean of readings taken from 4 animals.) Treatment commenced 24 hours before infection and continued twice daily for 2 days.

post-infection samples showed conclusively that each ferret was infected and produced an adequate level of serum antibody.   This perhaps represents an ideal antiviral situation whereby symptoms and viral replication are reduced but enough viral replication occurs to provide subsequent protection through antibody.

Ferret	Treatment	Virus Isolation Day		
		+2	+3	+4
1	BRL 5907	–	–	–
2	Aerosol	–	–	–
3	Twice Daily	–	+	–
4		+	+	+
5	Untreated	+	+	–
6		+	+	+
7		+	+	–

<u>Table 1</u>   Effect of aerosol treatment with BRL 5907 on virus isolation from nasal washings of ferrets infected with 300 EID$_{50}$ A/Hong Kong/68 (H3N2).   Treatment commenced 24 hours before infection and continued twice daily for 2 days.

The BRL 5907 in both the quoted experiments was presented to the animal in the form of a small particle aerosol directly to the respiratory tract. We have previously shown (Boyd, M.R. and Planterose, D.N., in preparation) that influenza infected mice treated in this way with BRL 5907 will be protected much better than if the interferon inducer is given by a systemic route.

RIBAVIRIN

It was of interest, therefore, to test the broad spectrum antiviral Ribavirin (ICN 1229) administered as an aerosol to influenza infected ferrets (4). The ribavirin was kindly supplied by Dr. R.W. Sidwell of I.C.N. Pharmaceuticals. Table 2 shows the results of an experiment in which rectal temperatures taken at frequent time points were plotted in the form of a six-point moving average. The figures quoted show the numbers of ferrets whose temperatures remained within 1% confidence limits for three Ribavirin dose levels and untreated controls.

Although a clear dose related response is indicated, each ferret produced a normal antibody level after the infection, again showing reduction of symptoms with continuing virus replication.

NASAL AIRWAY RESISTANCE

As an additional measure of respiratory distress in infected ferrets, we have been attempting to use the technique devised by Dr. Haff of Smith, Kline and French for measuring nasal airway resistance (5). We have modified the technique by using a rubber

Table 2   Treatment of ferrets with small particle aerosol of Ribavirin. Treatment was carried out twice daily for 2 days commencing 3 hours before infection with 30 EID_{50} A/Hong Kong/68 (H3N2). Figures show the number of ferrets whose rectal temperature remained within 1% confidence limit throughout the experiment.

Treatment	Conc.	Ferrets remaining within 1% confidence limits
Untreated	-	0/3
Ribavirin Aerosol	0·5%	0/3
	1·0%	2/3
	5·0%	3/3

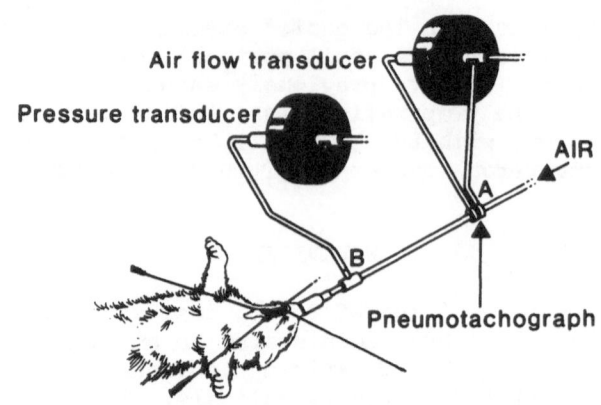

<u>Figure 2</u>   Apparatus for the measurement of nasal airway resistance
in ferrets

cuff placed around the ferret nostrils and use a Penthrane vapor-
iser to induce anaesthesia. This has the advantage of avoiding
the often serious problem of the ferret sneezing violently while
anaesthetised. The apparatus is illustrated in Figure 2 and the
output from the two pressure transducers is recorded on a Devices
dual-channel recorder. Within limits the pressure developed varies
linearly with the input airflow and uninfected ferrets provide nasal
resistance readings which vary little from day to day.

During an influenza infection, whether by intranasal instillation or by transmission, the nasal airway resistance can increase
by as much as five hundred percent. Usually a two or three-fold
increase is found either 48 or 72 hours after infection (Table 3).
Since nasal resistance could well be a measure of the amount of
virus damage to the nasal mucosa, its measurement could be a good
indication of the usefulness of an antiviral agent.

In conclusion, we have presented data to show that topical
treatment with an interferon inducer, BRL 5907 has a beneficial
effect on both temperature and virus excretion in influenza
infected ferrets. Furthermore, aerosol treatment of ferrets with
Ribavirin also reduces the febrile response due to infection.
Treatment with both agents allowed complete antibody conversion.

Finally, we have confirmed that measurement of airway resistance provides a potentially useful test for the evaluation of
antiviral compounds.

Table 3   Nasal airway resistance of ferrets before and after
intranasal infection with 10^4 EID_{50} A/Port Chalmers/73 (H3N2) virus.

Ferret	Airway resistance (mm H_2O/l/min)		
	Pre infection	Post infection	
		Day+2	+3
F1	45,44	85	121
F2	70	140	119
F3	30,47	101	130
F4	46	277	247
F5	48,54	40	98

REFERENCES

1.   Smith, W., Andrewes, C.H. and Laidlaw, P.P.
     A Virus Obtained from Influenza Patients. Lancet, 2, 66 (1933).

2.   Francis, T. and Stuart-Harris, C.H.
     Studies on the Nasal Histology of Epidemic Influenza Virus
     Infection in the Ferret. J. Exp. Med., 68, 789 (1938).

3.   Sharpe, T.J., Birch, Pamela J. and Planterose, D.N.
     Resistance to Virus Infection During the Hyporeactive State
     of Interferon Induction. J. Gen. Virol., 12, 331 (1971).

4.   Sidwell, R.W., Huffman, J.H., Khare, G.P., Allen, Lois B.,
     Witkowski, J.T. and Robins, R.K.
     Broad Spectrum Antiviral Activity of Virazole: 1-β-D-ribo-
     furanosyl-1,2,4-triazole-3-carboxamide. Science, 177, 705
     (1972).

5.   Wardle, J.R. Jr., Familiar, R.G. and Haff, R.F.
     A Technique for Measuring Nasal Airway Resistance in Ferrets.
     J. Allergy, 40, 100 (1967).

EFFECTS OF PYRIMIDINE DERIVATIVES ON RNA

DEPENDENT RNA POLYMERASE OF MENGOVIRUS INFECTED FL CELLS

E.M. TONEW AND B. FAHLBUSCH

Academy of Sciences of German Democratic Republic
Research Centre for Molecular Biology and Medicine
Central Institute for Microbiology and Experimental
Therapy, Jena, GDR

MATERIALS and METHODS

Virus: Mengovirus strain, plaque purified as previously described
be TONEW and TONEW (1971).

Cell culture and enzyme assay for virus-induced RNA polymerase
as described by TONEW et al (1974).

Nucleoside triphosphate medium and incorporation of the radioactive precursor: as described by TONEW et al (1974).

Separation of Mengovirus RNA species by 4 M LiCl precipitation:
The various species of viral RNA synthesized of presence of
actinomycin D or and inhibitors by the mitochondrial-microsomal
fraction (MMF) of Menfovirus-infected FL cells in nucleoside
triphosphate medium were deproteinized by the SDS-phenol
method according to SCHERRER and DARNELL (1962).

Acrylamide gel electrophoresis of viral RNA: was carried out with
2.6% composite acrylamide gels (agarose 0.5%, acrylamide 2.1% and
0.5% SDS in the gels) at pH 8.3, according to PEACOCK and DINGMAN
(1968). 0.1 samples were electrophoresed for 2 hours at 3.5 mA/gel.
The gels were sliced into 1.5 mm fractions, solubilized and counted
for radioactivity as described by WALL and Taylor (1969).

Extraction of cellular ribonucleates: FL cell ribosomal RNA
(rRNA) was isolated by a modification of the method of SCHERRER
and DARNELL (1962) according to ZIOLA and SCARBA (1974). The cells
were labelled with ^{3}H-uridine as precursor.

RESULTS

Antiviral activity of the pyrimidine derivatives AWD 625
(2.8-bis-(N-methyl-N-ethylamino)-4.8-bis (diethylamino)-pyrimide-
/5.4/-pyrimidine): the agar diffusion plaque-inhibition test
performed with 50 mm of the pyrimidine compounds showed moderate
plaque-free areas without cytotoxical zones. The one-step growth
cycle of Mengovirus carried out with concentrations of 100 uM for
substance AWD 625 and 50 uM for substance AWD 627 indicated a high
protection of virus-induced cytopathic effect and nearly complete
suppression of virus multiplication processes expressed as inhibition
about 99.9 and 99.4 per cent of infections virus yield (Table 1).

TABLE 1

THE ANTIVIRAL ACTIVITY OF THE PYRIMIDINE DERIVATIVES AWD 625
AND AWD 627 IN AGAR DIFFUSION PLAQUE-INHIBITION TEST AND ONE-
STEP GROWTH CYCLE OF MENGOVIRUS INFECTED FL CELLS

Substance Nr.	toxicity	radius in mm inhibition areas	Concentration in uM	One-step growth cycle to control in Log $_{10}$	Inhibition in per cent to control
AWD 625	0	6	100	3.05	99.9
AWD 627	0	7	50	2.26	99.45

Influence on Mengovirus polymerase activity: the standard cell-free
system using Mengovirus-infected FL cells at the 5th h. p.i.
demonstrated in presence of the four triphosphates a good
incorporating ability after incubation at 37°C for 60-180 min.
On the other hand the same cell-free system without the labelled
triphosphates showed a diminution of viral RNA accumulation
respectively lower incorporation rates. The addition of the two
pyrimidine inhibitors to the standard MMF reaction mixture resulted
in a significantly difference in comparison to control in presence
of actinomycin D. Farther the addition of DMSO 5% obviously
influenced not the synthesis of Mengovirus RNA by the MMF.
(Table 2).

MENGOVIRUS POLYMERASE ACTIVITY IN PRESENCE OF PYRIMIDINE DERIVATIVES

Series	Mengovirus FL cells reaction mixture	cpm	Inhibition per cent
A	Control triphosphates ATP,CTP, GTP and ^{14}C-UTP	5698	0
B	Without ATP,CTP and GTP	2405	–
C	A+Substance AWD 625 (100 uM)	3163	43
D	A+Substance AWD 627 (50 uM)	2492	56
E	A+Solvent (5% DMSO)	5589	0.98

Analysis of polymerase synthesis product by polyacrylamide gel
electrophoresis: menogvirus RNA polymerase synthesis product
extracted from the MMF reaction mixture of the virus control
showed a standard profile, (Fig. 1). By treatment with pancreatic
RNase in concentrations of 10 and 20 ug/ml the ribonuclease
sensitive ssRNA disappeared completely, (Fig. 2). The identification of the profile was performed by LiCl precipitation of
viral specific RNA extracted from reaction mixture. The LiCl
precipitated pellet resolved in RNA as well as the supernatant
material give separately the appearence of two respectively
one peak of labell. An addition of 20 ug/ml RNase to the duplicate samples digested fully the ssRNA in the LiCl precipitated
material, (Fig.3 and 4). So the position of the three substantial
amounts of labell have been determined to be incorporated in all
three classes of viral RNA. By treatment of the reaction mixture
with the two pyrimidine derivatives it was observed a markedly
reduction of the last (Mengovirus ssRNA) peak. The diminution
of viral ssRNA accumulation by the addition of the two pyrimidine
derivatives amounted to 43 respectively 56 per cent. The precursor
incorporation rate in the RI and the RF Mengovirus RNA remained
apparently on the same level as in the control, (Fig.5). To
establish nearer this inhibition effect on other experiment was
started.

To a standard MMF reaction mixture of Mengovirus-infected FL
cells 20 ug/ml RNase and 1 per cent DOC were added. Thereafter
incubated for 160 min at 37°C together with either of the pyrimidine
derivatives as a function of time, (Fig. 6). This assay demonstrated
only small differences between treated and untreated samples at the
end of the incubation time.

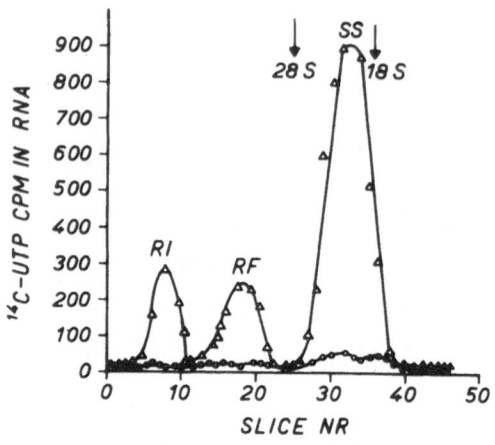

Fig. 1   Fig. 2

Composite electrophoretic profile of control Mengovirus
reaction mixture with all triphosphates.   The about 1 x 10^8
cells were disrupted with
DOC.   The reaction mixture was
incubated at 37°C for 60 min
in presence of actinomycin D.
Viral RNA was extracted and
deproteinized as described in
materials and methods.   Arrows
indicate localisation of 28 S
and 18 S ribosomal RNA.
___▲___   Total virus-specific RNA
synthesized in cell-free standard reaction mixture in presence of all four triphasphates
___O___ without unlabelled triphosphates

Composite electrophoretic profile of standard reaction mixture of Mengovirus-infected FL
cells treated with 20ug/ml or
10ug/ml RNase.   Virus-specific
RNA was extracted and deproteinized as described in materials
and methods.   The samples were
loaded onto agarose-acrylamide
gel and run under standard conditions.   Arrows indicate localisation of 28 S and 18 S
ribosomal RNA.
___▲___   Total Mengovirus RNA
synthesized in standard reaction mixture in presence of 20
/ug/ml RNase
___O___ and in presence of 10
/ug/ml RNase

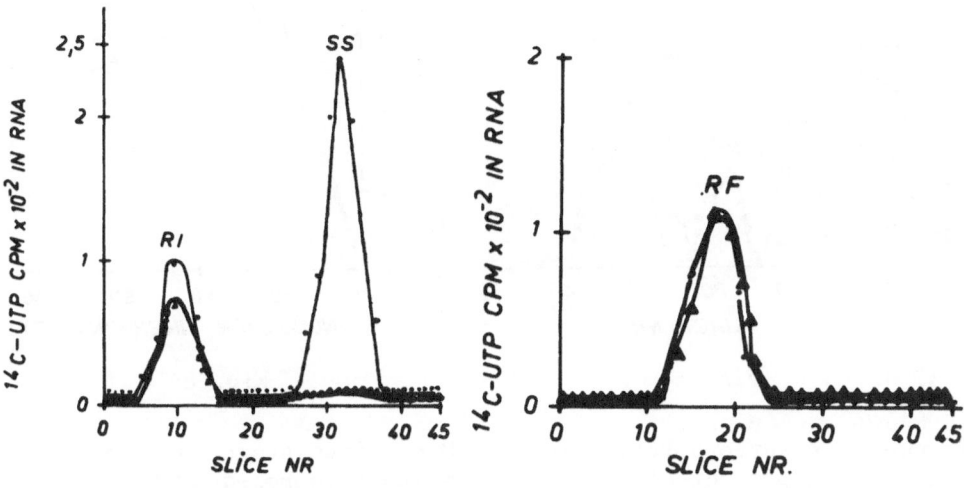

Fig. 3

Composite electrophoretic profile of precipitated with LiCl
extracted Mengovirus RNA in
presence of all triphosphates.
Duplicate samples were treated
with RNase and loaded onto
acrylamide gels.
__O__ Incorporation of Mengovirus
RNA of LiCl sediment
__A__ treated with 20 ∕ug/ml
RNase

Fig. 4

Composite electrophoretic profile of Mengovirus RNA precipitated with LiCl as described in
methods. The supernatante
and duplicate samples were treated with 20 ∕ug/ml RNase and
loaded onto acrylamide gels.
__▲__ Incorporation into the
soluble material
__O__ Incorporation into the
soluble material of LiCl precipitated supernatant treated
with 20 ∕ug/ml RNase

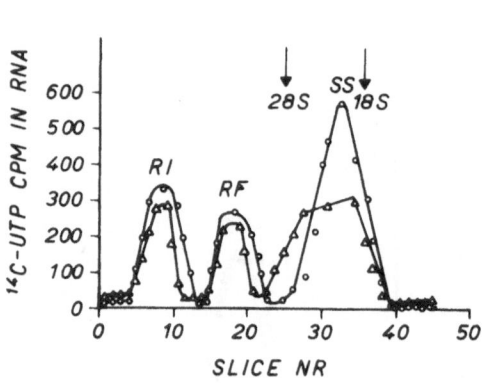

Fig. 5   Fig. 6

Composite electrophoretic profile of the product of substance AWD 625 and AWD 627 (100 and
50 µM) treated Mengovirus FL
cells standard reaction mixture.
After incubation time described
above the extracted viral RNA
was loaded onto agarose-acrylamide gels and run under standard conditions. Arrows indicate
localisation of 28 S and 18 S
ribosomal RNA.
___●___   Mengovirus RNA from
standard reaction mixture
treated with 100 µM AWD 625
___Δ___   treated with 50 µM
AWD 627

Mengovirus standard reaction
mixture composed of the ingre-
dients described in methods
+ 20 µg/ml RNase and 1% DOC.
After incubation of 37°C for
160 min at the indicated time
intervals the reaction were
precipitated. Duplicate
samples were treated as
follows: 1 and 2 added 100 or
50 µM AWD 625 and AWD 627,
3 untreated control.
___●___ - Incorporation of ^{14}C-UTP
into Mengovirus RNA in presen-
ce of 20 µg/ml RNase
___Δ___ the same mixture in presence of 100 µM AWD 625
___X___ the same mixture in presence of 50 µM AWD 627

DISCUSSION

In the present study it was indicated that the three classes of
Mengovirus RNA appeared in cell-free system of Mengovirus-infected
FL cells in the same manner as in Mengovirus-infected L and bovine
kidney cells, WALL and TAYLOR(1970). However in presence of the
pyrimidine derivatives AWD 625 and AWD 627 the production of
virus induced RNA has been influenced exclusively in the
accumulation of the amount of viral ssRNA. The synthesis of a
reduced level of Mengovirus ssRNA may be interpreted as a function
of suppression of viral RNA polymerase activity. The small
diminution of the incorporation rates of the precursor later than
40 min in the double-standard RNA in the time-dependent experiement
can be regarded as weak influenced by the inhibitors. An explanation
of the inhibition described here may be the forming of substance
complexes with protein or nucleic acids as it was established
for the isatinisothiosemicarbazones with model protein TONEW et al
(1974). It is also possible that these compounds interfere with
the pyrimidine nucleosides in their utilisation in cellular or
viral biosynthetic processes because the chemical structure belongs
to the pyrimidine analog. The way of this predominantely ssRNA
inhibition is still obscure and requests more distant study.

REFERENCES

1.   Scherrer, K.B. and Darnell, J.E. (1972).
      Sedimentation characteristics of rapedly labeled RNA from
      He-La cells.
      Biochem. Biophys. Res. Commun. $\underline{7}$, 486-490.

2.   Tonew, M. and Tonew, E. (1971).
      Antivirale Wirkung von Imidazol Derivation I.
      Die Hemmung der Vermehrung des Mengovirus in FL Zellen.
      Arch ges. Virusforsch. $\underline{33}$, 319-329.

3.   Tonew, E., Loeber, G., and Tonew, M. (1974).
      The influence of antiviral isatinisothiosemicarbazones on
      RNA dependent RNA polymerase in Mengovirus-infected FL cells.
      Acta Virol, $\underline{18}$, 185-192.

"IN VIVO" DEPRESSION OF EITHER ENDOTOXIN OR VIRUS-INDU-
CED INTERFERONS BY RIFAMPICIN AND RIFAMYCIN DERIVATIVES

E. RONDA, M.L. ALONSO, and I. BARASOAIN

Inst. "Jaime Ferrán" of Microbiology. C.S.I.C.

Joaquin Costa, 32 - Madrid - Spain

SUMMARY: Several experiments have been carried out in relation to
the influence of rifamycin molecules on the interferon production
when NDV and two bacterial lipopolysaccharides were employed as
inducers. The highest interferon level was obtained by NDV and all
the maximal peaks of yield appeared between 4 - 6 hr intervals.
Antibiotics clearly blocked the interferon depending on an appropiate timing of drug and inducer. The most effective time was the
injection of drug 4 hrs before the inducer had been administered.

INTRODUCTION: Since non viral agent inducers of interferon were
discovered, many efforts have been made to find out if they are
able to interfere with the viral infection (Merigan, 1973). On the
other hand, antibiotics inhibiting either protein synthesis or nucleic acids have also been tested in order to know their effects,
not only on viral infections, but on interferon yield. Chromomy-
cin A_3, rifamycin and rifampicin activities on Newcastle disease
virus (NDV) have been previously studied in an "in vitro" system
(Ronda and Alonso, 1973, 1974).

   In the present work we focused our interest on determining
the influence of three ansaminic molecules on biological systems
in which interferons are induced either by NDV or by two bacterial
lipopolysaccharides isolated from B. melitensis and P. aeruginosa
respectively.

MATERIAL AND METHODS: Viruses and cells. NDV, Italy strain. Stocks
were prepared by injecting 10 days-old chick embryos with 10^3 egg
DL_{50} into the allantoic sac. The allantoic fluid was collected
36 to 48 hours post-infection. Vesicular stomatitis virus (VSV),

Indiana C strain, was harvested from VSV-infected chick embryo cells yielding a titer of 10^8 plaque-forming units (PFU) per ml.

Primary chick embryo cells (CEC) and media were prepared as detailed in a previous paper (Ronda and Alonso, 1974).

Antibiotics. Rifampicin, rifamycin SV and AF/0-13 (Lepetit Lab.) were used. The names are those originally used by Maggi et al. (1966).

Lipopolysaccharides(LPS). The P.aeruginosa and B. melitensis lipopolysaccharides were obtained following two methods previously described (Westphal and Jann, 1965; Leong et al., 1970) and purified by column chromatography (Barasoain et al., 1975).

Animals. Unvaccinated male white Leghorn chickens aged 1 month and weighing 120 to 170 grs were used.

Interferon inducers. Groups of 10 chickens were injected into the wing vein or by intramuscular route (i.m.) with NDV (10^3 chick LD_{50}/0.3 ml); both LPS from P. aeruginosa or B. melitensis were injected intravenously (i.v.) at doses of 100 ng/100 gr body weight A pool of sera was made in each group and interferon titers at different intervals were determined.

Interferon induction in presence of antibiotics. The above experiment has been followed. Antibiotics were injected i.v. before (4 hr, 2 hr), simultaneously or after (2 hr, 4 hr) the inducer.

Interferon assay. Pools of sera from each group were used as interferon; those from injected birds with NDV were heated to 56° C for 30' to eliminate infectious virus. Sera were titrated in CEC using a modification of Dulbecco's plaque technique (Ronda and Alonso, 1974). Cultures of treated interferon CEC were challenged with 50 to 70 PFU of VSV as detailed in our above indicated work. Interferon titers expresed as units per ml of serum were recorded as the reciprocal of the highest dilution of serum which reduce by 50% the number of plaques counted in controls.

RESULTS AND DISCUSSION: In Fig. 1 four patterns of the interferon yields are depicted. As can be observed the maximal values are produced by NDV i.v. rather than for i.m. route while the lower levels were obtained with B. melitensis LPS as inducer. In all cases the peaks appeared between 4-6 hr intervals after inoculation of each inducer.

According to the maximal yield of circulating interferon at this time, chickens were exanguinated by cardiac punctures 6 hrs

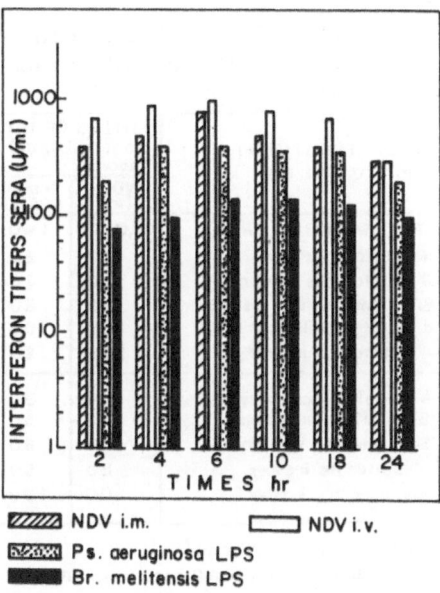

Fig. 1. Variations of the interferon yield in the sera collected at different times.

after the injection of interferon inducers.

Then, on this basis, the influence of three different ansaminic molecules were tested at variable timings of antibiotic drug and inducer. Results are enclosed in Table I, II and III. The success or failure of the interferon depression in the presence of such types of drugs rests in considerable measure on the appropiate timing of drug and inducer.

The maximun inhibition appears for the three antibiotics 4 and 2 hrs before the inducer was administered. Rifamycin SV showed the strongest inhibitory action even in treatment 4 hrs after the inducers. No great differences appear in the depressive activity between 1,000 and 500 ng. On the other hand we can see that interferon induction by NDV is more depressed than endotoxin-induced interferons.

B. melitensis LPS produces lower titers of interferon than P. aeruginosa LPS, being the former interferon more sensitive to the depressive action of the antibiotics.

TABLE 1. Effects and interaction of Rifamycin SV on interferon production, either with NDV or lipopolyccharides from B. melitensis or P. aeruginosa as inducers, in chickens.

TYPE OF TREATMENT AND DOSES USED		TITERS OF INTERFERON in sera (U/ml) different inducers		
		NDV (*)	B.melit. LPS(**)	P.aerug. LPS(***)
500ng of Rifamycin cin/100gr body weight in 0.3ml (i.v.)	CONTROL WITHOUT DRUG	1,000	140	400
	4 hr. before the inducer	0	20	100
	2 hr. before the inducer	<10	70	150
	Simultaneously with the inducer	60	80	200
	2 hr. after the inducer	100	100	250
	4 hr. after the inducer	256	120	300
1000ng of Rifamy-cin/100gr body weight in 0.3ml(i.v.)	4 hr. before the inducer	0	30	40
	2 hr. before the inducer	<5	50	80
	Simultaneously with the inducer	40	80	120
	2 hr. after the inducer	80	90	160
	4hr. after the inducer	100	100	250

(*) NDV ; 10^3 chick LD_{50} /0.3 ml (i.v.)

(**) B. melitensis LPS and (***) P. aeruginosa LPS;
100 ng /100 gr body weight in 0.3 ml (i.v.)

TABLE 2. Effects and interaction of Rifampicin on interferon production, either with NDV or lipopolyccharides from B. melitensis or P. aeruginosa as inducers, in chickens.

TYPE OF TREATMENT AND DOSES USED		TITERS OF INTERFERON in sera (U/ml) different inducers		
		NDV (*)	B.melit. LPS(**)	P.aerug. LPS(***)
500ng of Rifampicin /100gr body weight in 0.3ml (i.v.)	CONTROL WITHOUT DRUG	1,000	140	400
	4 hr. before the inducer	<10	60	70
	2 hr. before the inducer	80	80	90
	Simultaneously with the inducer	200	100	180
	2 hr. after the inducer	800	140	250
	4 hr. after the inducer	1,000	140	380
1000ng of Rifampi-cin/100gr body weight in 0.3ml (i.v.)	4 hr. before the inducer	<5	40	50
	2 hr. before the inducer	60	70	60
	Simultaneously with the inducer	180	100	120
	2hr. after the inducer	860	120	200
	4hr. after the inducer	1,000	120	400

(*) NDV ; 10^3 chick LD_{50}/0.3 ml (i.v.)

(**) B. melitensis LPS and (***) P. aeruginosa LPS;
100 ng /100 gr body weight in 0.3 ml (i.v.)

TABLE 3. Effects and interaction of AF/0-13 on interferon production, either with NDV or lipopolyccharides from B. melitensis or P. aeruginosa as inducers, in chickens.

TYPE OF TREATMENT AND DOSES USED		TITERS OF INTERFERON In sera (U/ml) different inducers		
		NDV (•)	B. melit. LPS(• •)	P. aerug. LPS(•••)
500 ng of AF/0-13 /100 gr body weight in 0.3 ml (i.v.)	CONTROL WITHOUT DRUG	1,000	140	400
	4 hr. before the inducer	0	30	20
	2 hr. before the inducer	<5	50	40
	Simultaneously with the inducer	100	80	70
	2 hr. after the inducer	250	90	160
	4 hr. after the inducer	700	100	250
1000 ng of AF/0-13 /100 gr body weight in 0.3 ml (i.v.)	4 hr. before the inducer	0	20	10
	2 hr. before the inducer	<5	40	30
	Simultaneously with the inducer	70	70	70
	2 hr. after the inducer	200	80	120
	4 hr. after the inducer	700	100	200

(•) NDV; 10^3 chick LD_{50}/0.3 ml (i.v.)

(••) B. melitensis LPS and (•••) P. aeruginosa LPS;
100 ng/100 gr body weight in 0.3 ml (i.v.)

Taking into account that the interferon is a major component in the host defensive response no inhibitory drugs should be administered with a profilactic purpose when an interferon induction is expected.

These antibiotics block several DNA-dependant polymerases of mammalian cells (Wehrli et al., 1968; Juhasz et al., 1972; Srb et al., 1974) and probably affecting in this way the interferon production (Ronda and Alonso, 1973, 1974), as well as the humoral and cellular immune responses (Sung, 1974; Paunescu, 1970; Dajani et al., 1973; Floersheim, 1973). However, the effect of these antibiotics could be due to an inhibitory action on the mitochondria (Gadaleta et al., 1970).

Such a triple biological system, as interferon-inducer-antibiotic is a very useful tool as an ecological model to study, experimentally, the antiviral defences.

These findings have led us to suggest that experimental virus induced tumors could be blocked using interferon inducers as LPS molecules that at the same time could act as immunosuppresant and in this regard further experiments are being planned.

Acknowledgements. This work was supported by Grant 612/46 from
III National Development Plan (Spain) (III Plan de Desarrollo).

REFERENCES

Barasoain, I., Rubio, N., Espinosa, M. and Portolés, A. (1975)
      z. Bakt. Infek. Paras. (in press).
Dajani, B.M., Kasik, J.E. and Thompson, J.S. (1973) Antimicrobial
      Ag. Chemotherap. 3, 451
Floersheim, G.L. (1973) Experientia 29, 1545
Gadaleta, M.N., Greco, M. and Saccone, C. (1970) FEBS Letters, 10,
      54
Juhasz, P.P., Benecke, B.J. and Seifart, K.H. (1972) FEBS Letters
      27, 30
Leong, D., Diaz, R., Milner, K., Rudbach, J. and Wilson, J.B.
      (1970) Infec. Immun. 1, 174
Maggi, N., Pallanza, R. and Sensi, P. (1966) Antimicrob. Ag .Chemo-
      therap. p. 765
Merigan, T.C. (1973) In N.B. Finter ed. "Interferons and interfe-
      ron inducers". Chapter 4, p. 45 North-Holland. Amsterdam,
      London.
Paunescu, E. (1970) Nature 228, 1188
Ronda, E. and Alonso, M.L. (1973) Abst. IV National Congr. of Mi-
      crobiol. C5 0 Granada. Spain
Ronda, E. and Alonso, M.L. (1974) Progress in Chemother (Athens)
      II, 1005
Srb, V., Puza, V., Spurna, V. and Keprtova, J. (1974) Experientia
      30, 484
Sung, S. Ch. (1974) Life Sciences 15, 359
Wehrli, W., Nuesch, J.; Knusel, F., Staehelin, M. (1968) Biochim.
      Biophys. Acta 157, 215
Westphal, O. and Jann, K. (1965) Methods in Carbohidrate chemistry,
      5, 83

INVESTIGATIONS UPON THE MODE OF ACTION OF COMPOUND 48/80 ON ss DNA

OF PHAGE ØX174

R. Dennin

Abteilung für Med. Mikrobiologie der Medizinischen

Hochschule, Lübeck, West Germany

The substance compound 48/80* is long known as a histamin releaser and still in the experimental phase of exploration (Kazimierczak et al; 4). Furthermore this substance turned out to be of interest in virology.

The investigations performed by Falke et al (1, 2) found compound 48/80 to be an inhibitor of virus penetration and the virus induced formation of giant cells in cultures of rabbit-kidney cells infected with certain strains of herpes virus hominis. Further results of these experiments demonstrated that compound 48/80 doesn't bother the virus replication inside the cell. These and other experiments had been carried out with complete viruses: that means with complex structures consisting of at least defined structures of proteins and double-stranded DNA. To elucidate one or more of the mechanism that might be involved in the interaction of this substance with parts of the viruses it should be of interest to run a somewhat simpler system.

For several aspects we have been working with an infection system called transfection. This system consists of isolated nucleic acid and a suspension of specially pretreated bacterial cells (Spheroplast) thus being penetrable by some kind of isolated nucleic acids. The transfection system used in all biological experiments to be described is that of Guthrie and Sinsheimer (3). The nucleic acid

* Mixture of mono-di- and trimers of p-methoxy-N-methyl-phenylethy-lamine (obtained through the courtesy of Burroughs Wellcome Co., Greenville, North Carolina, USA).

is the ss DNA of phage ØX174 and spheroplasts are derived from E. coli
C. In this system "inhibition" always means more or less suppression
of the occurence of pfu compared to untreated controls.

The first experiments carried out with the transfection system
showed that compound 48/80 is going to be inhibitory at concentrations of about 5 µg/ml. 20-40 ug compound 48/80/ml in the transfection
assay completely inhibits the formation of plaques. The DNA concentrations applied are about 2×10^{-3} µg ss ØX174 DNA/ml. It also
turned out that the action of compound 48/80 substantially is limited
to certain phases in the course of transfection.

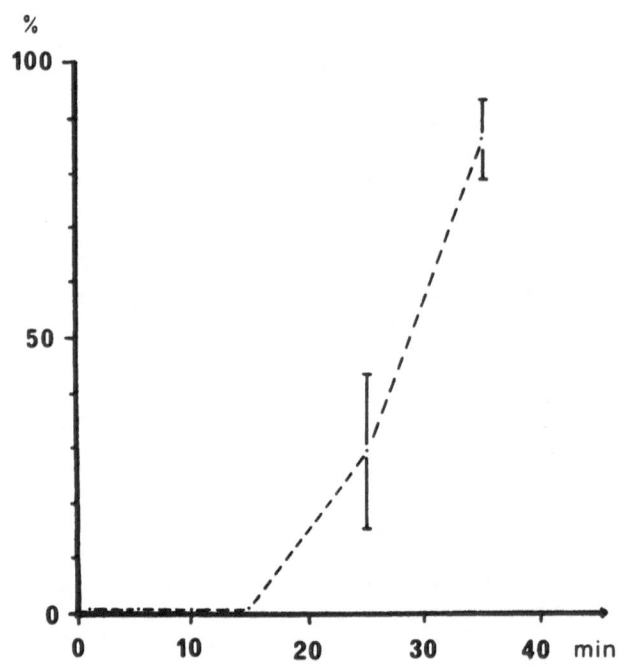

Fig. 1: Influence of compound 48/80 on the transfection
of E.coli K 12 (W6) spheroplasts with ss ØX174 DNA
(2×10^{-3} µg/ml); abscissa: time (in minutes) indicates
addition of compound 48/80 (40 µg/ml) to the assays
after transfection had been started;
the ranges indicate standard deviation;

The phases mainly concerned may include steps if the DNA applied
is   present mostly in the naked form that means: the DNA outside the
spheroplasts and as far as it is known from the relpication system
of phage ØX174 the synthetic steps of parental and progency replicative forms. We assumed that there might be a direct interaction
between compound 48/80 and the ss ØX174 DNA. The following
experiments now will demonstrate that indeed there is a drastic impact
on the ss ØX174 DNA. Fig 2 shows the results obtained by the method
of analytical buoyant density centrifugation in neutral buffered CsCl.

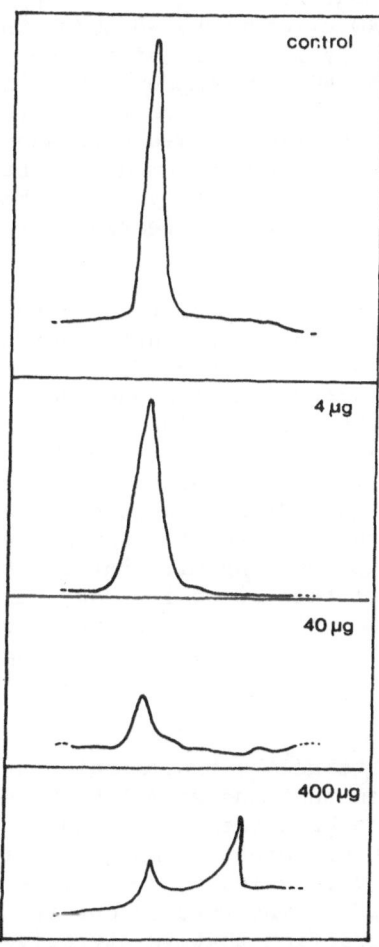

Fig. 2:   Tracings of analytical buoyant density runs in CsCl
2 µg ss ØX174 DNA/ml CsCl,ℓ 1.72 g/ml
buffer: 0.01 M Tris/HCl-0.01 M NaCl-0.001 M EDTA pH 8
44030 rpm - 24 h - 20° C.
Concentration of compound 48/80 /ml as indicated in the panels

The preceding procedure was mixing of the ss ØX174 DNA with compound 48/80 (final concentrations per ml are indicated in the figure). The assays were incubated at room temperature in any case for 5 minutes then dialysed for at least 4 h at 4°C in the same buffer as used for the buayant density runs. The samples then were prepared for the analytical runs. All UV-scannings were done at λ = 260 nm.

It can be seen that there is a drastic decrease of optical densit in the case of 40 ug compound 48/80/ml and 400 µg/ml respectively in the density region where normally the untreated ss ØX174 DNA (upper panel = control) with a density of ρ_{CsCl} = 1.725µg/ml is positioned. At the concentration of 40 ug compound 48/80/ml there is no hint of th remaining stuff in the analytical cell after the run has come to equilibrium. Only for the 400 µg compound 48/80/ml assay there is a rise in optical density at the meniscurs region (see the bottom of panel of fig. 2) that in addition showed a broadening that can be accounted for by diffusion of low molecular weight material. The density for the peaks in optical density that liked to be remaining ss DNA seems to be the same as the untreated control within the range of accuracy of this method.

Further analytical runs were performed by the band sedimentation technique. For techniqual and experimental reasons (see below) the ss ØX174 DNA concentration - calculated for 1 ml - in the initial solution that furthermore contained compound 48/80 was about 5-10 times higher than in the buoyant density CsCl runs. By increasing the DNA concentration in relation to compound 48/80 it should be possible to detect - if any - small differences in the sedimentation patterns o the DNA molecules. And indeed there was a slight increase in the sedimentation coefficients that tend to increase with the compound 48/80 concentration for up to 40 µg/ml. But if the compound 48/80 concentration is 400 µg/ml then no sedimentable material could be detected. All the applied optical density remained at the meniscus region and only a broad diffusion developed during the run.

DISCUSSION

The hints already obtained by biological testing compound 48/80 in the transfection system that the ss ØX174 DNA may be effected directly by this substance have been confirmed by means of analytical ultracentrifuge runs with different techniques. These physico-chemical studies evidently revealed a strong interaction of compound 48/80 with the ss ØX174 DNA. The results obtained so far allow the interpretation of an interaction that is strongly depending on the relation in concentration of DNA and compound 48/80. This interaction seems to range from a slight modification of the single stranded closed ØX174 DNA molecules at lower compound 48/80 concentrations resulting in the alteration of sedimentation coefficients up to a heavy impact at higher concentrations of compound 48/80 that may cause a serious impairment or even a destruction of the DNA molecules applied.

REFERENCES

1.   Falke, D. & K.J. Netter. Die Hemmung der Riesenzelbildung durch das sog. Compound 48/80 nach der infektion mit dem Herpesvirus hominis. 1. Die Wirkung auf die Virussynthese. Arch. ges. Virusforsch. 28, 308-324 (1969).

2.   Falke, D. Wechselseitige Dissoziierbarkeit von DNS-Synthese und Riesenzelbildung bei Herpesvirus hominis durch Cytosin-Arabinosid und durch Compound 48/80. 32. Tagung der Deutschen Gesellschaft für Hygiene und Mikrobiologie (1969) Münster i. W.; Bericht im Zbl. Bakt., 1. Abt. Orig. 212, 390-394 (1970)(Sanderdruck).

3.   Guthrie, G.D. & Sinsheimer, R.L. Observation on the infection of bacterial protoplasts with the deoxyribonucleic acid of the bacteriophage ØX174. Biochim. Biophys. Acta 72, 290-297 (1963).

4.   Kazimierczak, W. & Maslinski, C. Histamin Release from Mast cells by Compound 48/80. The Membrane Action of Zinc. Agents and Actions 4, 320-327 (1974).

ANTI-HERPES SIMPLEX VIRUS (HSV) EFFECT OF AMPHOTERICIN B METHYL
ESTER IN VIVO

H. SHIOTA, M.D., B.R. JONES, F.R.C.S., INSTITUTE OF

OPHTHALMOLOGY, LONDON and C.P. SCHAFFNER, M.D.

INSTITUTE OF MICROBIOLOGY, RUTGERS UNIVERSITY, N.J., USA

SUMMARY

Amphotericin B methyl ester (AME), semisynthetic derivative of
amphotericin B, was studied for its anti-herpes simplex virus (HSV)
effect in the rabbit cornea. It was highly active in preventing
HSV-lesions, and its antiviral effect was linearly related to the
logarithmic dose of AME. The antiviral activity was at least
additive with that of 5-iodo-2'-deoxyuridine (IDU). It is suggested
that AME should be active against IDU-resistant HSV and herpetic
kerato-uveitis. Possibilities of use of AME against other viral
diseases are discussed.

INTRODUCTION

Amphotericin B methyl ester is a semisynthetic derivative of
amphotericin B (Fig. 1) that possesses antifungal activity comparable
to that of the parent compound (Mechlinski and Schaffner, 1972).
It is less toxic and more soluble in water (Schaffner et al 1972;
Bonner et al 1972; Keim et al 1973). Recent study in vitro
(Stevens et al. 1975) shows that AME has antiviral activity against
sterol-containing lipid-enveloped viruses, although amphotericin B
does not possess antiviral activity. The purpose of this study was
to examine the antiviral activity of AME against HSV keratitis in
rabbits.

METHODS AND MATERIALS

Dutch rabbits weighing between 1.6 and 2.5 Kg were used. PH 8
strain of HSV was inoculated into the cornea using our technique of
multiple micro-trephination (Jones and Al-Hussaini 1963). Rabbits

Amphotericin B (AB) ; R_1 = H

Amphotericin B methyl ester (AME) ; R_1 = CH_3

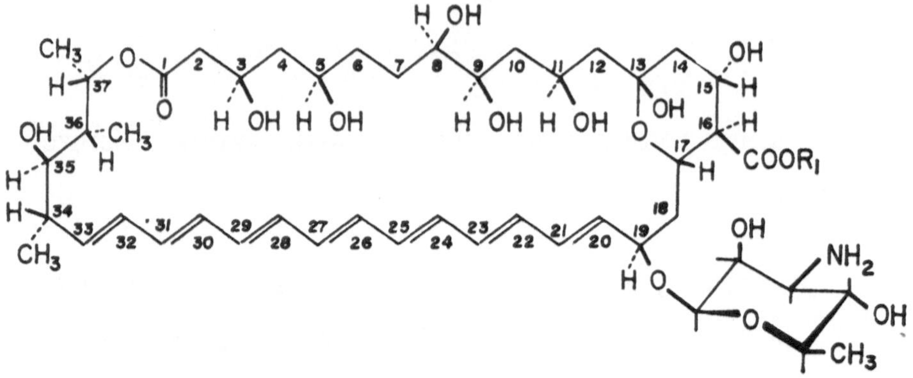

Fig. 1. The structure of amphotericin B and amphotericin B methyl ester.

were anaesthetised with I.V. pentobarbital sodium (30 mg/Kg) and given a retrobulbar injection of 0.5 ml of 1% lignocaine. One eye was closed with cellophane tape while the other was proptosed and inoculated. Four serial decimal dilutions were prepared with Eagle's minimum essential medium supplemented with 5% foetal bovine serum, 200 μmoles/ml of glutamine, 100 μg/ml of vancomycin and 50 μg/ml of streptomycin from a pool of HSV, having a titre of 1.15×10^6 plaque forming unit/ml. Each dilution was drawn into a fine glass capillary tube of 1.0 mm internal diameter, the upper end was then plugged with plasticine. An empty capillary tube was used to trephine through the corneal epithelium to mark the superficial stroma in the centre of the cornea. Similar trephinations were done with each of the four serial dilutions of HSV according to the plan in Fig. 2. After inoculation, the eye was left open for 30 seconds before the lids were closed with cellophane tape. This procedure was repeated on the other eye.

The solutions of various concentrations of AME hydrochloride were prepared by dissolving in sterile distilled water at room temperature and filtered through a millipore filter of 0.22 μm pore-size. If not used immediately, they were held at $+4^\circ$C for no more than four to nine days before use. In two experiments further dilutions were prepared from solutions remaining after an earlier experiment. They were held at $+4^\circ$c and used within 24 days of preparation of the original solutions.

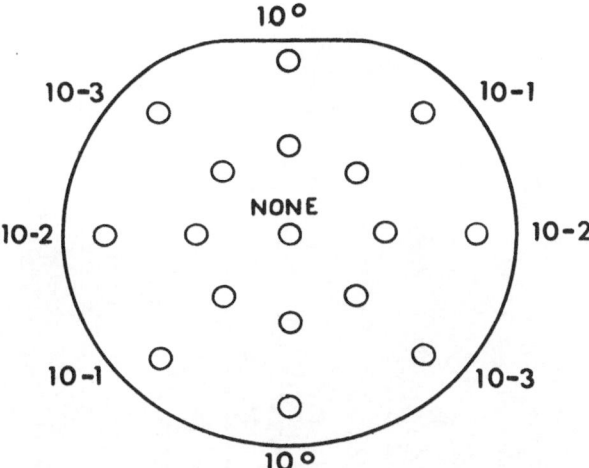

Fig. 2.   The plan of inoculation

The right eyes were treated with one or other concentration of
AME and the left eyes with a control; or vice versa.   Treatment
was started five minutes after inoculation, and continued hourly
during the daytime (10 applications between 10 a.m. and 10 p.m.)
for two days.   Each application consisted of one drop of 0.065 ml.

The eyes were examined 48 hours after inoculation, using a
Zeiss photo-slitlamp after applying 1% Rose-Bengal which stains
plaques of HSV-replicating cells in the corneal epithelium (Jones
and Patterson 1967).   The 50% corneal infectivity titre (CID_{50})
was calculated for right and left eyes by the method of Reed and
Muench (1938).

To examine the effect of adding either IDU or rifampicin, both
eyes of each rabbit were treated with 1% AME drops hourly as above.
In addition one eye was treated with either 0.1% IDU drops (with
0.002% phenyl mercuric nitrate as preservative) or 1% rifampicin
eye ointment or control, consisting of the appropriate inactive
vehicle.

RESULTS

On examination 48 hours after inoculation, the control eyes
exhibited large dendritic ulcers whose dimensions were in good accord
with the virus concentrations inoculated at each site.   However,
those treated with AME always showed fewer and smaller lesions than

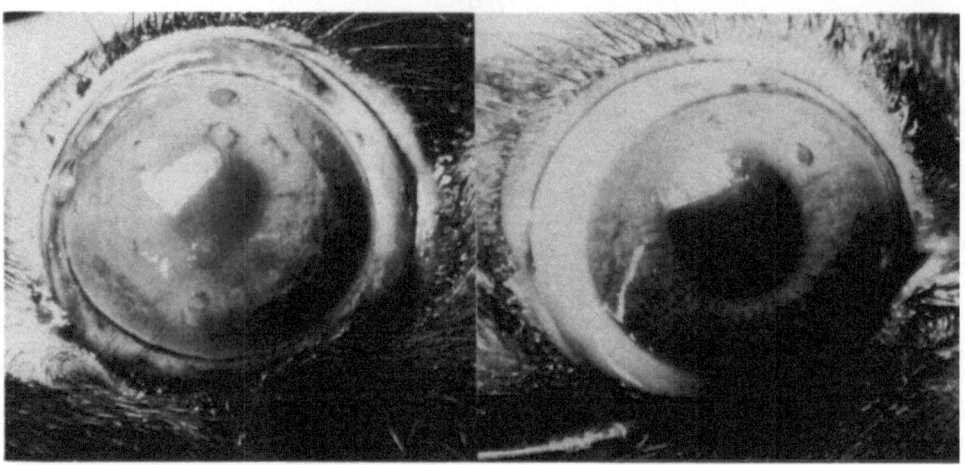

Fig. 3. Response of HSV keratitis in rabbit to AME therapy 48 hours
post-inoculation: (Left) control eye; (Right) treated eye with
4% AME drops given hourly (10 times by day) commencing 5 minutes
after virus inoculation.

the control eyes (Fig. 3). This antiviral effect was quantified by
calculating the log reduction in infectivity titre as between control
and treated eyes (Table 1). Comparison of right and left eyes in
individual rabbits thus obviates the effect of variation in the
infectivity titre between different rabbits.

    The antiviral effect was linearly related to the concentration
of AME in the drops applied within the range of 0.25% to 2% (Fig.4).

    The effect given by the standard clinically used concentration
of IDU drops (0.1% IDU) is shown for comparison (Table 1 and Fig.4).

    In order to determine whether the antiviral effect of AME is
the result of the first few applications of AME binding with un-
absorbed virus and inactivating it, a further experiment was done
in which three applications of 1% AME were made at 30 minute intervals, commencing 5 minutes after virus inoculation. As shown in
Table II, no significant antiviral effect was observed.

    In order to examine the effect of combining IDU with AME, 1%
concentration of AME was chosen (Table III). This 1% AME gave an
antiviral effect (0.95) in close agreement with the earlier result
(1.09). The addition of IDU produced a further inhibition of lesion
formation (0.68) that was of the same order as 0.41 given by the

TABLE I

ANTIVIRAL EFFECT OF VARIOUS CONCENTRATIONS OF AME

AGAINST HSV IN RABBIT CORNEA

10 times hourly (10 a.m. - 10 p.m.) for 2 days

Concentration of IDU or AME	No. of rabbits	Corneal Infectivity titre (Log CID_{50})		Antiviral Effect (Log reduction in titre)
		Control eyes	Treated eyes	
0.1% IDU	4	1.95	1.54	0.41
0.25% AME	4	2.24	1.67	0.57
0.5 % AME	4	2.31	1.53	0.78
1.0 % AME	4	1.43	0.34	1.09
2.0 % AME	4	2.32	0.79	1.53

TABLE II

ANTIVIRAL EFFECT OF 1% AME AGAINST HSV IN RABBIT CORNEA

3 applications only

Treatment (within 65 min. of inoculation)	No. of eyes	Corneal Infectivity titre (Log CID_{50})	Antiviral effect (log reduction in infectivity titre)
1% AME x 3	4	1.47	0.28
Placebo x 3	4	1.75	

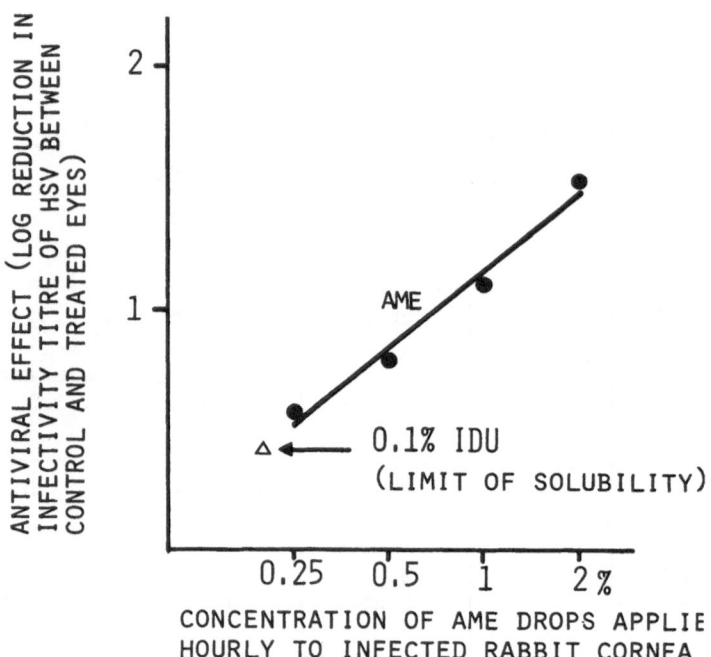

Fig. 4. Dose-response relation for antiviral effect of AME against
HSV in rabbit cornea: log reduction in infectivity titre given by
various concentrations of AME applied hourly (10 times by day)
commencing 5 minutes after virus inoculation. Effect of 0.1% IDU
drops given similarly is shown for comparison.

0.1% IDU drops when used alone. The antiviral effects of these two
agents are thus additive. A similar experiment to see whether AME
could confer anti-HSV effect on rifampicin gave a negative result
(Table IV).

DISCUSSION

These results indicate that topically applied AME has a true
dose-related antiviral effect against epithelial HSV-lesions in the
rabbit cornea, in a model that is a close analogue of human disease.
This effect extends at least one log higher than that given by the
most concentrated solution of IDU that can be used clinically.

Because its mode of action in binding to the sterol sites of
the lipid-envelope of HSV is different from that of IDU, it is to
be expected that AME will be effective against HSV that is resistant
to IDU, or other pyrimidine or purine nucleoside antivirals.

TABLE III

ASSESSMENT OF ANTIVIRAL EFFECT OF ADDING IDU TO AME
AGAINST HSV IN RABBIT CORNEA

10 times hourly (10 a.m. - 10 p.m.) for 2 days

Treatment (with drops)	No. of eyes	Corneal Infectivity titre (log CID_{50})	Antiviral Effect (log reduction in infectivity titre)
1% AME[*] + 0.1% IDU	4	0.32	0.68
1% AME[*] + Placebo	4	1.00	
0.1% IDU	4	1.54	0.41
Placebo	4	1.95	

* This solution of 1% AME had been stored at $+4^{o}$c for 22 days.

TABLE IV

ANTIVIRAL EFFECT OF ADDING RIFAMPICIN TO AME
AGAINST HSV IN RABBIT CORNEA

10 times hourly (10 a.m. - 10 p.m.) for 2 days

Treatment (with drops & ointment)	No. of eyes	Corneal Infectivity titre (log CID_{50})	Antiviral effect (log reduction in infectivity titre)
G. 1% AME + Oc. 1% rifampicin	4	0.65	0.14
G. 1% AME + Oc. Placebo	4	0.79	

Furthermore, the low toxicity with high solubility and penetration deep into the eye of topically applied AME (Jones 1975) together with the acceptability of intravenous administration, makes it likely that AME will be useful for therapy of deep herpes simplex keratitis and uveitis. It may also be valuable against deep diseases due to other lipid-enveloped viruses including varicella-zoster virus, cytomegalovirus, EB virus and influenza virus.

REFERENCES

Bonner, D.P., Mechlinski, W. and Schaffner, C.P. (1972), The Journal of Antibiotics, 25, 261.

Jones, B.R. and Al-Hussaini, M.K. (1963), The Transactions of the Ophthalmological Societies of the United Kingdom, 83, 613.

Jones, B.R. and Patterson, A. (1967), Excerpta Medica International Congress Series No. 163, 143.

Jones, D.B. (1975), Association for Research in Vision and Ophthalmology, In press.

Keim, G.R., Poutsiaka, J.W., Kirpan, J. and Keysser, C.H. (1973), Science, 179, 584.

Mechlinski, W. and Schaffner, C.P. (1972), The Journal of Antibiotics, 25, 256.

Reed, L.T. and Muench, H. (1938), American Journal of Hygiene, 27, 493.

Schaffner, C.P. and Mechlinski, W. (1972), The Journal of Antibiotics, 25, 259.

Stevens, N.M., Engle, C.G., Fisher, P.B., Mechlinski, W. and Schaffner, C.P. (1975), In press.

COMPARATIVE DRUG TRIAL IN CHOLERA

A.F.B. MABADEJE

DEPARTMENTS OF PHARMACOLOGY AND MEDICINE

COLLEGE OF MEDICINE, UNIVERSITY OF LAGOS, LAGOS, NIGERIA

INTRODUCTION

During the cholera epidemic which broke out in Nigeria at the end of December 1970, it was observed during in vitro sensitivity tests that the isolated species of Vibrio cholerae was sensitive to "Septrin" the Wellcome brand of co-trimoxazole. Tetracycline was the recommended drug of first choice. Permission was then sought from the Professor of Medicine to carry out a comparative trail of drugs in patients admitted to the Cholera Ward of the Lagos University Teaching Hospital. The trial began in January 1971 and it was prematurely terminated in April 1971.

MATERIALS AND METHODS

The criteria for admission into the trail included the following:
(a) Passing stool four or more times within 24 hours with or without vomiting.
(b) Presence of watery choleraic stool.
(c) Absence of vegetative forms of Entamoeba histolytica in fresh speciment of stool.
(d) No previous treatment with antibacterial agent since commencement of symptoms.
(e) No history of pregnancy if a female.
(f) Isolation of Vibrio cholerae from stool on day of admission.

All patients fulfilling (a) to (e) of the above criteria were admitted into the Cholera Ward and were randomly allocated into five treatment groups. Those from whose stool specimens V. cholerae were not isolated were dropped from the trial and

their places on the random table allocated to new arrivals. The
aim was to include a total of 100 petients in the trial equally
divided between the following five treatment groups A to E:

    Group A: Tab. Sulphadimidine 1G. six hourly
    Group B: Caps. Tetracycline 250 mg six hourly
    Group C: Caps. Chloramphenicol 250 mg six hourly
    Group D: Tab. Septrin 2 twelve hourly
    Each "Septrin" tablet contained 80 mg trimethoprim and
400 mg sulphamethoxazole.

    Group E: Tab. Placebo 2 six hourly.
    Each Placebo tablet contained 50 mg ascorbic acid.

    Specific treatment was begun only after rehydration but this
was usually within six hours. Specific treatment was stopped
when stool or rectal swab had been negative for V. cholerae on
two consecutive days.

    Stool or rectal swab was obtained daily from each patient and
cultured for V. cholerae. Intravenous fluids were administered
to all patients and oral kaolin and morphine mixture given until
stool frequency was reduced to two or less within 24 hours.
Intravenous infusion was stopped when stool frequency was four or
less per day. After two negative stool or rectal swab reports
each patient was given 15 G. magnesium sulphate on two
consecutive days in order to induce purgation. The patient was
discharged from the ward after two negative post-purgation stool
reports and was seen weekly for four weeks in the Out patient
clinic.

    Blood was obtained on admission and a full blood count as
well as estimation of electrolytes and urea was carried out.
These tests were repeated after rehydration.

BACTERIOLOGY

    Examination of stool and rectal swab specimens was carried
out in the Department of Microbiology. The methods employed
included dark-ground microscopy, culture in Alkaline Peptone
Water (pH 8.6) and T.C.B.S. medium. Biochemical and slide
agglutination tests were performed for confirmation and typing of
isolates.

RESULTS

    The trial had to be terminated prematurely when the Cholera
Ward was closed as a result of the Industrial Action by Hospital
doctors in May 1971. By the time the doctors resumed work

the epidemic had thinned down and it was no longer necessary to
reopen the Ward. Out of 57 patients analysed 29 were males and 28
were females. Table 1 shows the distribution into the five
treatment groups. There were 13 in A, 9 in B, 14 in C, 12 in D
and 9 in E.

The mean number of days for diarrhoea to stop $\pm$ S.D. was
respectively 3.5 $\pm$ 1.51 in A, 2.3 $\pm$ 1.00 in B, 3.7 $\pm$ 1.20 in C,
2.1 $\pm$ 1.16 in D and 5.7 $\pm$ 2.45 in E. Thus diarrhoea was of
signiricantly shorter duration in each of the four groups A to
D when compared with the placebo group. The mean number of days
$\pm$ S.D. for the first negative stool report was respectively
5.5 $\pm$ 1.13 in A, 3.6 $\pm$ 1.81 in B, 5.3 $\pm$ 0.99 in C, 3.6 $\pm$ 0.90 in
D and 6.9 $\pm$ 2.03 in E. This shows that those who received
tetracycline, chloramphenicol and Septrin had a significantly
shorter period of bacterial excretion than those who received
placebo. After purgation one patient in each of the tetracycline,
chloramphenicol and Septrin groups became stool positive while
two patients in the placebo group became stool positive. No side
effects attributable to the drugs were observed in this trial.
Of 100 patients admitted to the Cholera Ward during the period
64 had V. cholerae isolated from their stool. 7 patients were
excluded for not satisfying the criteria for inclusion. One
was a pregnant female, three had been given tetracycline before
reaching the ward and three died within six hours of admission.

Two other patients died after their stool became negative
for V. cholerae; one female in the tetracycline group died from
chronic renal failure with hypertension. Autopsy revealed
chronic nephritis. The other was a male in the sulphadimidine
group who died of hepatic cirrhosis.

DISCUSSION

Cholera has always travelled along human routes of
communication and once introduced into a susceptible community
with a low standard of sanitation, it usually thrives and
spreads rapidly (Barua and Cvjetanovic 1970). It was therefore
not surprising that the spread of cholera along West Africa
which began in Guinea in August 1970 ultimately reached Nigeria
by the end of December 1970 having passed through Ivory Coast,
Liberia, Mali, Ghana and Dahomey.

The epidemic strain in Nigeria was the El tor biotype and
Ogawa serotype of V. chlorae. Human beings in the incubation,
clinical or convalescent stage of the disease are the reservoirs
of the cholera vibrio. Since there may be as many as 10-100
asymptomatically infected individuals for every clinical case of
cholera it shows the iceberg phenomenon common in enteric
infections. Excretion of vibrios by cases and contact carriers
does not generally continue for more than 7-10 days but in areas where

TABLE 1:   SUMMARY OF RESULT IN THE FIVE TREATMENT GROUPS

	A SULPHADIMIDINE 1G. q 6 Hrs.	B TETRACYCLINE 250 mg q. 6 Hrs.	C CHLORAMPHENICOL 250 mg q. 6 Hrs.	D SEPTRIN 2 Tabs q. 12 Hrs.	E PLACEBO ASCORBIC ACID 100 mg q. 6 Hrs.
NUMBER OF PATIENTS	13	9	14	12	9
NUMBER OF MALES	6	3	11	6	3
NUMBER OF FEMALES	7	6	3	6	6
AGE RANGE (YEARS)	20-60	20-82	12-47	16-60	12-68
MEAN AGE (YEARS)	35.0	41.4	26.2	34.2	45.7
DAY DIARRHOEA STOPPED i.e. B.O. 2 per day	1-6	1-4	2-5	1-4	2-10
MEAN ± S.D.	3.5 ± 1.5	2.3 ± 1.00	3.7 ± 1.20	2.1 ± 1.16	5.7 ± 2.45
t	2.63	3.78	2.58	4.47	
p	0.05	0.05	0.05	0.05	
DAY FOR FIRST -ve STOOL	4-8	2-8	3-7	2-5	5-10
MEAN ± S.D.	5.5 ± 1.13	3.6 ± 1.81	5.3 ± 0.99	3.6 ± 0.90	6.9 ± 2.03
t	2.03	3.69	2.58	5.12	
p	0.05	0.05	0.05	0.05	
NUMBER +ve POST PURGATION	-	1	1	1	2
SIDE-EFFECTS	NIL	NIL	NIL	NIL	NIL
DEATHS	1	1	NIL	NIL	NIL

there is poor sanitation efforts should be made to reduce the risk
of spread by administering chemotherapy to patients and their close
contacts as well as vaccination of their neighbours.

The Lagos cholera Committee comprising Lagos University Teaching
Hospital members and officials of Federal and Lagos State Ministries
of Health recommended tetracycline as the drug of first choice to
be given intravenously to those vomiting and severely dehydrated
patients and orally subsequently after rehydration.

In other treatment centres where tetracycline was used the
average duration of stay in hospital was 3 days in the majority
of cases (Oni 1971, Salami 1972). However, it is not clear if the
stool became negative of if diarrhoea did stop before discharge.
In this trial both "Septrin" and tetracycline reduce the duration
of diarrhoea to 2.1 and 2.3 days respectively and both reduced
number of days for bacterial excretion to 3.6. Thus Septrin has been
shown to be as equally effective in cholera as tetracycline the
recommended drug of first choice.

SUMMARY
     A comparitive trial has been carried out on 57 cholera patients
randomly assigned into 5 treatment groups. Group A received
sulphadimidine, B tetracycline, C chloramphenicol, D cotrimoxacole
as "Septrin" and E Placebo as ascorbic acid. The mean number of
days for diarrhoea to stop was significantly shorter in each of
the other four groups when compared with the placebo group. Those
receiving tetracycline, "Septrin" and chloramphenicol had a
significantly shorter period of bacterial excretion than those
receiving tetracycline and "Septrin" fared better than those
receiving other drugs but there was no difference between those
receiving "Septrin" and tetracycline. Thus "Septrin" was shown
to be equally effective in cholera as tetacycline the recommended
drug of first choice.

ACKNOWLEDGEMENTS
     My thanks are due to Professor Mabayoje for permission to
carry out the trial, Professor Ogunbi for microbiological investigations, the Sisters and Staff Nurses of the Cholera Ward of
L.U.T.H., Burroughs Wellcome Nigeria Ltd. for the supply of
"Septrin" and Mr. 'Sola Olatidoye for secretarial assistance.

REFERENCES
     1. BARUA,D. and CVJETANOVIC, B. 1970: The Surveillance of
        Cholera. W.H.O. Chronicle 24, 41-46.

     2. ONI, O.O.A. 1971: Cholera Epidemic in Ibadan, January to
        March 1971. Nig. Med. J.I. 229-233.

     3. SALAMI, M.Y.L. 1972: Clinical and Epidemiological Aspects
        of Cholera Outbreak in Metropolitan Lagos. Nig. Med. J.2.
        149.155.

TRIMETHOPRIM RESISTANCE OF PATHOGENIC ORGANISMS PREVIOUS TO COMMON CLINICAL USE OF SULPRIM[R]

S.ORTEL,   Prof. Dr.sc.med.

Inst. of Med. Microbiology and Epidemiology

GDR 4o2 Halle (Saale), Leninallee 6

Summary. About 1ooo organisms (Esch. coli, Klebsiella, Pseudomonas, Enteritis-Coli, Proteus sp.,
Staph. aureus, Enterococci, Listeria monocytogenes)
isolated from different materials of inpatients in
1973 and 1974 before Co-Trimoxazole was available
were tested against TMP, SMZ and TMP/SMZ in the disk-
diffusion test. We found that the percentage of resistant strains against the TMP/SMZ-combination for
Esch.coli was only 1.3 %, in Klebsiella 4.8 % and Enterococci 2 %. As yet no resistant strain of Ent.
coli, Proteus, Staph. aureus and Listeria monocytogenes against TMP/SMZ was stated. The favourable potentiating effect could also be demonstrated with the
agar dilution method and the FIC-values. The resistant strains had only MIC-values to TMP between 3.12
and 5o µg/ml; TMP resistance (5o µg/ml) of 6 Klebsiella strains could not be transferred to Esch.coli
K 12.

Trimethoprim and its combination with Sulfamethoxazole, Co-Trimoxazole, is a synthetic drug which
is used for therapy in human beings already for about
8 years and since 4 years also in veterinary medicine
in many countries of the world. In GDR the Co-Trimoxazole drug Sulprim[R] (Polfa-Warsaw) is available
only since the end of 1974 for therapeutic purposes.
During the next years an increased use of this drug
is to be expected and we have to observe the resistance and the appearance of TMP-resistance factors.

Investigations of several authors from the last years
confirm this opinion (Darrell, Garrod, Waterworth
1968; Fleming, Datta and Grüneberg 1972; Hedges and
Datta 1972; Pinney and Smith 1973).

        Therefore the present situation of resistance
of different gram-positive and gram-negative organisms in a country in which TMP and its combination
with SMZ has not been used till now may be of interest.
In our investigations we tested as, yet in the diffusion test on Wellcotest-Agar and DST-Agar Oxoid with
test discs about 1ooo strains of different species
(Esch. coli, Klebsiella pneumoniae, Pseudomonas, Enteritis-Coli, Proteus sp., Staph. aureus, Enterococci and Listeria monocytogenes). These germs had
been isolated from human materials of inpatients of
the university hospitals in Halle in 1973 and the beginning of 1974 - thus during a period in which Co-
Trimoxazole not yet was available.

        Fig. 1 shows the species of pathogens and the
origin of the material from which the 1ooo organisms
had been isolated. In most cases the pathogens came
from samples of urine (Esch. coli, Pseudomonas, Enterococci), in the second place are samples of faeces
with Klebsiella and Enteritis-Coli; then follow swabs
of wounds (Staph. aureus), pus of ear and swabs of
conjunctiva (Staph. aureus), then sputum, bile, li-
quor and others.

        The results of the diffusion test are presented
in fig. 2. From fig. 2 we see that against TMP· alone
3.1 % of the tested Coli strains, about 1o % of the
Klebsiella and all strains of Pseudomonas must be regarded as resistant since they showed no inhibition

Organism	Urine	Fae-ces	Wound	Ear	Eye	Sputum	Bile	Food	Pleura	Trachea	Liquor	Meco-nium	Total
E. coli	271	–	5	–	–	5	8	–	1	–	–	–	290
Klebsiella	12	125	–	–	–	–	–	7	–	–	1	–	145
Proteus sp.	68	–	10	14	–	7	1	–	–	–	–	–	100
Pseudomonas	45	3	18	–	4	4	–	–	2	2	–	–	78
Enteritis - Coli	–	111	–	–	–	–	–	–	–	–	–	–	111
Staph aur	3	1	95	25	22	7	–	–	3	–	–	–	156
Enterococci	78	–	10	2	–	3	7	–	–	–	–	–	100
Listeria monocy.	–	36	–	–	–	–	–	–	–	–	–	4	40
Total	477	276	138	41	26	26	16	7	6	2	1	4	1020

Fig. 1
Origin of tested organisms

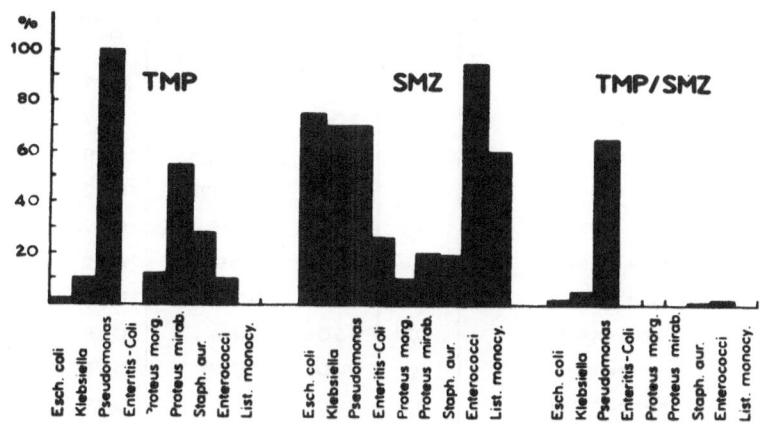

Fig. 2

Resistance of different organisms against TMP,
SMZ and TMP/SMZ in the diffusion test

zone on TMP-discs which were impregnated with 1.25 ug.
Indole-positive and indole-negative Proteus strains
showed a different resistance to TMP (12.5 % for Proteus morganii, 55 % for Proteus mirabilis). Staph.
aureus organisms were resistant in 3o % of the tested
strains and Enterococci in 11 %. Against Sulfamethoxazole (SMZ-discs with 23.75 ug/ml) most of the species, both gram-positive and gram-negative, showed
resistance. More favourable are here the results for
Proteus morganii (1o %), Proteus mirabilis (2o %) and
Enteritis-Coli (27 %). On the other hand, the combination of TMP and SMZ yielded a good potentiating action. Against Co-Trimoxazole no resistance could be
observed in 111 tested Enteritis-Coli, in 4o indole-
positive and 6o indole-negative Proteus strains, 156
strains of Staph. aureus and 37 List. monocytogenes
strains of different serotypes. Out of 29o Coli
strains only 4 (1.3 %) were resistant in the diffusion
test against the combination. In Klebsiella the value
was 4.8 % and in Enterococci 2 %. However, Pseudomonas
strains did not respond to the combination in about
67 %.

The potentiating action could also be demonstrated by investigations in plate dilution test against
TMP and SMZ and the combination of these drugs. Also
the FIC-values give distinct hints at the good synergistic action because it lays always below o.5 (Fig.
3). These results obtained from a large number of different organisms isolated from patients' material in

Organism	TMP	SMZ	TMP/SMZ	FIC
Esch. coli K 12	0,1	8	0,025 /0,5	0,31
Esch. coli 7	6,4	2000	1,6/32	0,27
Esch. coli 9	3,2	32	0,2/4	0,19
Esch. coli 466	25,0	2000	6,4 /125	0,32
Klebs. 1285	1,6	500	0,4/8	0,27
Klebs. 1294	0,8	16	0,05/1	0,12
Staph. SG 511	1,6	16	0,05/1	0,09
Staph. aur. 1254	0,8	500	0,2/4	0,25
Enterococcus 170	0,2	2000	0,05/1	0,25
Enteroc. 1213	1,6	2000	0,2/4	0,13

Fig. 3

MIC-values of different organisms to TMP, SMZ,
TMP/SMZ (1:2o) and FIC-indices

1973 and 1974 show that the starting situation with
regard to Co-Trimoxazole-therapy in GDR is very favourable and for many species of germs already good
results have been obtained.

In further investigations 225 selected strains
of different species of organisms were tested in the
plate dilution test against TMP for MIC-values. Fig.4
shows the results we obtained for the tested strains
(3o Coli, 48 Klebsiella, 64 Proteus sp., 57 Staph.
aureus and 26 Enterococci). This figure shows that
the values for resistant Coli and Klebsiella were on-

Organism		Number	0,05	0,1	0,2	0,4	0,8	1,6	3,12	6,25	12,5	25	50
E. coli		30	3	7	7	1	3	3	1	1	1	1	2
Klebsiella pneumoniae		48			4	6	17	10	3	2	2	3	1
Proteus	Indole +	7					1	3	3				
Proteus	Indole −	57			1		3	25	27	1			
Staph. aureus		57		1	3	25	11	16			1		
Enterococci		26	2	8	3	8		1	1		1		2
		225	5	16	18	40	35	58	35	4	5	4	5

Fig. 4

MIC-values (ug/ml) of TMP for 225 selected
bacterial strains

ly between 3.12 ug - 5o ug/ml, for Proteus at 3.12
and 6.25 ug/ml. As maximum values of TMP-resistance
we determined 5o ug/ml except for Pseudomonas; here
the values were more than about loo ug/ml. Thus we
found for resistant Coli-, Klebsiella- and Proteus-
strains values which were 125 to extremely 5oo times
greater than those found for the sensitive test Coli
strain K 12 which has a MIC-value of o.1 ug/ml. We
did not find any strain the resistance of which was
higher than 5o ug/ml except Pseudomonas.

Clinical data of inpatients and the MIC-values
of the lo isolated organisms against different chemotherapeutics and Trimethoprim are shown in fig. 5.
Patients in most cases had suffered from pyelonephritis and had not been treated with TMP/SMZ drugs before.
The isolated organisms had a multiple resistance
against those chemotherapeutics which are mostly used
in our country. The TMP-resistance was always combined
with a resistance against several antibiotics.

In order to investigate, whether the TMP-resistance in our TMP-resistant strains is present in the
plasmide we tested for the ability to transfer this

No.	Age (Year)	Sex	Hospital	Diagnosis	Material	Therapy with TMP/SMZ	organism	TMP-resistance relative to MIC of standard value E. coli (0,1 µg/ml)	TMP/SMZ	SMZ	Spectrum of resistance
1	57	♀	Uro-logy	chron. PN	Urine	no	E. coli	500x	res	res	STAFuSuTp
2	52	♀	Uro-logy	chron. PN	Urine	no	Kleb-siella	250x	res	res	SCTANaFuSuTp
3	1	♂	Chil-dren	Dys-pepsia	Fae-ces	no	Kleb-siella	125x	ms	res	CTAKSuTp
4	70	♀	Uro-logy	PN	Urine	no	E. coli	500x	res	res	CANaSuTp
5	1	♀	Chil-dren	Dys-pepsia	Fae-ces	no	Kleb-siella	125x	ms	res	SCTASuTp
6	10	♀	Chil-dren	PN	Urine	no	Entero-cocci	500x	res	res	STp
7	76	♂	Uro-logy	PN	Urine	no	Entero-cocci	500x	ms	res	STp
8	35	♂	Uro-logy	PN	Urine	no	Kleb-siella	500x	res	res	SCTANaSuTp
9	20	♂	Derma-tology	Epididy-mitis	Ure-thra	no	Staph. aureus	125x	s	ms	PTp
10	1	♂	Chil-dren	PN	Urine	no	E.coli	250x	res	res	CTANaFuTp

Fig. 5
Patients with TMP-resistant organisms

property to a recipient strain (Coli K 12). Our investigations were performed with 6 Klebsiella strains
showing a TMP-MIC-value of 5o µg/ml. We didn't succeed in obtaining a plasmide transfer of TMP, although this was possible with Chloramphenicol, Tetracycline, Ampicillin/Carbenicillin, Sulfonamide, resp.
Tetracycline alone in three cases. However, Fleming,
Datta and Grüneberg succeeded in TMP-transfer; but
their strain had a TMP-resistance-value which was
10.ooo times higher ($>$1ooo µg/ml) than that of the
test strain Coli K 12.

        Summarizing we can state by our investigations
done as yet that at the present time the situation of
Co-Trimoxazole-resistance of bacteria in the GDR,
where TMP-drugs are used not yet in greater quantities, is still very favourable and that in our hospitals strains with TMP-resistance-factors did not
appear as yet. The risk of an increasing resistance
by an intensified use of these drugs only can be
avoided by their careful employment in clear indications with the aid of sensitivity testing.

Literature

1. Darrell, J.H., Garrod, L.P. and Waterworth, P.M.
   (1968), J.clin.Path. XXI, 2o2-2o9

2. Fleming, M.P., Datta, N. and Grüneberg (1972),
   Brit.med.J. 1, 726

3. Hedges, R.W., Datta, N. and Fleming, M.P. (1972),
   J.gen. Microbiol. 73, 573-575

4. Pinney, R.J. and Smith, J.T. (1973),
   J.med.Microbiol. 6, 13-19

SUSCEPTIBILITY OF CHLORAMPHENICOL-RESISTANT STRAINS OF SALMONELLA TYPHI TO TRIMETHOPRIM/SULFAMETHOXAZOLE

Margaret Barnett Bushby and S.R.M. Bushby

Wellcome Research Laboratories, Research Triangle

Park, North Carolina 27709, U.S.A.

SUMMARY

The resistance of certain strains of Salmonella typhi to chloramphenicol is due to an R-factor which also confers resistance to sulfonamides. Typhoid fever, caused by these strains, responds to treatment with TMP/SMX, but, because of their resistance to SMX, the question arises as to whether the sulfonamide contributes to the efficacy of the treatment.

With each of the strains examined the MIC of TMP was halved by the presence of SMX and the zones of inhibition produced by a disc containing TMP were increased by the addition of SMX. Also, with each of the strains, the decreases produced in the growth rate by sub-inhibitory concentrations of TMP were increased by the presence of SMX. In experimental infections of mice, the protection afforded by TMP was increased by SMX.

The combination trimethoprim/sulfamethoxazole (TMP/SMX) is generally regarded to be as effective as is chloramphenicol for the treatment of typhoid fever. It is effective in cases due to chloramphenicol-resistant strains (Linh 1974; Lampe et al 1974; Brown et al 1975) but as these strains are also resistant to sulfonamides the question arises as to whether patients infected with them would not respond equally as well to treatment with timethoprim alone as with the combination.

With respect to other infections, it has been recommended that the combination should not be used unless the causal organism is sensitive to both components but, as the principle claim for the combination is that it widens the spectrum of activity of the individual antibacterials, the recommendation conflicts with the claim. The widening of the spectrum of activity is due to synergy and it occurs because the resistance to the single components is not absolute. To appreciate how synergy can occur, in the presence of partial resistance, the mechanism of action of these antibacterials should be recalled.

Both drugs interfere with the biosynthesis of the folate coenzymes and thus ultimately affect the biosynthesis of proteins and nucleic acids. The sulfonamide acts as a competitor for para-aminobenzoic acid in the formation of dihydropteroic acid by dihydropteroate synthetase. This acid is condensed with glutamic acid to form dihydrofolic acid, which is then reduced to tetra-hydrofolic acid by dihydrofolate reductase. It is at this reduction step that TMP acts through binding with the dihydrofolate reductase. SMX and TMP therefore act in the same biochemical pathway and the enhancement of activity from their simultaneous administration is due to their actions being sequential.

The blocking of the enzyme dihydropteroate synthetase by sulfonamides and of dihydrofolate reductase by TMP is competitive, and the amount of inhibitor needed to reduce the biosynthesis of dihydropteroic acid or tetrahydrofolic acid to levels below those essential for growth depends on the amount of substrate present. Because the sulfonamide acts before TMP, its role in the dual action is merely to reduce the amount of dihydrofolic acid against which TMP competes. If the competition between TMP and dihydrofolic acid were linear, then the effects of the dual action would be no more than additive but, because the competition by TMP increases relatively with decreases in dihydrofolic acid, the effects are synergic.

In the case of clinically sulfonamide-resistant strains, the dihydrofolate biosynthesis by the majority, if not all of them, is reduced by therapeutic concentrations of the drugs but not to an extent which affects their growth. However, because of the non-linearity of the competition between trimethoprim and dihydrofolic acid, even a relatively small reduction in folates by sulfamethox-azole causes a significant decrease in the minimum effective concentration of trimethoprim.

To return to the sulfonamide-resistant strains of Salmonella typhi, we determined the sensitivities of 10 strains to TMP in the absence and presence of SMX in vitro.

Table 1. Sufonamide-resistant *Salmonella typhi*

Effects of x5 and x19 SMX on
minimum inhibitory concentration of TMP

Strain	Minimum Inhibitory Concentration - μg/ml		
	TMP alone	TMP + x5 SMX	TMP + x19 SMX
S4200 S4206 S4201 S4202 S4197 S4199 S4203 S4205 S4198	0.16	0.08 + 0.39	0.08 + 1.48

Medium:- Mueller Hinton Agar (Difco)

Table 2. Sufonamide-resistant *Salmonella typhi*

Effects of x19 SMX on zone of inhibition
produced by 1.25 μg TMP susceptibility disc

Strain	Diameter of Zone - mm		
	TMP 1.25 μg	SMX 23.75 μg	TMP 1.25 μg + SMX 23.75 μg
S4200	30	6	36
S4206	27	6	34
S4201	26	6	35
S4202	26	6	33
S4197	25	6	32
S4199	25	6	31
S4203	26	6	32
S4204	27	6	33
S4205	27	6	32
S4198	25	6	32

Medium:- Wellcotest Sensitivity Test Agar

Table 3.　Sufonamide-resistant *Salmonella typhi*

Effects of 30 µg SMX per ml on inhibition of growth by TMP

Strain	% Inhibition by TMP - µg/ml					
	0.03		0.01		0.003	
	Alone	+SMX	Alone	+SMX	Alone	+SMX
S4200	97	98	95	97	93	96
S4206	94	97	93	95	86	96
S4201	87	96	81	94	71	90
S4202	83	96	71	89	50	82
S4197	83	97	81	92	63	89
S4199	74	96	61	85	47	86
S4204	72	96	65	86	45	78
S4205	71	96	59	97	36	75
S4198	71	97	54	84	38	74

Medium:-　Oxoid Sensitivity Test Broth

Incubation:-　12 hours at 37°

Inhibition read turbidimetrically

Table 4.　Experiment in Mice

Organism　*Salmonella typhi* - S4205

Inoculum　10^9 organisms in 0.5 ml 4% hog mucin, intraperitoneally

Treatment　Drugs administered orally to groups of 6 mice, immediately after infection, 6 and 24 hrs. later.

Drug		% Survival	Average Day Survival
TMP	SMX		
5	1.25	83	5.8
5	-	33	2.3
1.25	2.5	50	3.8
1.25	-	0	1.7
0.62	2.5	50	4.0
0.62	1.25	67	4.8
0.62	-	17	1.2
-	2.5	0	<0.17
-	1.25	0	<0.17
-	0.62	0	<0.17
-	-	0	<0.17

Table 1 shows that the minimum inhibitory concentration of TMP was the same for each of the strains and that this concentration was halved by the presence of 5-times and 19-times the concentration of SMX. Table 2 shows that the diameters of the zone of inhibition produced by 6 mm discs containing 1.25 ug of TMP were increased when 23.75 ug of SMX was present; the increases varied among the strains, ranging from 5 to 9 mm. Further evidence of synergy was sought by comparing the amount of growth of these strains in a fluid medium after 12 hours' incubation in the presence of 0.03, 0.01 and 0.003 ug TMP per ml, along and with 30 ug SMX per ml. Growth was read turbidometrically. Table 3 shows the percentage inhibition produced by TMP along and the percentage increase of this inhibition by the presence of SMX. Although from these results it is apparent that the sensitivities of the strains to these sub-effective concentrations of TMP vary, with each strain the sensitivity is increased by SMX.

Evidence of the increased sensitivity to TMP, demonstrated by each of the three in vitro methods, was sought in infected mice. Although the mouse is not a good model for exploring the potentialities of trimethoprim for the treatment of infections in man, because in it the half-life of trimethoprim is very much shorter, being only about one half, it is the only model available. The organisms suspended in hog mucin were injected intraperitoneally and although several of the strains were tested, none proved lethal except when approximately 10^9 organisms were injected. Under these conditions the infection was very acute with death occurring overnight so it in no way resembled the natural infection in man. However, TMP afforded some protection and this was enhanced by the presence of SMX. Table 4 shows the results obtained with one of the strains.

In conclusion therefore, although these chloramphenicol-resistant strains are sulfonamide-resistant, their susceptibility to TMP is enhanced by the presence of SMX; so, as with other TMP-sensitive - SMX-resistant organisms, there is a rational basis for treating patients with typhoid fever due to chloramphenicol/sulfonamide-resistant strains with the combination rather than with TMP alone.

(These strains were kindly supplied by Dr. Virginia Vaquez, Mexico City).

ACTIVITY OF TRIMETHOPRIM AND SULPHONAMIDES AGAINST PSEUDOMONAS AERUGINOSA

Daphne Gray and J.M.T. Hamilton-Miller

The Royal Free Hospital

Pond Street, Hampstead, London NW3 2QG

Infections with Pseudomonas aeruginosa, although relatively uncommon under normal conditions, may cause serious clinical problems because of the considerable intrinsic resistance of this species. This applies especially to urinary tract infections, where oral therapy, such as with co-trimoxazole (Brumfitt & Pursell 1972), is highly desirable. Ps.aeruginosa is generally regarded as being resistant to co-trimoxazole, which is not therefore used for the treatment of urinary tract infections of such aetiology. However, we have noticed that a high proportion of Ps.aeruginosa isolated at this Hospital appear to be sensitive to a 300 µg. disk of "triple sulphonamides". Consequently, we decided to investigate further the activity of different sulphonamides against Ps.aeruginosa and also the occurrence of synergism between trimethoprim (tm) and sulphamethoxazole (SMZ).

MATERIALS AND METHODS

Antimicrobial Agents

Trimethoprim lactate, SMZ and sulphadimidine (SDM) were generously given by the Wellcome Foundation, Roche Products and Imperial Chemical Industries Ltd., respectively. Sulphadiazine (SDZ) was obtained as a solution containing 1 gm in 4 ml. (sulpha-diazine for injection, B.P., May & Baker Ltd.). Aqueous solutions containing 15 mg./ml. of either SMZ or SDM were made by adding the minimum amount of conc. NaOH solution. It was possible to prepare a solution of SMZ containing 150 mg./ml. by suspending the solid in 40% (v/v) propylene glycol and adding 10 M NaOH dropwise.

Antibiotic sensitivity disks containing 25 µg. SMZ, 300 µg.
"compound sulphonamide" (sulphathiazole, SDM and sulphamerazine),
2.5 µg. tm and 25 µg. co-trimoxazole (23.75 µg. SMZ + 1.25 µg. tm)
were obtained from Oxoid Ltd.

Bacterial Strains

82 strains of Ps.aeruginosa, isolated from urine specimens
sent to this Department, were tested. The strains were identified
by the methods of Phillips (1969).

Microbiological Methods

MIC of the sulphonamides and tm were determined, separately,
by the plate dilution method, using Sensitest agar (Oxoid).
Bacteria were grown overnight in Hartley's digest broth (Southern
Group Laboratories), diluted 1 to 1000 in water, and inoculated in
batches of 25 strains with a multiple inoculator. Plates were read
after overnight incubation at 37C, the end-point being taken where
at least 99.9% inhibition of the initial inoculum was noted.

Synergy testing was performed by carrying out MIC determinations
with serial dilutions of tm made in various concentrations of SMZ.
Isobolograms were constructed from the results, and synergism was
quantified in terms of fractional inhibitory concentrations.

Disk sensitivity testing was done using Sensitest agar, plates
being inoculated with 1 to 1000 dilutions of 6-hour cultures.

RESULTS

Disk Sensitivities

All the strains tested were resistant to tm, SMZ and co-
trimoxazole. However, 69 of the 82 strains (84%) were sensitive
to the "compound sulphonamide" disk.

MIC of Sulphonamides and Tm

MIC were determined for 81 strains for tm, and for 71 for the
sulphonamides. The results are shown in Table 1.

11 of the 13 strains which were resistant to the "compound
sulphonamide" disk were tested for MIC; all had MIC of 1 mg./ml.
or greater for SMZ and SDZ. For SMZ the mean MIC for these strains
was 16.4 mg./ml.

Table 1.   Activity of three sulphonamides and trimethoprim against
          <u>Ps.aeruginosa</u>

Antimicrobial Agent	MIC (μg./ml.)						
	31.3	62.5	125	250	500	1000	>1000
Sulphadiazine	6	17	20	14	3	3	8
Sulphamethoxazole	4	7	18	16	5	8	12
Sulphadimidine					1	1	69
Trimethoprim		19	12	23	14	7	6*

   * all these strains had MIC 2000 μg./ml.

       Discounting the highly resistant strains, it can be seen that
SDM is of very low activity, while SDZ (mean MIC = 116.4 μg./ml.)
was significantly more active (P < 0.01) than SMZ (mean MIC =
268 μg./ml.).   The activity of tm resembles that of SMZ, the mean
MIC being 214.8 μg./ml.   There was a good correlation (correlation
coefficient = 0.506, P < 0.001) between sensitivities to tm and to
SMZ among the individual strains.

Synergistic activity of Tm and SMZ

       Using 8 of the highly resistant strains, which had MIC of SMZ
> 2.5 mg./ml., we were unable to demonstrate significant synergism
between the components of co-trimoxazole.   On the other hand, with
all 22 of the less resistant strains (MIC for SMZ < 1 mg./ml.) which
we tested marked synergism was noted.   For these 22 strains, mean
MIC for tm and SMZ, acting alone, were 108 μg./ml. and 227 μg./ml.,
respectively.   When the two drugs were tested in combination,
however, mean MIC were reduced for each drug by some ten-fold;
thus, mean values of MIC in combination were 11.4 μg./ml. tm +
16.9 μg./ml. SMZ.

DISCUSSION

       <u>Ps.aeruginosa</u> strains make up about 2% of the bacterial
species isolated from urine samples at this Hospital, and all
appear to be resistant to the conventional co-trimoxazole disk.
Our results suggest that, for most of these strains, this
resistance is an artefact created by the use of an inappropriate
disk (tm : SMZ ratio of 1 : 20).   MIC for SMZ for the strains we
tested fall into two clear-cut groups - ≥ 2000 μg./ml. for the
minority population (16%) resistant to the "compound sulphonamide"
disk, and a mean of about 200 μg./ml. for the rest.   The latter

group had a mean MIC of tm of about 100 µg./ml.   Such concentrations
of SMZ and tm cannot readily be achieved in the urine;   however,
due to the high degree of synergy observed with the majority of the
strains (the MIC of each compound being reduced by about ten times)
and the fact that in urine the SMZ : tm ratio is approximately 2 : 1
(data of Kaplan et al 1973), these organisms will be susceptible to
the levels of tm and SMZ present in the urine during therapy with
co-trimoxazole.

Bushby and Barnett (1967) failed to find synergism between tm
and SMZ against Ps.aeruginosa, but they used the 1 : 20 ratio; their
findings, however, caused Fowle (1968) to suggest that co-trimoxazole
was not indicated for any Ps.aeruginosa infections.   Ritzerfeld and
Hasch (1972) and Simmons (1970) both reported some degree of
synergy between tm and SMZ, but the former used a 1 : 20 ratio, and
the latter's strains were extremely sensitive to SMZ (MIC ≾ 12.5
µg./ml.), and so may not be representative.

Our findings show that Ps.aeruginosa may be put into the same
class, in regard to their sensitivity to co-trimoxazole, as
gonococci (Phillips et al 1970) and Bacteroides fragilis (Phillips
and Warren 1974): all three bacterial types are relatively
resistant to tm, and are sensitive to the combination by virtue of
the high degree of synergy which can be demonstrated.

SUMMARY

Our findings suggest that a high proportion (> 80%) of
Ps.aeruginosa strains isolated from urinary tract infections will
be inhibited by concentrations of tm and SMZ likely to be found in
the urine during treatment with co-trimoxazole. A convenient marker
for these strains is their sensitivity to a 300 µg. disk of
"compound sulphonamide".

REFERENCES

Brumfitt, W. and Pursell, R.   1972 Brit.med.J., 2, 673.
Bushby, S.R.M. and Barnett, M.   Proc.5th.Int.Congress Chemotherapy
    (Vienna, 1967), A 1-6, 753.
Fowle, A.S.E.   1968 Brit.med.J., 2, 557.
Kaplan, S.A., Weinfeld, R.E., Abruzzo, C.W., McFaden, K., Lewis, M.
    and Weissman, L.   1973 J.inf.Dis., 128S, 547.
Phillips, I.   1969 J.med.Microbiol., 2, 9.
Phillips, I., Rimmer, D., Ridley, M., Lynn, R. and Warren, C.
    1970 Lancet, 1, 263.
Phillips, I. and Warren, C.   1974 Lancet, 1, 827.
Ritzerfeld, W. and Hasch, B.   1972 Chemotherapy, 17, 348.
Simmons, N.A.   1970 J.clin.Path., 23, 757.

MICROBIOLOGICAL AND CLINICAL STUDIES WITH CO-TRIMOXAZOLE

M. Aguirre, J.M. Alés, F. Lahoz & R. Vela

Fundación Jiménez Díaz

Madrid-3.- Spain

The antimicrobial drug Co-trimoxazole presents a wider spectrum of activity as compared with the action of each one of its two components when utilized individually.Co-trimoxazole is active upon the majority of pathogenic bacteria among which are those that today constitute great probleme, specially related to hospital infections, which we will discuss in this paper.

Results obtained with Co-trimoxazole in 3,700 antiobiograms performed in 1,974 with the following antimicrobial drugs:Benzyl-penicillin, ampicillin, cloxacillin, carbenicillin, cephalothin, cephaloridine, cephalexine, vancomycin, fucidin, lincomycin, streptomycin, kanamycin, neomycin, aminosidine, gentamicin, tobramicin, colistin, rifamycin, tetracycline, chloranphenicol, erythromycin, novobiocin, fosfomycin, nitrofurantoin, nalidixic acid, oxolinic acid, sulphonamide, co-trimoxazole, are presented:

Co-trimoxazole in antibiograms

	Index of sensitivity	Index of benignity	Index of specificity
Staphylococcus aureus	91	78	1.2
Proteus mirabilis	65	60	1.1
Escherichia coli	81	57	1.4
Pseudomonas aeruginosa	18	38	0.5
Klebsiella	67	54	1.2
Enterobacter	75	54	1.4
Providencia	0	0	0

369

The index of sensitivity with co-trimoxazole, equivalent to the percentage of bacterial strains sensitive to the antimicrobial drug are shown in the first column. The indez of benignity, that is, the number of bacteria sensitive to this drug, compared with the sensitivity to the rest of the antimicrobial agents tested, is presented in the second column. The index of specificity, resulting from the division of the index of sensitivity by that of the benignity, are the results presented in the third column.

This data demonstrates the positive value of co-trimoxazole, except in the cases of infection by Pseudomona and Providencia.

We have studied 83 cases of respiratory infection in which the following bacteria were isolated: Haemophilus influenzae, Klebsiella pneumoniae. Staphylococcus aureus, Aerobacter aerogenes, Proteus mirabilis, Escherichia coli. Pseudomonas aeruginosa, Diplococcus pneumoniae. All of these cases were treated during 7 days with a total dose of 320 mgs. of Trimethoprim and 1,600 mgs. of sulphametoxazole by day, in divided doses every 12 hours. Cultures of the sputum were repeated three days after the termination of tretment wit the results de 80.7 % of negative culture.

Clinical results were evaluated simultaneously by determining the body temperature, cough, characteristic of the sputum, etc. with the results: Good 67 cases, fair 10 cases, bad 6 cases. In one case, treatment was interrupted because of the appearance of exanthema and in another case because of gastric intolerance. One other case presented mild gastric discomfort.

We also treated in a similar way, 58 cases of urinary infection, where cultures presented the following: Escherichia coli, Proteus mirabilis, Proteus indol +, Aerobacter aerogenes, Pseudomonas aeruginosa, and in which the cultures obtained three days after terminating treatment, presented 76.4% of negative culture

Clinical results are: Good 48 cases, fair 3 cases, bad 7 cases. No data is present about two cases which did not complete treatment because of gastric symptoms.

We cultured urine of paraplegyc patients with indwelling catheter, were we found a disappearance of the bacteria or an im-

portant diminution in the number of colonies in the urine. This
has an evident importance on the possible complications related to
 catheterized patients.

        In all cases treated, we determined before and after admi-
nistration of co-trimoxazole, blood counts, alkaline phosphatase,
TGO, TGP, creatinine, urea, glucose and routine urinalysis, without
observing any significant alteration of normal values.

        Because of the possible effect of co-trimoxazole upon the
folate, we determined the blood values of folate, and vitamine B_{12}
and index of Herbert, without observing any anormal variations.

        In view of the data obtained, and because of the conve-
nient form of administration and minimal effects of co-trimoxazole,
we beñieve that this antimicrobial agent has an important place in
actual antimicrobial therapy.

COTRIMOXAZOLE AS AN ALL-PURPOSE ANTIBACTERIAL AGENT

J. C. Gould and B. Watt

Central Microbiological Laboratories

Western General Hospital, Edinburgh

Previous experience with the use of a restrictive and rotational antibiotic policy has been encouraging, (Forfar et al, 1966; Gould, 1975; Keay et al, 1967; Samuel and Gould, 1967). The possible benefits are the control of ecological pressure in hospital wards by withdrawing the selective pressure of certain antibiotics so that there is less chance for the survival and propagation of antibiotic resistant strains. In this way the period of usefulness of important antibacterial agents may be increased. Clinical staff may also welcome the resulting simplification of choice of drug, and mistakes in administration are less likely.

This report summarises experience with such a type of antibiotic policy in a small general medical and surgical hospital of 100 beds, when cotrimoxazole was the antibacterial agent of choice for all infections. Relatively small amounts of this antibacterial agent had been used in treatment during preceding years (Gould 1975) and the frequency of isolation of cotrimoxazole-resistant strains of bacteria from patients lesions and from the environment was relatively low. Accordingly both clinicians and bacteriologists agreed that it was a suitable agent to succeed the cephalosporins (cephalexin) which had been used as the drug of choice during the previous phase of the investigation. The cephalosporins were withdrawn when the cotrimoxazole was introduced as the drug of choice.

The choice of a general all-purpose antibacterial

agent depends not only upon its antibacterial spectrum
but also on its toxicity, acceptability, and whether or
not it can be administered parenterally as well as
orally, since there are a number of patients,
particularly those who are post-operative, who require
parenteral administration at least for a few days.
For this purpose a parenteral preparation of cotrimoxazole
(Bactrim infusion, Roche) was made available for this
clinical trial.

        Discussion with clinical colleagues agreed that all
patients with an infection meriting chemotherapy would
receive cotrimoxazole, 2 drapsules, 3 times a day for
7 days (each drapsule contained 80 mgm trimethoprim and
500 mgm sulphamethoxazole) unless there was any special
indication to alter the dosage.   Where parenteral
therapy would be indicated, cotrimoxazole for intravenous infusion was used in a dosage of 10 ml twice
daily, increased to 15 ml twice daily in severe
infections, and administered in not less than 125 ml of
fluid for each infusion (Bactrim infusion, Roche - each
5 ml contains 80 mgm trimethoprim and 400 mgm sulphamethoxazole in a vehicle containing 40% propylene glycol
at pH 10.5).   This cotrimoxazole preparation is compatible with most routine infusion fluids but ad-mixture
with amino-acid or other parenteral feeding fluids was
avoided.   Contra-indications to cotrimoxazole were any
allergy to the drug, liver damage or blood dyscrasias
or any specific clinical or bacteriological reason
which made the clinical outcome of treatment doubtful.
Also patients admitted with an infection under treatment
continued on the chemotherapy they were receiving.
Further patients who were failing to respond to treatment
were changed to alternative therapy which was directed
by clinical and/or bacteriological information available.

        Evaluation of the trial was made by bacteriological
examination of material from patients under treatment
whenever available and by clinical assessment and
recovery.   Detailed bacteriological and clinical pro-
formata were completed for each patient as treatment
proceeded.   Strains of bacteria isolated from patients
with infection, from members of attendant staff and
from the environment were examined, identified and had
detailed sensitivity tests carried out.   These
observations were similar to those carried out during
the year preceding the trial (1971-72) and during the
first phase with cephalosporin in use (1972-73), so
that a reasonable comparison could be made between the
results.   In the event this second phase of the trial

has continued for a period of two years (1973-75).

The types of bacteria isolated from patients infections are shown in Table 1. The number of infections treated with chemotherapy during the year preceding the trial was 158; during the first phase it was 176, but over the two years of cotrimoxazole use, only 224 were treated. This represents a fall in the number of treated infections, particularly respiratory tract infections admitted to the medical hospital. There was no appreciable change in the number of post-operative infections. The proportion of the different organisms isolated showed no significant change over the two periods. It must be remembered that as this is an acute hospital the majority of infections were either contracted outwith the hospital or developed as a result of auto-infection. There was little bacteriological evidence of cross-infection except in a few surgical patients. Thus antibiotic resistance is not a major problem as shown by the proportion of resistant strains isolated (Table 2). The proportion of anti-biotic and cotrimoxazole-resistant strains from patients is not significantly altered since before the trial commenced. Most of the strains resistant to both the cephalosporins and cotrimoxazole were Pseudomonads and coliform bacilli of a basically resistant type and there was no evidence of the emergence of resistance in treated cases except when replacement with one or other of these refractory types of organism occurred. It is encouraging that the proportion of ampicillin and tetracycline-resistant strains isolated from the environ-ment has fallen during the first and second phases of this trial; admittedly the proportion of cephalosporin-resistant organisms from the environment has increased, possibly due to the use of cephalexin during the first cycle, but this proportion can be expected to fall in subsequent years. The two years of cotrimoxazole usage has not altered the frequency of isolation of cotrimoxa-zole-resistant strains from the environment.

Cotrimoxazole has thus been used for two years in the majority of patients presenting with infection in a general hospital. It has proved itself active in most cases of infection including those of the respiratory tract, urinary tract, soft tissues, post-operative wounds and infections of the biliary tract. The number of instances when it had to be withdrawn because of failure of response was small.

TABLE 1

BACTERIA ISOLATED FROM LESIONS

Bacteria	Year before trial	During two years of cotrimoxazole
Staph.pyogenes	50	76
Staph.albus	4	13
Streptococcus		
α-type	1	7
β-type	15	16
γ-type	16	28
anaerobic	3	4
Pneumococcus	42	55
Haemophilus	58	85
Esch.coli and other coliforms	87	162
Proteus	13	21
Pseudomonads	5	10
Clostridium	4	8
Bacteroides	7	7
Neisseria	0	1
	305	493
No. of infections per year	158	112

TABLE 2

PERCENTAGE OF RESISTANT STRAINS ISOLATED

	Source of organism			
	Patients lesions		The environment	
Antibiotic	Before trial	During trial	Before trial	During trial
Cephalexin	14.8	15.7	11.9	17.1
Ampicillin	12.0	12.5	20.2	12.4
Cotrimoxazole	3.1	3.9	7.2	6.4
Tetracycline	21.0	20.1	15.2	9.3

The in vitro preparation was successfully used and presented no administrative problem although obviously more attention than with other parenteral antibiotics. No toxic effects either local or general were observed. The oral preparation was generally acceptable; during the second year a "soluble" oral preparation was used, but was not preferred by the patients. There were some patients who had epigastric pain, anorexia or nausea following dosage with cotrimoxazole but this was rarely severe and probably no more common than with other oral antibiotic preparations. A few patients developed rashes and in those, the drug was withdrawn and the rashes disappeared. No general toxicity nor side effects were observed and no incidental observation of adverse effect in haemopoietic response of any patient.

It is concluded that cotrimoxazole is an effective general purpose antibacterial agent with a low incidence of side effects which can be safely used orally and parenterally. It is effective against most of the bacteria causing infections in acute medical and surgical hospitals and the incidence of resistance remains low with no evidence during this trial, when there was more intensive use of cotrimoxazole, of this resistance increasing. To maintain this situation however it is recommended that care be taken to limit intensive use to phases, as in this trial, or to carry out very careful laboratory monitoring to detect cotrimoxazole resistance, so that steps to limit the spread of such strains can be undertaken.

We wish to thank the clinicians and nursing staff concerned for their co-operation. We gratefully acknowledge generous supplies of Bactrim from Roche Products Limited, and advice from Dr. Ian Lenox-Smith.

REFERENCES

Forfar, J.O., Keay, A.J., Maccabe, A.F., Gould, J.C. and Bain, A.D. Liberal use of antibiotics and its effect in neonatal staphylococcal infection, with particular reference to erythromycin. Lancet 2: 295-300 (1966).

Gould, J.C. The use of cephalosporins in a general hospital antibiotic policy. Proceedings of a Conference on the Cephalosporins, Stratford, 1975. In the press.

Keay, A.J., Syme, J. and Barnes, P.M. Cephaloridine in the treatment and prophylaxis of infection in the newborn. Postgraduate Medical Journal (August Supplement) 43: 105-9 (1967).

    Samuel, M.E. and Gould, J.C.   Bacteriological studies in a nursery during a trial with cephaloridine. Postgraduate Medical Journal (August Supplement) 43: 109-12 (1967).

TREATMENT OF HUMAN BRUCELLOSIS WITH DOXYCYCLINE AND TRIMETHOPRIM - SULFONAMIDE

L. Telegdy and Julia Kéri

Central Infectious Hospital

1097 Budapest, Hungary

SUMMARY

19 patients with different forms of brucellosis of bovine origin were treated with doxycycline (Vibramycin) 200 mg daily combined with trimethoprim - sulfonamide. Treatment was carried out for three weeks and was repeated when necessary. In subacute and chronic cases ACTH or prednisolone was also given and if a delayed type allergy was demonstrated a desensibilisation with specific antigen was also applied. No relapse or getting chronic had been noted in four acute cases with these doses, and two patients had relapsed with 100 mg doxycycline daily, after a good initial response. All five cases of subacute relapsing brucellosis had a complete recovery. No improvement had been achieved using antibiotics only in a case of chronic brucellosis and transitory regression of the symptomes in further severe cases can be attributed to additional therapy.

Human brucellosis in Hungary is not a frequent disease, though it still occurs among veterinary surgeons and dairy farm workers, due to bovine infection. The intracellular persistancy of brucellae, the developing delayed type hypersensitivity to the bacterial antigens, resulting in relapses and a tendency of chronicity, represent a difficult task in the therapy. Antibiotics are the more effective the earlier they are administered. This therapy must be adjuvated with corticothrophine or prednisolone in relapsing, asubacute stadium and in chronic brucellosis. When a delayed type allergy is demonstrated, it is worth attempting a desensibilisation with killed brucella suspension (Olderhausen, 1969).

Table 1.   Our Therapeutical Pattern in Treatment of Brucellosis

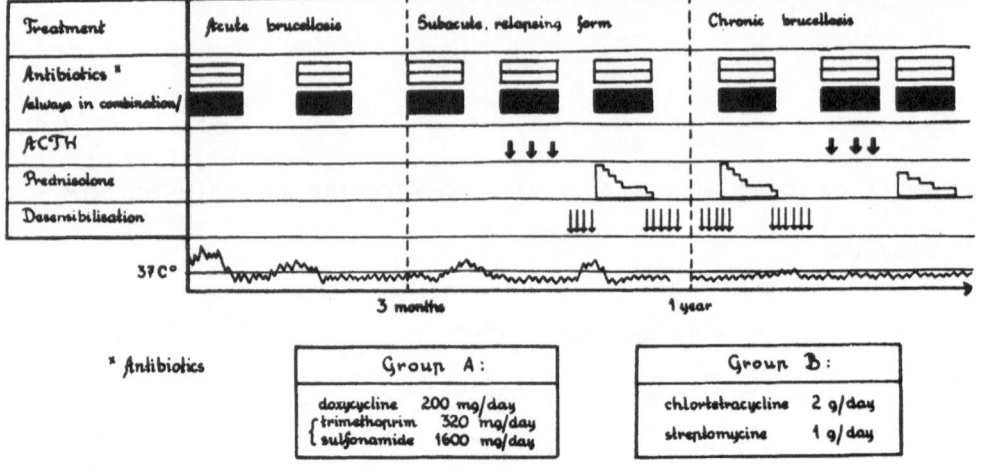

* Antibiotics

Group A:	
doxycycline	200 mg/day
{ trimethoprim	320 mg/day
{ sulfonamide	1600 mg/day

Group B:	
chlortetracycline	2 g/day
streptomycin	1 g/day

Table 2.   Clinical Results in the Treatment of Brucellosis

	Group A	Group B
Acute brucellosis		
Nº of Patients	6	32
Complete recovery	4	16
Relapses	1	14
Chronic outcome	1	2
Subacute-relapsing form		
Nº of Patients	5	13
Complete recovery	5	1
Relapses continue	none	10
Chronic outcome	none	2
Chronic brucellosis		
Nº of Patients	8	17
Complete recovery	none	none
Transitory improvement	7	13
No effect of therapy	1	4

Our therapeutical scheme in different stadiums of bracellosis is shown in the 1st table.

Antibiotics were given alsways in combination in acute, subacute and chronic stadium as well. Treatment was continued for three weeks and was repeated in the same dosage when it was necessary.

Till 1973, we treated 62 cases with chlortetracycline (Tetr.) and streptomycine (Strm) according to the WHO/FAO principles on the therapy of brucellosis (1964)(Group "B" in table 1). We observed gastrointestinal side-effects in half of the patients during the long-term treatment with Tetr. There was a risk of neurotoxicity using 30 gm or more Strm. in a patient.

After the encouraging experiences of Schafei and Luka (1973), in the treatment of brucellosis with doxycycline (Dox.), as well as Lal (1970) and Daikos et al (1973) with trimethoprim – sulfonamide (TMS.), since 1973 we have administered these two drugs in combination (Group "A" in the table, 19 patients). The high sensitivity of brucellae to both durgs and the high tissue concentration of Dox. (Wittenau and Delahunt, 1966) are the benefits for which we considered this combination as a "drug of choice" in the treatment of brucellosis.

We observed that in febrile periods of the disease the fever ceased on the 3rd – 4th day, organ manifestations as hepatomegaly, orchitis, arthralgia, etc. usually disappeared after a three-week treatment. No side-effect attributable to Dox. was observed, and one case of transient leukopenia could br ascribed to TMS

We achieved significantly better results with the Dox.+ TMS pattern, in comparison with the Tetr. +Strm. combination. Our clincial results can be seen in the 2nd table.

Acute brucellosis: no relapse or chronicity had been noted in 4 patients using 200 mg Dox. daily, combined with 320 mg trimethoprim and 1.600 mg sulfonamide daily. Using 100 mg/day Dox. in the same combination, we observed after a good initial response a development of osteomyelitis brucellosa in a patient, and a relapse in a further case. In the group "B" treated with Tetr. +Strm., half of the patients (16/32) suffered one or more relapses and two of them showed symptomes of chronicity in spite of the repeated treatment.

Subacute, relapsing brucellosis: all the five patients
recovered completely after the therapy with Dox.+TMS. While in
the group "BP only one patient out of 13 had recovered.

Chronic brucellosis: as there is no certain evidence of
bacterial activity in each case of this stadium, and symptomes
registered may be attributed to sensitisation with brucellae, it
is difficult to evelute the effectiveness of the therapy in
chronic brucellosis. We had not obtained any improvement in one
case using Dox. +TMS and transitory regression of the symptomes
in further 7 cases may be due to complex therapy. This is the
case also in group "BP. However, the supposed presence of the
pathogen indicates that in this stadiu, - besides other therapeutical measures - antibiotics (preferably Dox.+TMS) should be used
as well.

REFERENCES

1.   Daikos, G.L. et al (1973), J. Infect. Dis 128, Suppl. 731

2.   Lal, S. and Modawal, K. (1970), Brit. med. J. 3, 256.

3.   Olderhausen, H.F. (1969), in: Gsell, O. and Mohr, W.: Infektions-
      krankheiten 11/1, Springer, Berlin 539.

4.   Schafei, A.Z. and Luka, W.S. (1973), Brit. med. J. 3, 50.

5.   WHO/FAO Expert Committee on Brucellosis (1964), WHO Techn.
      Rep. Ser. No. 289.

6.   von Wittenau, M.S. and Delahunt, C.S. (1966), J. Pharmacol.
      exp. Ther. 152, 164.

TRIMETHOPRIM/SULFAMETHOXAZOLE SYNERGY AND PROSTATIS

S.R.M. Bushby and Margaret Barnett Bushby

Wellcome Research Laboratories

Research Triangle Park, North Carolina 27709, U.S.A.

SUMMARY

TMP/SMX is often effective in the treatment of bacterial prostatitis, but, because of the concentration of TMP in the prostatic fluid of dogs is four times that in plasma and the concentration of SMX in this fluid is only one-tenty of that in plasma, the question arises as to whether SMX contributes to the efficacy.

The ratio of TMP to SMX in plasma of man is around 1:20 but, based on observations in dogs, it is only 2:1 in the prostatic fluid. Although synergy between TMP and SMX occurs over a wide range of ratios, the 2:1 ratio is strikingly different from the 1:20 in the plasma which, based on maximum reduction in MIC, is near optimal for the majority of pathogenic bacteria. Therefore, the MIC of TMP and SMX, singly and together, in the ratios of 2:1, 1:1 and 1:2 have been determined for 24 strains of bacterial species likely to cause prostatitis. Four strains were sulfonamide-resistant and these were the only ones which did not show synergy with the combinations.

Chronic bacterial prostatis, which is considered to be a cause of recurrent urinary infections in men (Meares and Stamey, 1968; Stamey et al, 1970), is rarely cured by treatment with any of the antibacterials commonly used for these infections. According to Winningham et al (1968) these antibacterials fail because they do not penetrate in adequate concentrations into the prostatic fluid to eliminate the infection completely. From studies in dogs they concluded that the reason for the antibacterials not penetrating into this fluid is due to their unsuitable physical properties. These investigators proposed that an effective antibacterial for the treatment of prostatis should be lipid soluble with basic properties, have a pK_a of 8.6 or greater and possess optimal biological activity at a pH of 6.6

Reeves and Ghilchik (1970), because Bushby and Hitchings (1968) had reported a considerable degree of diffusion of trimethoprim (TMP) into body fluids, measured the concentration of this antibacterial in the prostatic fluid of dogs; they found the concentration to be 2 to 3 times that present in plasma. Robb et al (1971) using TMP and its close analogue, diaveridine, for testing the hypothesis that a weak base can attain concentrations in prostatic fluid which are in excess of simultaneously measured plasma levels, confirmed that TMP was present in this fluid at concentrations some 3 to 4 times those present in plasma. Both groups of workers, therefore, suggested that TMP, in conjunction with a sulfonamide, in order to take advantage of synergy, should be used for the treatment of bacterial prostatitis.

Clinical experience with the trimethoprim-sulfamethoxazole combination is confirming these forecases (Meares, 1973 and 1975; Drach, 1974; Meares and Stamey, 1975) but for eradication of the infection, treatment may have to be prolonged. Doubts about the value of including sulfamethoxazole (SMX) in the treatment have been raised on the grounds that SMX does not show the same selective penetration into prostatic fluid. Winningham and Stamey (1969) showed that the concentration of SMX in prostatic fluid was only about one-tenth of that present in plasma and this finding agrees with that of Robb et al (1971). Thus, it is argued that the ratio of concentrations of TMP:SMX in the prostatic fluid is far removed from the optimum ratio for producing maximum synergy which is about 1:20 (Bushby, 1973).

Much stress has been given to the need for the drugs to be present in optimum ratio at the sites of infections but it cannot be stressed too strongly that the effect on the organism is the same over a wide range of ratios and that the optimum ratio is merely the one with which the effect is produced by the lowest concentration of each drug. With other ratios the minimum effective concentration of one of the components will be less but the concentration of the other component will be greater than occurs with the optimum ratio. The need for attaining this optimum ratio only arises when there is a problem in reaching adequate concentrations of the drug at the infection site, a situation that rarely occurs.

Table 1.   Potentiation of TMP by SMX

Ratios — 2:1, 1:1 & 1:2

Organism	MIC µg/ml		FIC[*] Index		
	TMP alone	SMX alone	TMP:SMX 2 : 1	TMP:SMX 1 : 1	TMP:SMX 1 : 2
Escherichia coli S5471	0.06	3	0.505	1.02	1.04
Escherichia coli S5377	0.25	12	0.505	0.501	0.52
Escherichia coli S5351	0.06	>384	>1.01	>1.01	>1.01
Escherichia coli S3663	0.5	12	0.51	0.502	0.504
Escherichia coli S5102	0.25	>384	>1.01	>1.01	>1.01
Escherichia coli S5093	0.25	>384	>1.01	>1.01	>1.01
Escherichia coli CN314	0.12	3	0.51	0.52	0.54
Escherichia coli ATCC25922	0.25	6	1.02	0.52	0.54
Klebsiella pneumoniae S5466	0.5	24	0.505	0.51	0.502
Klebsiella sp. S5379	0.5	12	0.51	0.52	0.54
Klebsiella sp. S5378	0.5	12	0.51	0.52	0.54
Klebsiella sp. S3661	0.5	6	0.52	0.54	0.58
Klebsiella sp. S4921	0.5	>384	>1.01	>1.01	>1.01

$$* \text{ FIC (Fractional Inhibitory Concentration)} = \frac{\text{MIC of drug in combination}}{\text{MIC of drug alone}}$$

Table 2.   Potentiation of TMP by SMX

Ratios - 2:1, 1:1 & 1:2

Organism	MIC µg/ml		FIC*Index		
	TMP alone	SMX alone	TMP:SMX 2 : 1	TMP:SMX 1 : 1	TMP:SMX 1 : 2
Proteus mirabilis S5540	1.0	0.75	0.41	0.285	0.285
Proteus mirabilis S5462	1.0	0.75	0.41	0.285	0.205
Proteus mirabilis S5363	1.0	1.5	0.33	0.41	0.285
Proteus mirabilis S3662	1.0	0.75	0.41	0.205	0.205
Proteus mirabilis S3731	2.0	1.5	0.205	0.285	0.222
Proteus vulgaris CN329	1.0	0.75	0.205	0.285	0.455
Staphylococcus aureus CN491	0.5	6	0.52	0.54	0.29
Staphylococcus aureus ATCC25923	0.5	1.5	0.58	0.41	0.41
Staphylococcus aureus S5447	1.0	6	0.27	0.29	0.165
Staphylococcus aureus S5515	0.5	6	0.52	0.54	0.29
Staphylococcus aureus S5407	0.5	3	0.54	0.58	0.33

*FIC (Fractional Inhibitory Concentration) $= \dfrac{\text{MIC of drug in combination}}{\text{MIC of drug alone}}$

However, in order to document this contention, we have compared the in vitro antibacterial activities of TMP and SMX, alone and in the ratios that they would be expected to be present in prostatic fluid if the drugs behave in the same way in man as they do in the dog. The concentrations of TMP and SMX are usually about 2 ug/ml and 40 ug/ml, respectively, i.e. 1:20 in plasma. Therefore, if the concentrations of TMP and SMX in the prostatic fluid are, respectively fourfold higher and tenfold lower than in the plasma, then the concentrations in the prostatic fluid will be 8 ug TMP per ml and 4 ug SMX per ml, i.e. in the ratio of 2:1. The ratios in which we determined the minimum inhibitory concentrations of the two drugs were 1:2, 1:1 and 2:1.

Tables 1 and 2 show the results with 24 organisms likely to cause urinary infections. The activities of the single drugs are expressed as the minimum inhibitory concentrations (MIC) and those of the combinations as fractional inhibitory concentrations (FIC) indices. This index is the sum of the MIC of each of the drugs in the combination expressed as a decimal fraction of the MIC of the respective drug when acting alone. Indices below 1.0 denote synergy and the lower the index, the greater is the synergy. The observed indices show that, even with the 2:1 ratio, with only 5 of the 24 strains was there no evidence of synergy; with 1 of these 5 strains synergy did occur with a 1:1 and 1:2 ratios and the other 4 strains were resistant to >384 ug SMX per ml.

The suggestion that SMX is unnecessary in the treatment of prostatitis is based on the results of kinetic studies in normal dogs. Whether or not the drugs behave similarly in man, especially when the prostate is inflamed, is not known for certain because it is not possible to avoid urinary contamination of prostatic fluid without surgical intervention. However, at the Trimethoprim/Sulfamethoxazole Symposium held in Boston, an unidentified speaker (1972) reported that prostatic fluid was obtained from a young man with urinary diversion (bilateral ureterostomy) and that the TMP concentration in it was 2 to 3 times that in the plasma. So, in this young man TMP behaved similarly to the way that it does in the dog but the prostate of this man was, presumably, not infected.

In conclusion, synergy does occur with ratios of TMP and SMX that are present in the prostatic fluid of dogs. Therefore the same rational basis for using the combination, rather than either drug singly, applies for chronic prostatitis as it does for other infections.

REFERENCES

Bushby, S.R.M. and Hutchings, G.H. (1968), Brit. J. Pharmacol., 33, 72.

Bushby, S.R.M. (1973), J. Inf. Dis. Suppl., 128, S442.

Drach, G.W. (1974), J. Urol., 111/5, 637.

Meares, E.M.Jr., and Stamey, T.A. (1968), Invest. Urol., 5, 492.

Meares, E.M.Jr. (1973), J.Inf.Dis.Suppl., 128, S679.

Meares, E.M.Jr. (1975), Canad,Med.Assoc.J.Suppl., 112,22S.

Meares, E.M.Jr. and Stamey, T.A. (1975), Letter submitted to J.Amer.med.Assoc.

Reeves, D.S. and Ghilchik, M. (1970), Brit.J.Urol., 42, 66.

Robb, C.A., Carroll, P.T., Tippett, L.O. and Langston, J.B. (1971) Invest.Urol., 8, 6, 679.

Stamey, T.A., Meares, E.M.Jr. and Winningham, D.G. (1970) J.Urol., 103, 187.

Winningham, D.G., Nemoy, N.J. and Stamey, T.A. (1968), Nature, 219, 139.

Winningham, D.G. and Stamey,T.A. (1970), J,Urol., 104, 559.

THE CONCENTRATION OF SULPHAMETHOXAZOLE AND TRIMETHOPRIM IN HUMAN PROSTATE GLAND

W. Oosterlinck, R. Defoort and G. Renders

Department of Urology - Akademisch Ziekenhuis

B-9000 Ghent - Belgium

SUMMARY

Sulphamethoxazole and trimethoprim concentrations were measured in I9 enucleated human prostate glands. For sulphamethoxazole the ratio plasma concentration to that of the prostate varied from I.25 to 3.29. The trimethoprim concentrations were 2 to 3 times higher than in the plasma. These results are compared with the data of the literature. It seems obvious that the association SMZ-TMP is very useful in the treatment of chronic bacterial prostatitis.

In chronic bacterial prostatitis most anti-microbial drugs are ineffective for eradication of the infecting organisms from the prostatic fluid. Dunn and Stamey (I967) detected only minimal diffusion of nitrofurantoin into prostate fluid. Stamey et al.(I970) found that ampicillin, penicillin-G, cephalothin, kanamycin, oxytetracycline, polymyxin-B and nalidixic acid were nearly undetectable in the prostate fluid of the dog. Winningham and Stamey (I970) found an adequate therapeutic level of some sulphonamides in the prostatic fluid of the dog. Hessl and Stamey (I97I) concluded from theoretical and experimental data that of the tetracycline derivates only tetracyclinehydrochloride, if administered intravenously, has the potential of achieving significant inhibitory concentration against Gram-negative bacteria

in prostatic fluid. Their observations were in disagree-
ment with those of Fabre et al.(I97I) who found good
concentrations of doxycycline in the homogenized human
prostate gland.

At any rate one may conclude that the anti-bacterial arsenal for the treatment of chronic prostatitis
is very restricted. In the following study we measured
the concentration in human prostate gland of the combination of sulphamethoxazole (SMZ) and trimethoprim (TMP)
in order to define its possible role in the treatment
of chronic bacterial prostatitis.

METHODS and RESULTS

Nineteen patients, suffering from benign prostate
hypertrophy, received the drug combination before pro-
statectomy (enucleation). Their age varied from 59 to
8I years. Six of them received 400 mg SMZ + 80 mg TMP
by a single intramuscular injection about four hours
before operation; five others received the drug combination in 2 tablets, each containing 400 mg SMZ and 80 mg
TMP, also four hours before operation; the third group
(8 patients) received 2 tablets 2 times a day, for four
days, with the last intake some four hours before the
operation.

Bloodsamples were taken at the same time as enucleation of the prostate. Prostate and bloodsamples were
frozen immediately and kept at -20°C until just before
analysis. TMP was determined by the spectrofluorimetric
method of Schwartz et al.(I969; Schwartz, I972) and free
(active) and total sulphonamides by the method of Bratton
and Marschall, modified by Rieder (Rieder,I972).

The SMZ and TMP determinations in plasma and prostate are listed in table 1.

The highest concentrations of SMZ and TMP are
reached after the repeated dose. The prostate was better
impregnated with SMZ after four days : the plasma/pro-
state ratio varied from I.25 to 3.29. TMP is 2 to 3 times
more concentrated in the prostate than in the plasma.
These high concentrations are reached already after four
hours. After four days of treatment the SMZ/TMP ratio
varied from 2 to 8.

Table 1 : all concentrations are expressed in /ml. $\bar{X}$ = mean value.

	SMZ (active)			TMP			Prostate
	Plasma	Prostate	Plasma/Prostate	Plasma	Prostate	Plasma/Prostate	SMZ/TMP
I amp. intra-muscul.	12,1	3,16	3,82	0,41	0,81	0,50	3
	13,5	5,06	2,66	0,46	1,34	0,34	3
	23,2	6,51	3,56	0,51	1,67	0,30	3
	21,2	-	-	0,54	2,47	0,21	-
	18,2	5,33	3,41	0,22	1,67	0,13	3
	17,8	5,87	3,03	0,26	1,34	0,19	4
	$\bar{X}$ = 17,8	$\bar{X}$ = 5,19	$\bar{X}$ = 3,29	$\bar{X}$ = 0,40	$\bar{X}$ = 1,55	$\bar{X}$ = 0,28	$\bar{X}$ = 3,7
2 tabl.	17,8	4,61	3,86	1,37	3,13	0,43	1
	27,1	13,40	2,02	0,93	3,17	0,29	4
	32,9	10,00	3,29	1,18	5,00	0,23	2
	30,6	-	-	0,97	2,41	0,40	-
	2,26	0,45	5,02	0,43	0,47	0,91	0,95
	$\bar{X}$ = 26,2	$\bar{X}$ = 7,11	$\bar{X}$ = 3,55	$\bar{X}$ = 0,98	$\bar{X}$ = 2,84	$\bar{X}$ = 0,45	$\bar{X}$ = 2
2 x 2 tabl. during 4 days	108,2	50,1	2,15	2,53	5,84	0,43	8
	66,6	52,8	1,55	2,96	5,82	0,50	7
	40,8	15,2	2,68	1,91	5,09	0,37	2
	63,2	19,2	3,29	2,68	5,57	0,48	3
	58,0	23,6	2,45	1,73	4,11	0,42	5
	80,6	64,5	1,24	2,82	7,73	0,36	8
	43,4	-	-	0,73	4,29	0,12	-
	66,3	29,1	2,27	3,91	5,91	0,66	4
	$\bar{X}$ = 65,9	$\bar{X}$ = 34,9	$\bar{X}$ = 2,23	$\bar{X}$ = 2,39	$\bar{X}$ = 5,54	$\bar{X}$ = 0,42	$\bar{X}$ = 5,3

DISCUSSION

Research seems to show that the concentrations of
SMZ and TMP, measured in the enlarged, enucleated prostate are representative for the concentrations of both
products in the acini of the prostate gland in adult
men.

The factors determining diffusion into the prostate gland (lipid solubility, pKa and degree of ioni-
sation, proteinbinding) are excellent for TMP (Stamey
et al., I970). Reeves and Ghilchik (I970) were the first
to draw attention to the high concentrations of TMP
(two to three times higher than in serum) in the prostate fluid of the dog. Robb et al.(I97I) affirmed these
experiments and found concentrations as high as I6,2
times the plasma levels. Granato et al.(1973) obtained
comparable results.TMP concentrations in human prostatic
tissue and prostatic fluid were first measured through
a microbiological method by Nielsen and Hansen (I972).
They found the concentrations of TMP "at a therapeutically active level with respect to the majority of those
bacteria usually occurring in urinary tract infection".
We found TMP concentrations in the human prostate 2 to
3 times higher than in the plasma.

Winningham and Stamey (I970) and Robb et al.(I97I)
found a plasma concentration of SMZ IO times higher than
that of prostatic fluid. The prostate concentration of
SMZ in our study was more favourable. The ratio of plasma concentration to that of prostate varied from I.2. to
5.0.

Carroll et al.(I97I) established the anti-bacterial
effectiveness of the SMZ-TMP association in the prostate
fluid of the dog and suggested the possibility of therapeutic application to chronic bacterial prostatitis.
Schirren and Schaller (I97I) reported on the prolonged
high concentrations of SMZ/TMP in the human sperma fluid.

Although we found high concentrations of TMP in the
prostate, its ratio to SMZ is not optimal. Nevertheless
the ratio SMZ/TMP is sufficient to obtain a synergism
of both components against a wide variety of microorganisms and especially Gram-negative bacteria. (Böhni,
I969).

Communications, mentioning clinical trials of SMZ/ TMP in bacterial prostatitis are rather seldom. Stamey (I972) wrote about I3 patients of whom 2 seemed to be cured after I4 days of therapy. Hirdes and Schönfeld (I973) described excellent results in 25 of 32 patients. Drach (I974) reported of initial success in I4 of I8 patients, but relaps following therapy occurred in 8 of them. Clinical research is especially hindered by the difficulties in establishing the exact diagnosis of bacterial prostatitis.

The relevance of our results in association with other data of the literature for the treatment of bacterial prostatitis seems obvious.

REFERENCES

Böhni E. (I969) Schweiz. Med. Wschr. 99, I505-I5IO.
Böhni E. (I969) Chemother. suppl. ad Vol.I4, I-2I.
Carroll P.T., Robb C.A., Tippett L.O. and Langston J.B. (I97I) Invest. Urol. 8, 686-694.
Drach G.W. (I974) J. Urol. III, 637-639.
Dunn B.L. and Stamey T.A. (I967) J. Urol. 97, 505-507.
Fabre J., Milek E., Kalfopoulus P., Mérier G. (I97I) Schweiz. Med. Wschr.IOI, 625-633.
Granato J.J., Gross D.M. and Stamey T.A. (I973) Invest. Urol. II, 205-2IO.
Hessl J.M. and Stamey T.A. (I97I) J. Urol. IO6, 253-256.
Hirdes W.H. and Schönfeld J.K. (I973) Trimethoprim - Sulphamethoxazole in bacterial infections. Eds. L. Bernstein and A. Salter. London, Churchill Livingstone p.II3
Nielsen M.L. and Hansen I. (I972) J. Urol. and Nephrol. 6, 244-248.
Reeves D.S. and Ghilchik M. (I970) Brit. J. Urol.42, 66-72.
Rieder J.(I972) Chemother. I7, I-2I.
Rieder J.(I972) unpublished data.
Robb C.A., Carroll P.T., Tippet L.O. and Langston J.B. (I97I) Invest. Urol. 8, 679-685.
Schirren C. und Schaller D.(I97I) Androl.3, 24.
Schwartz D.E., Koechlin B.A. and Wenifeld R.E. (I969) Chemother. suppl. ad vol.I4, 22-29.
Schwartz D.E. (I972) unpublished data.
Stamey T.A.(I972) Urinary infections. Baltimore, Williams and Wilkins Co. p. I99.
Stamey T.A., Meares E.M. and Winningham D.G.(I970)J.Urol.

IO3, I87-I94.
Winningham D.G. and Stamey T.A.(I973) J. Urol. IO4,
559-563.

ACKNOWLEDGMENT

We wish to thank Prof. Rieder, Department of Experimental Medicine, F. Hoffmann-La Roche and Co. Ltd, Basle, for his technical cooperation in ensuring the determination of SMZ and TMP in the prostate gland.

LONG TERM TREATMENT WITH THE COMBINATION SMZ/TMP* IN CHILDREN WITH URINARY TRACT INFECTIONS

Leon Bernstein Hahn & Carlos A. Barclay

Instituto Nacional de Rehabilitacion del Lisiado
Servicio de Urologia y Departamento de Investigaciones
Clinicas, Productos Roche, Buenos Aires, Argentina

The results of a long-term treatment of 34 children with chronic urinary tract infections, with the combination SMZ/TMP were reported. Twenty-six were females and 8 males and they all had congenital urinary tract obstructions or anomalies. Eight out of them underwent over a year's treatment; the other 26 between one and twelve months. The dosage schedule was 20 mg per Kg SMZ and 5 mg Kg TMP twice daily. 67.5% remained with sterile urine cultures; 17.7% developed re-infections and 14.8% recurrences. General tolerance was excellent and the authors point out the absence of deterioration or impairment in renal function tests.

Chronic infection of the urinary tract is often associated with significant anatomic or functional abnormalities. When the functional abnormalities can be eradicated the hope of cure is reasonable; when they cannot, cure is infrequent. Because of the growing nature of children's kidneys, it has been stressed the need of suppressive therapy in those patients with chronic bacteriuria.

For the last ten years we have been using (Bernstein Hahn, 1969; Bernstein Hahn et al, 1970 and 1971) the combination sulphametoxazol (SMZ) plus trimethoprim (TMP) in the treatment and prophylaxis of urinary tract infections.

* Bactrim - Marca Registrada. Productos Roche S.A.Q. e I., Buenos Aires, Argentina.

Table 1.   Data regarding the evolution of 34 children with
           urinary tract infection after long term treatment with
           SMZ/TMP.

BACTERIOLOGICAL RESPONSE		DURATION OF TREATMENT	FOLLOW-UP PERIOD(MONTHS)			
			3	6	9	12
POSITIVE 11/34 32,5%	REINFECTIONS 6/34 17,7%	3	POS	—	—	—
		3	POS	—	—	—
		6	POS	POS	—	—
		12	NEG	NEG	POS	NEG
		12	POS	NEG	NEG	POS
		12	NEG	NEG	POS	NEG
	RECURRENCES 5/34 14,8%	6	NEG	POS	—	—
		6	POS	NEG	—	—
		12	NEG	NEG	POS	NEG
		12	NEG	POS	POS	NEG
		12	POS	NEG	NEG	NEG
PERMANENT STERILE 23/34 67,5%		3	7	—	—	—
		6	—	6	—	—
		12	—	—	—	10

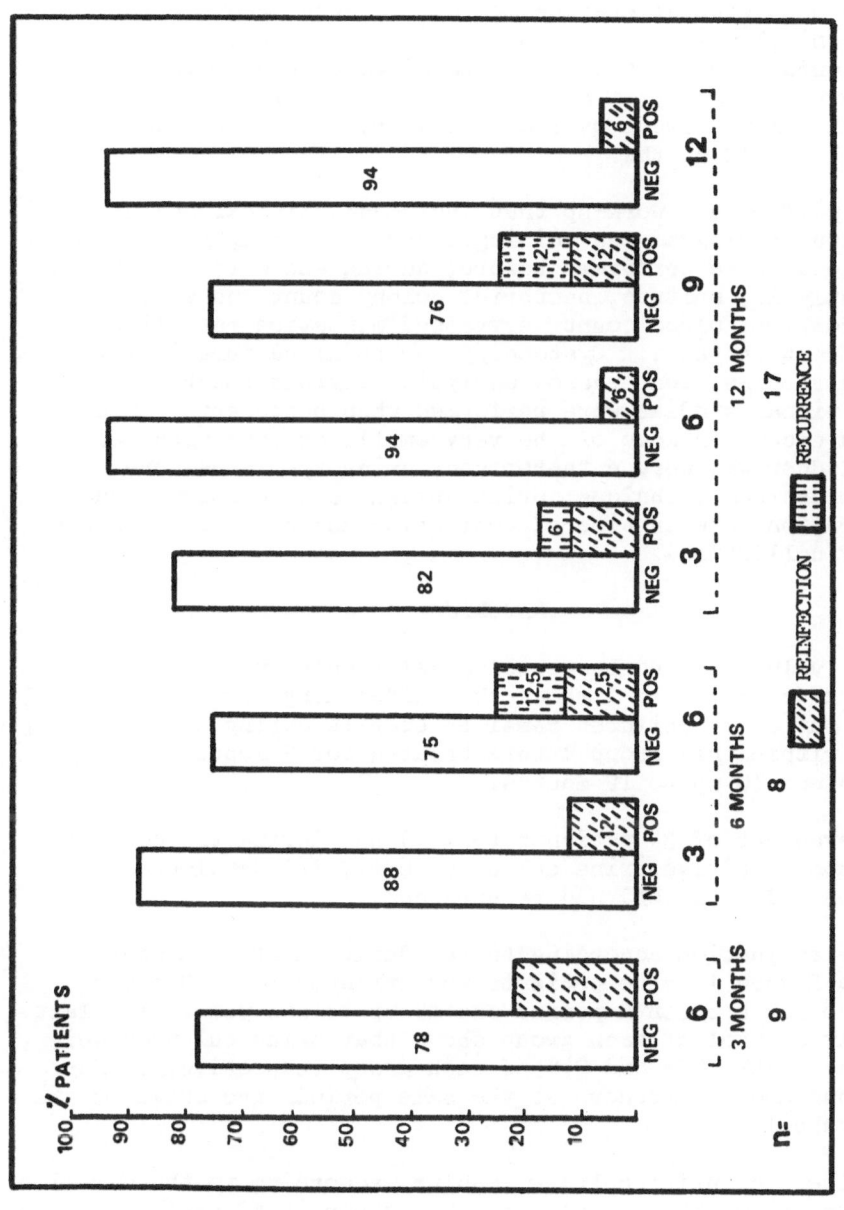

Figure 1. Pattern of urine culture follow-up in 34 children with urinary tract infection after long term treatment with SMZ/TMP.

MATERIAL AND METHODS

Thirty-four children, 26 females and 8 males between 2 to 14 years old, with an average age of 5.8 were treated. They all had congenital urinary tract obstructions or anomalies most of them secondary to neurological congenital disease. The dosage schedule was 20 mg/Kg of SMZ and 5 mg/Kg TMP every 12 hours. Eight of them underwent over a year's treatment; the other 26 between 1 and 12 months.

We performed a work-up that included: clinical evaluation, intravenous pyelogram and voiding cystourethrography. The following tests were performed before, during and after treatment: urine analysis, culture, bacterial colony count and sensitivity tests, complete blood count, erytrosedimentation rate,liver and kidney function tests. Cystoscopy, urethral calibration, voiding pressure studies, bone marrow analysis, thyroid function tests and additional studies were performed when necessary. In most children except in some of the very small, or some with neurogenic bladder who were cathe&erized, urine specimens were obtained by the midstream technique; urine specimens were stored under refrigeration between time of collection and culture (within 6 hours of collection).

RESULTS

In evaluating the bacteriological results we arrived to the following data: Table 1 shows that after long-term treatment 23 (67.5%) out of 34 children remained sterile during the follow up period; within this group 7 were treated for 3 months, 6 up to 6 months and 10 up to 12 months.

Eleven out of 34 patients (32.5%) had during the control period some positive urine cultures; 6 (17.7%) developed re-infection and 5 (14.8%) had recurrences.

The evaluation according to the duration of treatment is shown in Figure 1; nine patients were treated for a 3 month period, 8 for a 6 month period and 17 up to one year. The last quarterly control of each group shows that urine cultures were negative in 78%, 75% and 94% of each group respectively. Re-infections and recurrences at the same periods are shown in the same Figure 1.

Pattern of urine culture results, according to the duration of treatment for the overall group is shown in Figure 2. At the 3, 6 and 12 months control more than 82% were stile while in the 9 month control this percentage reached up to 76.

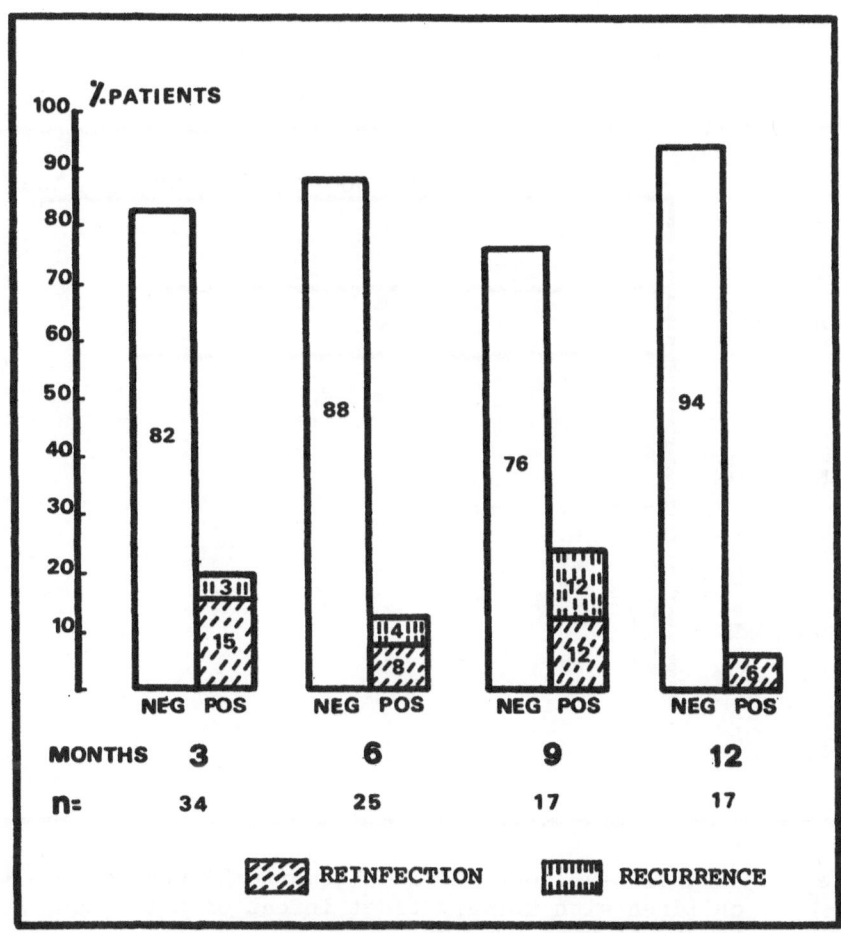

Figure 2.   Pattern of urine culture results according to the duration of treatment in 34 children with urinary tract infections after long term treatment with SMZ/TMP.

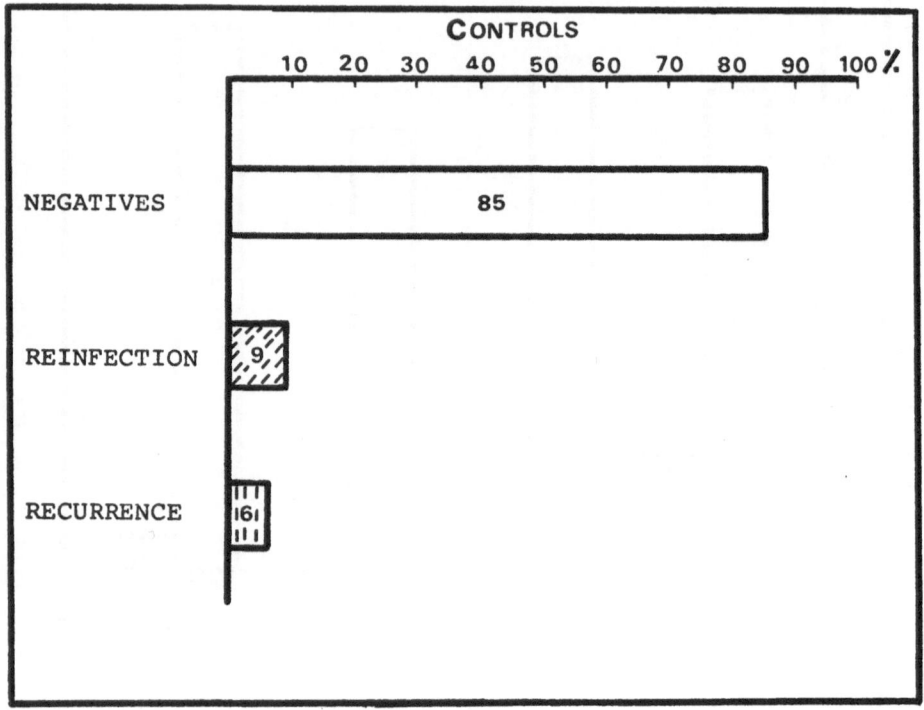

Figure 3.   Accumulative controls in 93 quarterly periods in 34
            children with urinary tract infection after long term
            treatment with SMZ/TMP.

Table 2. Effect of a long term treatment with SMZ/TMP on the
          bacteria cultured from urine specimens of 34 children
          with urinary tract infection.

BACTERIA	BEFORE TREATMENT	AFTER TREATMENT		
		PERMANENT STERILE	REINFECTION	RECURRENCE
ESCHERICHIA COLI	23	17	4	2
PROTEUS	5	2	–	3
AEROBACTER AEROGENES	2	1	1	–
E.COLI + PROTEUS	1	1	–	–
E.COLI+PROTEUS+ STREP.FAECALIS	1	–	1	–
KLEBSIELLA	1	1	–	–
PSEUDOMONAS AERUGINOSA	1	1	–	–
TOTAL	34	23	6	5
%	100	67,5	17,7	14,8

In considering the accumulative controls in 93 quarterly periods we found according to Figure 3 that 85% were negatives and 15% positives (9% re-infection and 6% recurrences).

Table 2 shows that, as expected, E.coli was the bacteria most frequently cultured following by different Protsus p. and A. aerogenes. The therapeutic activity against E.coli was significant.

SIDE EFFECTS

Tolerance was excellent; complete blood count, liver and kidney function tests and bone marrow smears failed to reveal drug induced abnormalities.

DISCUSSION

The control of urinary tract infection in children with congenital abnormalities is an increasing problem for pediatricians and urologists alike.

The possibility of employing a drug for a long-term period with efficacy and good tolerance is a positive advantage in this field.

The combination SMZ/TMP fulfils this condition, because of its efficacy and absence of significant side effects. On the other hand the possibility of using it in patients with renal insufficiency (Barclay et al, 1974) according to a special dosage schedule is currently under research in pediatric patients.

In 5 children studied up to now, we did not find any deterioration or impairment in renal function according to the kidney function tests performed before, during and at the end of treatment.

REFERENCES

Barclay, C.A., Bernstein Hahn, L., Mizgan, D. and Lamonaca, A. (1974), Prensa Med. Arg., 61 No.2, 68-76.

Bernstein Hahn, L. (1969) Paraplegia, 7, 96-101.

Bernstein Hahn, L. (1969) Tribuna Med., 4, 87.

Bernstein Hahn, L. and Sember, M.E. (1970), IIIrd International Congress, Asiatic Federation of the International College of Surgeons, Isfahan, Iran.

Bernstein Hahn, L., Quesada, E. and Turtela, F. (1971), XIII International Congress of Pediatric, Wien, 29.8 - 4.9.

LONG-TERM LOW-DOSAGE CO-TRIMOXAZOLE IN THE MANAGEMENT

OF URINARY TRACT INFECTION IN CHILDREN

J.M. SMELLIE, R.N. GRÜNEBERG, A. LEAKEY, W.S. ATKIN

University College Hospital, London

Wellcome Foundation, London

Long-term low-dosage prophylaxis is used in childhood
urinary tract infection to prevent recurrence after the initial
infection has been eradicated. Its use is indicated (1) in
children whose kidneys are liable to damage from repeated
infections, that is, those with vesico-ureteric reflux and
chronic pyelonephritis (children with obstruction of the lower
urinary tract having been identified and treated surgically) and
(2) in children even with normal urinary tracts who are troubled
by repeated symptomatic infections. (Normand & Smellie, 1965).
For this purpose a drug is required which is effective, well
tolerated,   free from side effects and does not induce drug
resistance. We have shown nitrofurantoin to be an efficient
prophylactic drug (Grüneberg et al, 1973) but as it occasionally
causes nausea we have also studied co-trimoxazole.

Children and Methods. Our results are presented of the
prophylactic use of co-trimoxazole in 130 children aged 1-12 years
originally seen in a hospital out-patient department, with
symptomatic urinary tract infection. There were 17 boys and 113
girls. Any with neurological defects, lower urinary tract
obstruction or raised serum creatinine were excluded from the
study.

The urine of all children was sterile on starting
prophylaxis. Investigation with intravenous pyelogram (I.V.P.)
and micturating cystourethogram (M.C.U.) revealed no significant
abnormality in 61 children, vesico-ureteric reflux of varying
severity in 57 (44 with unscarred kidneys and 13 with established
renal scarring). 12 children had an abnormality of structure such
as a horseshoe kidney but no reflux or obstruction.

The duration of prophylaxis and follow-up was based on these findings. A dose of 10 mg sulphamethoxazole (SMX) and 2 mg trimethoprim (TMP)/kg/day was given, either twice daily or in one evening dose, preferably in tablet form. Children with normal radiology received a prophylactic dose for 6-12 months, those with abnormal radiology without obstruction or reflux for 12-24 months, each depending upon the previous history of repeated infection; follow-up off treatment was continued for at least 1 year. Prophylaxis was continued in children with reflux until 1 year after reflux had disappeared and if chronic pyelonephritis was present, until the kidneys were fully grown. Children with reflux were followed for 2 years after stopping and those with chronic pyelonephritis indefinitely. During treatment the children were trained to void 2-hourly and twice at bedtime if there was reflux, to drink plenty, avoid bubble-bath and regulate the bowels.

Rectal swabs and urine samples were collected initially and after 2, 4 and 8 weeks and 3-monthly throughout treatment and if symptoms returned. The children were seen at the same intervals after treatment was discontinued. Urine samples were either refrigerated at $4^{\circ}C$ or plated immediately by a surface viable counting technique. Only rectal swabs showing faecal staining were accepted for culture. Standard two-film follow-up I.V.P. and M.C.U. were repeated after 2 years in children with reflux or with repeated infection.

Results
Efficacy of Treatment.
All children received at least 6 months and up to 72 months of low-dosage prophylactic co-trimoxazole. During treatment there were no further infections in either the group with normal radiology or in the group without obstruction or reflux during 1,017 months of treatment (Table I). There were, however, 6 infections during treatment among 57 children with reflux, 3 with and 3 without chronic pyelonephritis during approximately 1,600 months' treatment. This represents a very low recurrence rate of approximately 1 in 22 years. The infecting organism appearing during treatment differed in each child from the preceding organism, indicating that these were fresh or re-infections (Table 2). All were caused by organisms resistant to SMX and 5 of the 6 were resistant to TMP. The corresponding rectal swabs showed either a similar organism or that aerobic coliform organisms had been eliminated from the faecal flora. All of these patients were girls and no relationship was found between further infection and age, sex, preceding treatment or duration of treatment.

Although the infecting organisms were resistant to TMP and SMX, all but one were sensitive to either or both ampicillin and nitrofurantoin so that they were easily amenable to full dosage treatment with another regular antibacterial drug after which low

TABLE 1. INFECTIONS DURING PROPHYLAXIS WITH LOW-DOSAGE CO-TRIMOXAZOLE. (*Chronic Pyelonephritis)

Radiological findings	Number of children	Child-months of therapy	Number of infections
I Normal	61	713	0
II Abnormal without obstruction or reflux	12	304	0
III Reflux no C.P.*	44	1173	3
IV Reflux with C.P.	13	447	3
Total	130	2637	6

dosage prophylaxis was resumed. Within 3 months, culture of rectal swabs from these children yielded either no coliforms or the flora which had been resistant was once again sensitive, so that co-trimoxazole could be re-introduced as an effective prophylactic drug.

Of the 130 children treated, 63 were followed up off treatment, from the time of stopping treatment either until reinfection or for at least 6 and up to 42 months, the average observation time off treatment being 10 months. A further infection developed in 27 (42%) of those followed (Table 3).

TABLE 2. INFECTIONS DURING PROPHYLACTIS TREATMENT WITH CO-TRIMOXAZOLE.

	Preceding Infection			Time (mths) after starting treatment	Details of recurrence					
					Urine			Rectal Swab		
	Organism		Sensitiv. TMP SMX		Organism		Sensitiv. TMP SMX	Organism		Sensitiv. TMP SMX
FB	Esch.coli	NG	S S	9	Str.faecalis		R R	No coliforms		
DD	Esch.coli	O75	S S	19	Str.faecalis		R R	No coliforms		
JD	Esch.coli	O4	S R	25	Str.faecalis		M R	Esch.coli	S	R
JL	Esch.coli	O75	S S	26	Str.faecalis		R R	No coliforms		
DT	Esch.coli		not done	26	K.oxytocum		R R	K.oxytocum	R	R
AA	Pr.morganii		S S	62	Esch.coli	NG	R R	Esch.coli	R	R

NG = non groupable

TABLE 3.   INFECTIONS AFTER STOPPING PROPHYLACTIC CO-TRIMOXAZOLE
IN 63 CHILDREN.

	Radiological findings	Children with infections	Children with no infections	Total followed
I	Normal	21	26	47
II	Abnormal without obstruction or reflux	2	4	6
III	Reflux no C.P.*	4 +	6	10
IV	Reflux with C.P.	-	-	-
	Total	27 +	36	63

* chronic pyelonephritis
+ includes 3 children who stopped therapy in error

19 of these 27 (70%) infections occurred within 3 months
of stopping treatment and all but one within 1 year. 17 children
were virtually symptomless and only 1 girl, with normal radiology,
was febrile and off colour. The risk of developing further infection
appeared unrelated to age, sex or duration of prophylaxis.

Serological data was available in two-thirds of the further
infections and each of these also was shown to be a reinfection.
As before there was a close correlation between urinary and faecal
organisms and their serology and resistance pattern. In contrast
to the reinfections during treatment, however, 26 of these 27
reinfections were sensitive to TMP and half to SMX.

Among 47 children with normal radiology who were followed off
prophylaxis, 21 developed further infections. In 10 children
with reflux initially, treatment was discontinued. 3 of these
stopped through misunderstanding while their reflux persisted and
all had a fresh infection within 2 months. Reflux stopped
spontaneously in the other 7 children and there was no further
infection in 6 during follow-up.

The recurrence of infection after completion of treatment is
an indication of persisting impairment of the bladder defences,
allowing re-invasion and multiplication of organisms there. These
reinfections do not therefore represent a failure of the drug but
rather indicate that the underlying cause of the original urinary
infection persists. For example, all 3 children who mistakenly

stopped prophylaxis while their reflux persisted, had a re-
infection with a sensitive organism within 2 months of stopping,
whereas only 1 of the 7 girls who stopped treatment when reflux
was no longer present had a reinfection, 2 years later. It is
also of some interest that in all but 3 of the radiologically
normal children who had an infection after stopping treatment,
this coincided with other physical illness, or with domestic
stress or holiday resulting in reduced parental supervision of
the child.

Compliance in the regimen was good and the drug was taken readily.
We tested the urines of children attending the clinic, at random
and without forewarning of parent or child, and found evidence of
co-trimoxazole in the urines of 50 among 54 children tested.

Toxicity. Side effects were minimal. Sleepiness was observed in
5 children and a rash in 2. During prophylaxis with this dosage
of co-trimoxazole, serial estimations of platelets were made in
40 children and leucocyte counts in 72. No platelet counts below
180,000 per cu.mm. or leucocyte counts of less than 4,000 per cu.
mm. were recorded.

Induction of Resistance

During at least 6 months' prophylaxis per child and a total
of 2,637 months, only 6 children among 130 developed reinfections,
with organisms resistant to SMX and TMP but sensitive to other
regular antibacterials, and thus easily amenable to full-dosage
treatment. The resistant bowel flora had been replaced within 3
months by one sensitive to SMX and TMP.

27 of the 63 children followed after stopping treatment
developed reinfections. 26 were sensitive to TMP and half of
them to SMX and the rectal flora were similarly sensitive. In
many of these the supportive measures in which the child had been
trained during treatment appeared to have lapsed.

Induction of resistant organisms did not therefore prove to
be a problem in the long-term management of these children (some
of whom were on continuous therapy for up to 72 months).

Renal Growth and Vesico-ureteric Reflux

In 55 children who had serial cystograms during therapy,
reflux improved in 35, stopping in 21. Renal growth was
satisfactory in all but 3 of the 54 in whom it was assessed.
Each of these 3 had established scarring and further renal growth
was slow.

Conclusion

This study has shown that:-

1.   Low-dosage co-trimoxazole is an effective prophylactic for childhood urinary tract infection during treatment, as has been found by others. (Zoethout, 1973; Forbes & Drummond, 1973).

2.   Using a dose of 10 mg SMX and 2 mg TMP/kg/day resistant organisms were rarely encountered.

3.   No serious toxic effects occurred.

4.   After prophylactic treatment was stopped further infections occurred in 40% of the children followed, most of them within the first 3 months. They were usually reinfections, with urinary and faecal organisms sensitive to TMP and half to SMX suggesting continued impairment of the bladder defences.

5.   Satisfactory renal growth took place, and improvement in reflux continued while prophylactic co-trimoxazole was taken.

References

Forbes, P.A. & Drummond K.N. (1973). J.Inf.Dis. 128, S626.

Gruneberg, R.N., Smellie, J.M. & Leakey, A. (1973). In Urinary Tract Infection. Proc.2nd Nat.Sympos. p.131, ed. Brumfitt, W. and Asscher, W.A. Oxford Univ. Press.

Normand, I.C.S. & Smellie, J.M. (1965). Brit.Med.J. 1, 1023.

Zoethout, H.E. (1973). In Trimethoprim/sulphamethox azole in bacterial infections, p.175. Ed. Bernstein, L.S. & Salter, A.J., Churchill Livingstone, Edinburgh.

A DOUBLE-BLIND STUDY OF SULFAMETHOXAZOLE-TRIMETHOPRIM
vs. ITS COMPONENTS IN CHRONIC URINARY TRACT INFECTIONS

Christopher Demos, M.D., John Pinderhughes, M.D.

and Marion Oakes, A.B.

Hoffmann-La Roche, Nutley, N.J., USA

Additional data have been received from twenty-three
hospitals participating in the multi-center study to
assess the efficacy and safety of the antimicrobial
combination, trimethoprim-sulfamethoxazole (TMP-SMZ).
All studies were carried out according to the protocol
set forth in the earlier paper by Gleckman.*

Materials and Methods

Adult male and female patients who had chronic urinary
tract infections, and who had not received antimicrobial
agents for one week preceding were entered into the
study. The study group consisted of those asymptomatic
patients who have chronic significant bacteriuria or
patients who had recurrent symptomatic disease associated
with significant bacteriuria. The only organisms acceptable according to protocol were members of the
Enterobacteriaceae family. In this study the definition
of significant bacteriuria is as follows: a colony count
of at least 10^5 organisms/ml in each of two clean voided
urine specimens collected within a week.

Patients in any of the following categories were excluded
from the study: individuals under 16 years of age;
patients with known or suspected idiosyncrasies to
sulfonamides or trimethoprim; patients with indwelling
catheters; women who are pregnant or breast feeding;
patients with decreased renal function manifested by an
abnormal glomerular filtration rate; patients with known
folate states; patients with known glucose-6-phosphate

dehydrogenase deficiency, elevated levels of transaminase,
depression of hematocrit, total white count, neutrophils
and platelet count and patients with systemic lupus
erythematosus.

Standard microbiological methodology was utilized for
identifying the organisms.

Preliminary Evaluation

After significant pretreatment bacteriuria with one or
more members of Enterobacteriaceae family was established
and baseline laboratory values were within limits set
forth in the protocol, the investigator recorded the
complete medical history and physical examination results
for each patient. An intravenous urogram was performed
and patients were assigned to one of three treatment pro-
grams according to random selection. The three forms of
treatment were prepared as tablets with identical appearance to comply with the double-blind requirements. The
tablets contained either 500mg sulfamethoxazole (SMZ),
100mg trimethoprim (TMP) or 400mg SMZ and 80mg TMP.
Neither the investigator nor the patient was aware of
the identity of the medication. Two tablets, 30 minutes
before the breakfast and evening meals, were administered
for ten days.

Follow-up Studies

Patients were instructed to return at 48 hours, one, two,
five, nine and twelve weeks after the initiation of
therapy. At each visit, laboratory tests were performed
and the investigator was requested to report and evaluate
each new subjective symptom, physical finding and abnormal
laboratory result.

Results

The median age in years, percentage males, percentage of
patients with gross abnormalities of the urinary tract
for the TMP-SMZ, TMP and SMZ groups were 53, 54, or 55;
44, 45, and 53; 57, 56, and 59 respectively. The total
number of patients evaluated for efficacy was 512
(TMP-SMZ = 181, TMP = 162 and SMZ = 169). The organisms
isolated before treatment are shown below:

Organisms isolated before treatment	TMP-SMZ	TMP	SMZ
Escherichia Species	118	105	104
Klebsiella-Enterobacter	33	37	41
Proteus Species	36	24	24

Table 1 indicates the response to therapy of all evaluable patients in each treatment group at 10, 42 and 75 days after administration of therapy. A patient response was considered to be successful when the patient had a sterile urine or less than 10,000 organisms/ml of urine at the stated intervals after therapy. The Fisher Exact Probability Test demonstrates that Bactrim (TMP-SMZ) is significantly more effective than either of its components in eradicating chronic urinary tract infections. The p values for the comparison of Bactrim and sulfamethoxazole are <0.002 at 10, 42 and 75 days after therapy. The p values for the comparison of Bactrim and trimethoprim are <0.05 at days 10 and 42 after the onset of therapy and at day 75 the value is 0.065.

Table 1 - All Evaluable Patients

DAY	TMP-SMZ %	TMP %	SMZ %	P VALUE 1 vs. 2	1 vs 3
10	86.0 (179)	74.7 (162)	56.8 (160)	0.006	0.000
42	55.3 (170)	43.3 (157)	33.3 (165)	0.019	0.000
75	47.6 (166)	38.6 (153)	28.1 (160)	0.065	0.000

Table 2 shows the response to therapy in the patients with gross abnormalities of the urinary tract (complicated patients) and demonstrates that Bactrim is significantly more effective than either of its components with a p value of <0.001.

Table 2 - Complicated Patients

DAY	TMP-SMZ %	TMP %	SMZ %	P VALUE 1 vs. 2	1 vs 3
10	90.2 (102)	67.0 (91)	52.0 (100)	0.000	0.000
42	57.1 (98)	34.1 (88)	28.6 (98)	0.001	0.000
75	51.0 (98)	28.7 (87)	21.1 (95)	0.001	0.000

Adverse Effects

More patients were evaluated for adverse effects than for efficacy because of the protocol requirements. The 671 patients evaluated were quite evenly distributed

Table 3

Number and Percentage of Patients with Laboratory
Abnormalities*

Laboratory Abnormality	Bactrim		Trimethoprim		SMZ	
	#	%	#	%	#	%
SGOT	18	7	13	5	10	4
SGPT	2	0	0	0	2	0
Alk. Phos.	5	2	5	2	2	0
Bilirubin	1	0	1	0	0	0
Anemia	2	0	4	1	1	0
WBC decreased	6	2	4	2	5	2
Eosinophilia	0	0	0	0	1	0
Thrombopenia	2	0	9	3	7	3
Serum Creatinine	9	3	3	1	0	0
BUN	2	0	2	0	1	0
Total Adverse Reactions	47		41		29	
Total Patients with Adverse Reactions	37	16	33	14	25	11
Total Patients Treated	227		227		217	

*those reactions classified as being possibly or
probably related to drug

among the treatment groups; TMP-SMZ 227, TMP 227, SMZ
217. Those adverse effects deemed probably or possibly
related to the antibacterial agents are reported here.

The clinical adverse effects were not life threatening.
The incidence of rash was four (two per cent), four (two
per cent) and three (one per cent) in the TMP-SMZ, TMP
and SMZ groups respectively. Nausea and vomiting occurred
in seven (three per cent), nine (four per cent) and four
(two per cent) of the patients and the total number of
patients with reactions was twelve (five per cent),
thirteen (five per cent) and ten (four per cent) in the
TMP-SMZ, TMP and SMZ groups respectively. Diarrhea,
dizzy spells and lethargy occurred in less than one
per cent of patients. Monilial vaginitis occurred in
one patient on SMZ.

Abnormal laboratory findings in the three patient groups
are shown in Table 3. The liver function test abnormalities were only slightly elevated and returned to normal
on cessation of therapy. There were no patients in
whom more than one test of liver function was abnormal.
The changes in white blood cells were of a mild degree
and returned to normal after treatment. Thrombopenia
occurred about equally in the TMP and SMZ patients. The
creatinine elevations were not felt to be clinically
significant.

Conclusion

The data from this multicenter, prospective, double
blind study show conclusively that TMP-SMZ is a more
effective agent than either of its components in the
treatment of chronic urinary tract infections. The p
values for the response in patients with abnormalities
of the urinary tract is highly significant up to 75
days after termination of treatment with the combination
as compared to the component groups. The clinical
adverse effects were not of a serious nature.
Laboratory abnormalities were also of a mild degree
and returned to normal after cessation of treatment.

*   Gleckman, R.A., J.infect.Dis., 1973, 128, (Suppl.)
    S647-S651

A NEW COMBINATION OF TRIMETHOPRIM AND A SULPHONAMIDE (SULPHA-DIAZINE) IN URINARY TRACT INFECTIONS, A DOUBLE-BLIND STUDY

A. Lövestad, B. Gästrin, and R. Lundström

Departments of Infectious Diseases and of Clinical
Bacteriology, Central Hospital, Eskilstuna, Sweden

The common problem of urinary tract infections (UTI) make every attempt to improve current therapy worthwhile. Trimethoprim-sulphamethoxazole (co-trimoxazole) and sulphalene have been shown to be useful drugs in the treatment of UTI. In order to decrease the dosages of trimethoprim as well as sulphonamide, sulphadiazine was chosen in the combination with trimethoprim with the purpose of diminishing possible side reactions without losing the clinical efficacy. This was regarded as possible as the concentration of unmetabolized sulphadiazine in the urine is much higher than that of sulphamethoxazole after medication of equal doses of the drugs. It should be emphasized that A 2166 was composed for the use in UTI exclusively. Thus a controlled study was started comparing the combination trimethoprim-sulphadiazine with co-trimoxazole and with sulphalene, a long-acting sulphonamide.

MATERIAL AND METHODS

Fifty-nine adult, mainly female ambulant patients with clinical signs of UTI were admitted to following three groups by random.
1 Co-trimoxazole: 2 tablets twice daily (trimethoprim 320 mg/day and sulphamethoxazole 1,600 mg/day)
2 Sulphalene: 4 tablets the first day (400 mg) followed by 1 tablet daily (100 mg)
3 ASTRA 2166: 1 tablet twice daily (trimethoprim 180 mg/day and sulphadiazine 820 mg/day)
Group 1 and 2 comprised 20 patients each and group 3 19 patients. Semi-quantitative bacterial analysis of urine specimens

from mid-stream samples was performed on day 0, 7, 14 and 35
after the start of the treatment. At the same time determinations of the blood count, urine microscopy, SGOT, and serum
creatinine were performed. On day 7 and 14 the serum and urine
concentrations of trimethoprim, sulphalene, sulphadiazine and
sulphamethoxazole were determined.

The microorganisms isolated from the pretreatment
urine sample of the 59 patients were E.coli, 34; coliforms, 5;
Staph albus, 4; enterococci, 2; streptococci, type B, 1. Thirteen patients were found not to have significant bacteriuria
when admitted to the study and could thus not be evaluated regards the clinical effect.

RESULTS

Regards clinical and bacteriological criteria 46
patients were assessable. Fifteen patients were treated with
A 2166, 14 with co-trimoxazole and 17 with sulphalene. Reap-
pearence of the same bacteria in the urine 3 weeks after completion of the treatment was considered as a relapse. Bacteriuria with another species at this occasion was defined as a
new infection. No significant bacteriuria 3 weeks after the
treatment was defined as cure.

Both A 2166 and co-trimoxazole showed a cure rate of
86 % whereas sulphalene showed only 47 %. The difference was
significant on the 5 % level. (Table 1)

Table 1. Therapeutical results.

Drug	No. of patients with significant bacteriuria	Relapse	New in-fection	Cure rate
A 2166	15	1	1	86 %
Co-trimoxazole	14	2	0	86 %
Sulphalene	17	6	3	47 %
Total	46	9	4	

Laboratory findings regards hemoglobin, blood counts,
and SGOT did not show significant alterations in either group
of patients.

Serum creatinine, however, showed a temporary increase in the patients treated with A 2166 and co-trimoxaxole, but did not excess normal limits (fig 1).

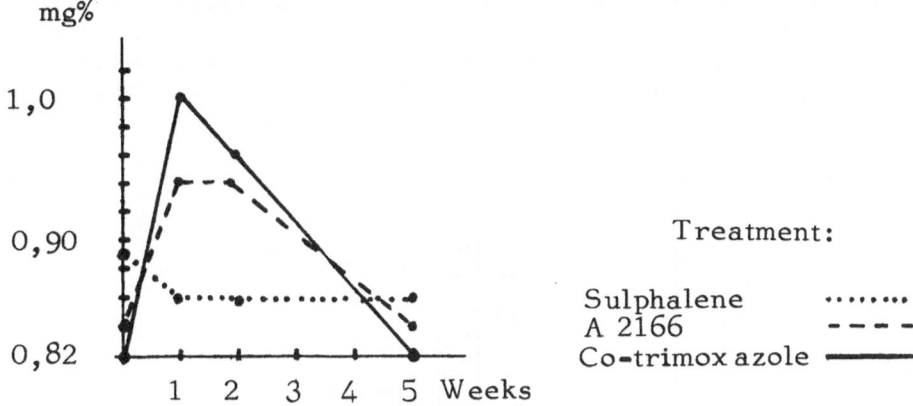

Fig 1. Mean serum creatinine levels during and after 2 weeks of treatment.

Concentrations of not protein-bound sulphonamide were determined before and 2 hours after administration of drug on days 7 and 14 after initiation of treatment (Figs 2 and 3). As seen in the figures, sulphalene showed low levels, as expected,

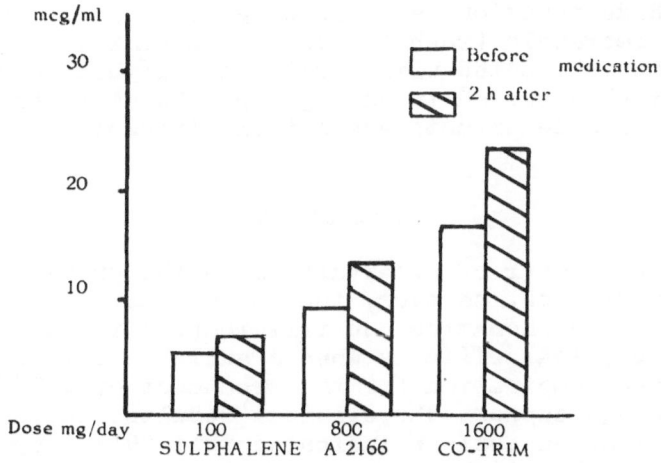

Fig 2. Concentration of not proteinbound sulphonamide in serum on the 14th day of treatment.

according to the low dosage. For A 2166 and co-trimoxazole the
serum levels corresponded well to the dosage. The urine level,
however, shows a much higher value of unmetabolized sulphonamide of A 2166 than for co-trimoxazole in spite of the lower
dosage of sulphonamide. The serum and urine levels of trimethoprim were higher in the co-trimoxazole than in the A 2166 group,
corresponding to the dosage. These determinations indicated
that the prescriptions had been followed satisfactorily.

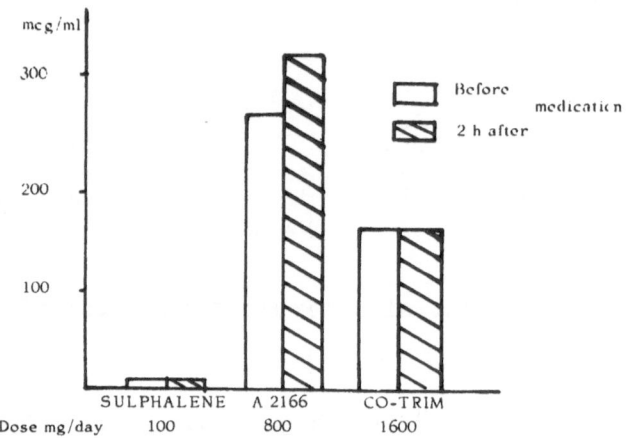

Fig 3. Concentration of unmetabolized sulphonamide in urine on
the 14th day of treatment.

        Side reactions were observed in 5 patients treated
with co-trimoxazole (rash 4, nausea and vomiting 1), whereas
of the patients treated with A 2166 and sulphalene only one
case with rash occurred in each group. The difference of the
incidences of side effects was not significant.

                        DISCUSSION

        The number of observations in the present series is
small. It indicates, however, that a substantial decrease of
the dosage of sulphonamide and trimethoprim is possible without losing clinical efficacy when a suitable sulphonamide is
chosen in the combination for the treatment of UTI. The laboratory findings support the clinical results. Comparison with
the long-acting sulphalene indicated that this drug was inferior to the combinations, apparently in part due to a lower
dosage of sulphonamide and corresponding lower serum and urine
concentration.

A significant increase of the serum creatinine was observed for the patients treated with A 2166 as well as for those who got co-trimoxazole but not for those treated with sulphalene. This is in concordance with our findings in an earlier study, a regular, temporary increase of serum creatinine occurred. According to Pompeius (2) who also observed an equal elevation of serum creatinine this depends on a temporary blockade of the tubular secretion of serum creatinine.

SUMMARY

ASTRA 2166 has been composed for the treatment of UTI. In a double-blind study comprising 59 patients, 20 were treated with co-trimoxazole, 20 with sulphalene and 19 with ASTRA 2166. Treatment with ASTRA 2166 and co-trimoxazole was superior to the treatment with sulphalene. The serum concentrations during treatment were well corresponding to the dosage given. The urinary concentrations of unmetabolized sulphonamide showed significantly higher levels for ASTRA 2166 compared with co-trimoxazole, whereas low concentrations were found in the urine of the patients treated with sulphalene.

BIBLIOGRAPHY

(1)   Lövestad, A., Sabel, G., Stefansson, M., Gästrin, B., and Lundström, R.: Trimethoprim - sulphamethaxole and nitrofurantoin in urinary tract infections, a controlled clinical study. Progress in Chemotherapy. Proceedings 8th International Congress of Chemotherapy 1973. Vol II, p.234. Hellenic Soc. Chemotherapy, Athens 1974.

(2)   Pompeius, R., et al: J. Urol. (to be published).

COMPARATIVE CLINICAL TRIAL OF PARENTERAL CO-TRIMOXAZOLE

IN MAJOR RESPIRATORY INFECTIONS.

M. Janousek, L. Corbeel, P. Stenier

Clinique St Pierre

Avenue Reine Fabiola

B-1340 Ottignies (Belgium)

The introduction of the trimethoprim-sulphamethoxazole combination (generic term : co-trimoxazole) heralded a certain renewal
of antibiotic therapeutics. It is indeed not merely a matter of
the administration of two drugs whose respective spectra more or
less complete each other, but that of a synergic correlation in
which the two constituents are reciprocally potentiated. This
synergy phenomenon seems to result from the fact that the 2 constituents point of impact is situated at 2 consecutive levels in
the metabolic sequence leading to tetrahydrofolic acid, an essential factor for the synthesis of certain nucleotidic compounds
indispensable to the survival and development of very many bacterial species.
A diagrammatic reminder of this fundamental metabolic sequence
would perhaps be useful (1) :

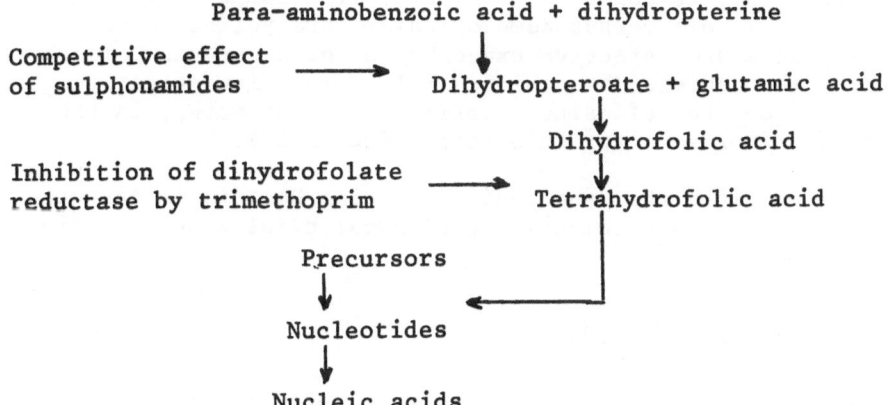

This potentiation phenomenon is demonstrated by the lesser bacteriostatic and bactericidal concentrations obtained when the two
drugs are mixed in the seeded culture medium, as compared to the
corresponding values when they are used separately. For instance,
with a strain of Klebsiella pneumoniae (2) :

Klebsiella pneumoniae 85

  Minimum bacteriostatic concentration (γ /ml)
      Sulphamethoxazole alone   :   3,12
      Trimethoprim alone   :   0,312
      SMZ + TM : 0,39 (8 x less) + 0,039 (8 x less)

  Minimum bactericidal concentration (γ /ml)
      Sulphamethoxazole alone   :   50
      Trimethoprim alone   :   0,625
      SMZ + TM : 0,78 (64 x less) + 0,078 (8 x less)

The same is found to be true in vivo, for instance in the mouse
experimentally infected with Haemophilus influenzae (3) :

  50 % curative dose (mg/kg, by mouth) :
      Sulphamethoxazole : 70,6
      Trimethoprim   :149
      SMZ + TM   : 4,4

At the same time, in theory at least, the presence of the 2 constituents lessens the probability of resistances being developed.
Moorhouse and Farrel sought in vain to find the emergence of resistant strains of the Enterobacteria present in a group of patients receiving oral co-trimoxazole during 5 days (4). However,
the appearance of co-trimoxazole resistances transmittable by a
cytoplasmic factor R has already been described (5).

In the past (6), we conducted a double blind comparative study of
oral co-trimoxazole versus demethylchlortetracycline in patients
suffering an acute infective exacerbation of a chronic pulmonary
affection (bronchitis, bronchiectasis). That investigation gave
grounds for our belief, since confirmed by many works, in the value of co-trimoxazole for this indication (7-12).

We have been given the opportunity of using Bactrim in parenteral
form for conducting a comparative clinical trial along the lines
of our previous study.

METHOD - SELECTION OF CASES

The patients admitted to this trial were suffering from acute infective exacerbations of chronic bronchitis requiring antibiotic treatment parenterally because of the gravity of the attack or because of digestive disorders that contra-indicated oral administration. These patients were randomly divided into two groups, according to the order of their inclusion in the trial and to a random numerical table. One group received co-trimoxazole, the other sigmamycine. Concomittant use of other antibiotics was excluded, but the other therapeutic elements (respiratory aid, heart stimulants, etc.) were used according to need.

Dosage had been decided as follows :

Co-trimoxazole : 2 ampoules morning and evening intramuscularly or by perfusion in 250 ml of 5 % dextrose solution (direct intravenous injection is not recommended because of possible irritation of the vein wall by the drug). One ampoule of Bactrim contains 400 mg of sulphamethoxazole and 80 mg of trimethoprim in 5 ml of solution.

Sigmamycine   : also administered intramuscularly or by perfusion, 300 mg to 1 g daily.

In either group, co-trimoxazole or sigmamycine was to be stopped after a few days in the event of failure or serious intolerance, and then replaced by a different antibiotic.

RESULTS

The observations covered 50 patients : 26 in the co-trimoxazole group and 24 in the sigmamycine. The effects of the treatment were assessed in the light of clinical criteria, primarily the sputum (diagram 1) and secondarily coughing (diagram 2) and dyspnoea (diagram 3). At the end of the treatment an overall clinical judgment was formed on each case, summing up all the elements of information (table 1).

DISCUSSION

The evolution is decidedly favourable and parallel in both groups when one compares the situations at the start and at the end of treatment, as regards sputum, cough and dyspnoea. The overall clinical assessment (table 1) reveals a certain superiority of co-trimoxazole, which does not however reach the habitually accepted significance threshold of p = 0.05.

In our first double blind comparative study of co-trimoxazole
versus demethylchlortetracycline (oral administration), we reached similar conclusions, i.e. a certain, but not significant,
superiority of co-trimoxazole. At that time we believed that
had the number of patients been greater the significance threshold would have been crossed. Since this second trial was carried out according to the same evaluation criteria, from curiosi-
ty and while aware that this operation could be criticized as regards strictly orthodox statistical procedure, we added together
the results of the two studies in order to obtain a 2 x 2 con-
tingency table (table 2).
Applied to these data, the value of the Chi Square is 4,23 for
1 degree of freedom, i.e. the null hypothesis of an absence of
difference between the two groups, can be rejected at the threshold of p. $< 0,05$.

TABLE 1 : Results

	Co-trimoxazole	Sigmamycine
Excellent	7 (27 %)	–
Good	17 (65 %)	18 (75 %)
Unsatisfactory	2 (8 %)	6 (25 %)
Total of cases	26	24

TABLE 2 : Results of the two studies

	Co-trimoxazole (oral + parenteral)	Control drug (oral + parenteral)
Positive results (excellent to good)	39 (85 %)	28 (64 %)
Negative results	7 (15 %)	16 (36 %)
Total	46	44

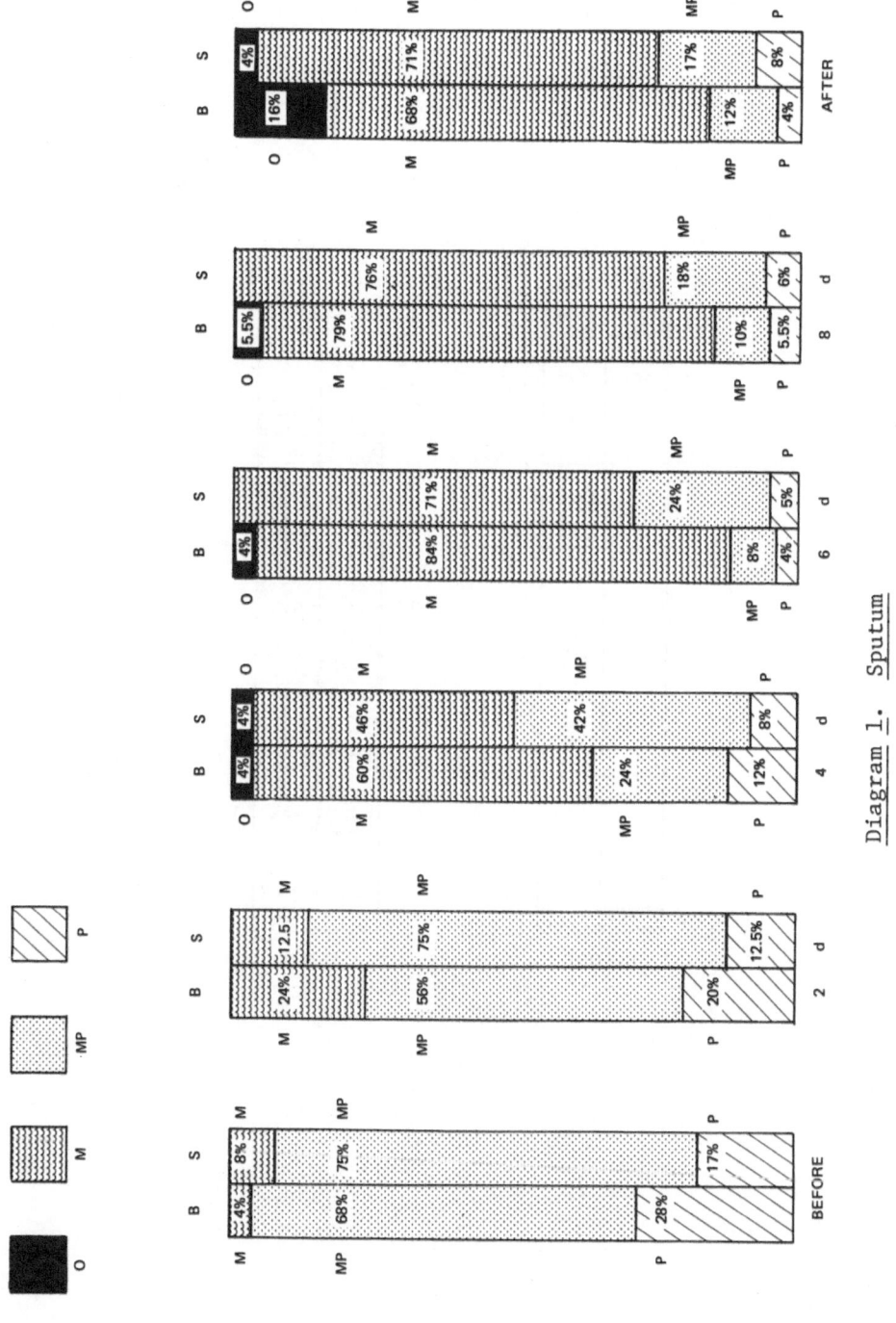

Diagram 1. Sputum

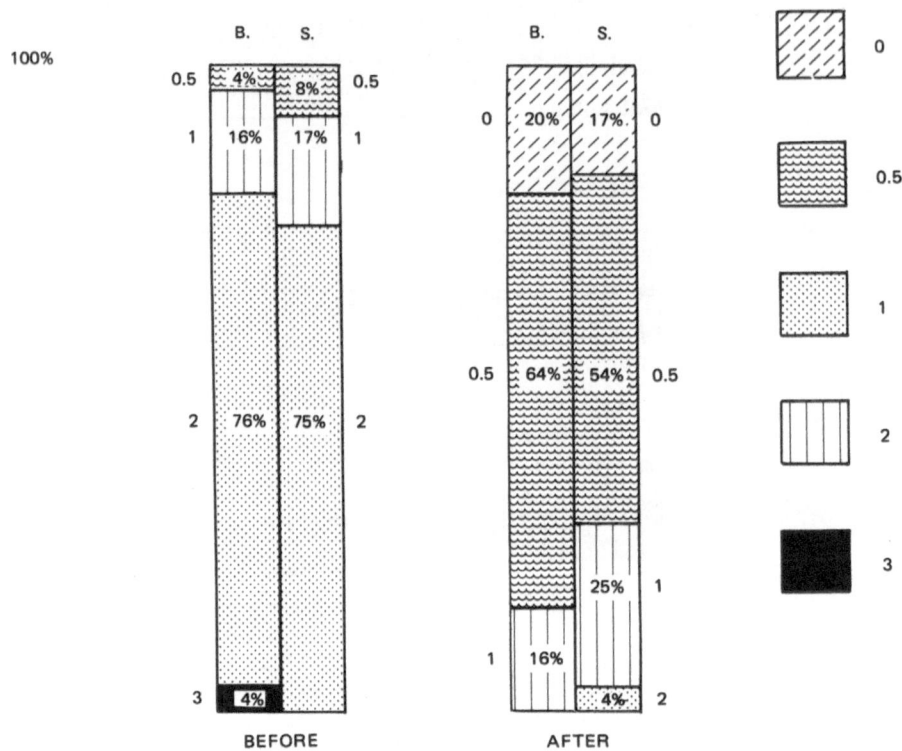

Diagram 2. Cough

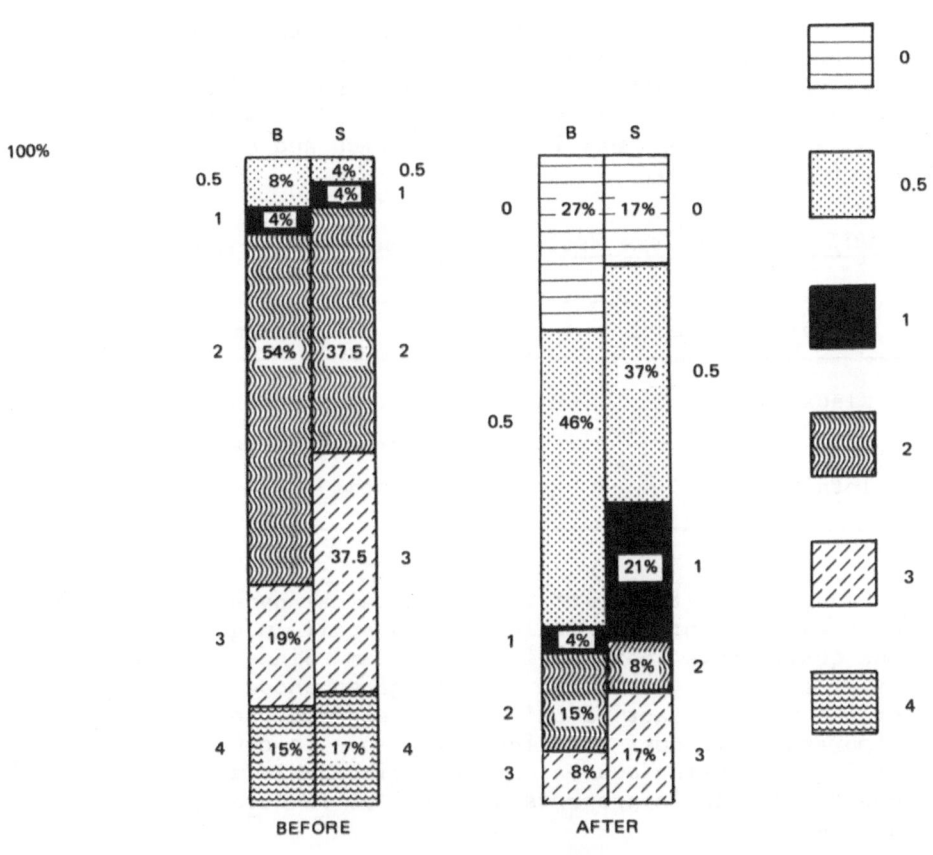

Diagram 3. Dyspnoea

In actual fact it is not easy to pinpoint the impact of an antibiotic in a clinical picture where the infective element is only
one part, whereas this antibiotic is itself integrated in a body
of therapeutic measures such as respiratory aid, physiotherapy,
heart stimulants, etc. The bacteriology of sputum, where it is
collected by natural means, does not seem to us to be of great
help, in view of the contamination problems that further compli-
cate the bacteriological modifications caused by the many previous antibiotic treatments. In those cases where we considered
the treatment to have failed, for one of the two patients receiving co-trimoxazole we found a Klebsiella once, and for the other
we could find no identifiable organism in spite of an obviously
infective syndrome; in the six cases of failure with sigmamycine,
Pseudomonas aeruginosa was isolated 4 times and a Proteus mirabilis twice (table 3).

TABLE 3 : Organisms isolated in cases considered failures

Co- trimoxazole		Sigmamycine	
Klebsiella	1 x	B. pyocyaneus	4 x
?	1 x	Proteus mirabilis	2 x
Total	2	Total	6

In the end, it was the criteria of a clinical nature that gave
the best evaluation; they included an overall judgment and above
all the qualitative appreciation of sputum. Since there did after
all exist a randomly selected control group whose only apparent
difference was the fact of being given sigmamycine instead of
co-trimoxazole, it does seem logical to use to conclude that,
everything else being equivalent, co-trimoxazole appears to influence the patient's progress at least as favourably as sigmamycine does.

TOLERANCE

Local tolerance is good, both by intravenous (perfusion) and by
intramuscular administration (table 4).
One case of generalized rash was seen in the co-trimoxazole group.
As regards biological tolerance, no deviation was noted in the
haemograms effected at the start and end of treatment, or in the
biological analyses concerning hepaticand renal function.

TABLE 4 : Local tolerance

	Co-trimoxazole	Sigmamycine
Intravenous		
Good	13	13
Poor	-	1 (phlebitis)
Total	13	14
Intramuscular		
Good	17	17
Poor (pain)	2	2
Total	19	19

CONCLUSIONS

The value of oral co-trimoxazole in respiratory infections has
been well established, as evidenced by many control studies
(7-12). This comparative clinical trial of co-trimoxazole in
parenteral form also demonstrates its value in serious respiratory infections that require a parenterally administered antibiotic drug. We do however consider that it would be useful to complete this investigation by a bacteriological study where the causal microorganisms are isolated by means of transtracheal punc-
ture.

REFERENCES

1. STRULLER Th. : Progress in Drug Research (1968), 12, 495
   E. Jucker.

2. BOEHNI E. : Chemotherapy (1969), Suppl. 14, 1-83

3. BOEHNI E. : The Chemotherapeutic activity of combination of
   trimethoprim and sulfamethoxazole in infections of mice.
   Postgrad. med. J. (1969), Suppl. 45, 18

4. MOORHOUSE E.C., FARREL W. : Effect of co-trimoxazole on faecal
   enterobacteria : no emergence of resistant strain.
   J. med. Microbiol. (1973), 6, 249.

5. BUSHBY, S.R.M. : Trimethoprim-sulfamethoxazole : in vitro
   microbiological aspects.
   J. infect. Dis. 1973, Suppl. 128, S442.

6. CORBEEL L., STENIER P. : Etude clinique en double anonymat de
   l'association sulfamethoxazole-trimethoprime dans les infections
   pulmonaires chroniques.
   V. Internationaler Kongress für Infektionskrankheiten,
   Wien 31 Aug.-5 Sept. 1970.

7. HOWELLS CH.L., TYLER L.E. : A comparative trial of ampicillin,
   tetracycline and a combination of trimethoprim and sulfamethoxazole in the treatment of respiratory infections.
   Brit. J. clin. Pract. 1971, 25, 2

8. JILG S. : Erfahrungen mit Bactrim Roche bei der Behandlung
   akuter und chronischer Infektionen des respirationtraktes.
   Med. heute 1971, 20, 3, 5

9. BRUNINX M., DE KOSTER J.P., GOLARD P., LIBERT P., MINETTE A.
   MOTTARD L., REMARCLE P., ROBIENCE Y., SCHMITZ P.   et
   VEREERSTRAETEN J. : Administration à titre prophylactique du
   Bactrim dans la bronchite chronique : étude clinique et biolo-
   gique à double insu.
   Acta tuberc. pneumol. belg. 1973, 64, 483

10. HUGHES D.T.D. : Use of combinations of trimethoprim and sulfa-
    methoxazole in the treatment of chest infections.
    J. infect. Dis. 1973, Suppl. 128, S701

11. PINES A. : Trimethoprim-sulfamethoxazole in the treatment and
    prevention of purulent exacerbations of chronic bronchitis.
    J. Infect. Dis. 1973, Suppl. 128, S706.

12. SANFORD CHODOSH, BERTRAM EICHEL, CHARLES ELLIS, TULLIO C.
    MEDICI and L. JACK FALING : Trimethoprim–sulfamethoxazole
    compared with ampicillin in acute infections exacerbations
    of chronic bronchitis. A double blind cross-over study.
    J. infect. Dis. 1973, Suppl. 128, S710.

List of Contributors

Aguirre, M.
Ales, J.M.
Allen, L.B.
Alonso, M.L.
Altorfer, W.
Arfaa, F.
Arkangelskaya, N.V.
Atkins, W.S.

Barasoain, I.
Barclay, C.A.
Beeson, M.F.
Benazet, F.
Bennett, J.E.
Boelart, J.
Bogdanova, N.S.
Boyd, M.R.
Brown, F.
Bryceson, A.
Bucknall, R.A.
Bushby, M.B.
Bushby, S.R.M.

Cartier, J.R.
Cartwright, R.Y.
Cerisola, J.A.
Cook, P.D.
Corbeel, L.

Daneels, R.
Defoort, R.
Demos, C.
Dennin, R.
Duma, R.J.

Fahlbusch, B.
Farahmandian, I.
Felix, H.
Firinu, A.
Flore, O.
Florent, J.
Fomina, A.N.
Friebertshauer, G.E.

Garriques, I.L.
Garzia, A.
Gaskin, H.
Gastrin, B.
Ginsberg, T.
Glasky, A.Y.

Goldblum, P.
Goosen, M.A.L.
Goosen, T.J.
Gould, J.C.
Gray, D.
Grinev, A.N.
Gruneberg, R.N.

Hahn, L.B.
Hall, A.P.
Hamilton-Miller, J.M.T.
Hay, J.
Holker, J.W.
Holt, R.J.
Huffman, J.H.
Hutchinson, A.

Itoh, M.

Janousek, M.
Jennings, R.
Jeunet, F.
Johnson, C.
Jones, B.R.
Jones, D.B.

Katz, E.
Keri, J.
Kerridge, D.
Klitchak, S.M.
Krause, E.

La Colla, P.
Lahoy, F.
Leakey, A.
Ledesma, O.
Loddo, B.
Lovestad, A.
Lundstrom, R.
Lunel, J.
Lugones, H.

Mabadeje, A.F.B.
Mancy, D.
Mandel, G.Z.
Mandour, A.M.
Margalith, E.
McGehee, R.F.

Nikolaeva, I.S.

433

Oakes, M.
Okazaki, N.
Ohno, Y.
Omram, L.A.M.
Oosterlinck, W.
Ortel, S.
Oxford, J.S.

Palese, P.
Paxton, L.
Perine, P.L.
Perrin, D.D.
Peters, W.
Petterson, T.
Phair, J.P.
Pinderhughes, J.
Polak, A.
Potter, C.W.

Raeter, W.
Rahman, A.M.A.E.
Reders, G.
Reed, S.E.
Revanker, G.R.
Robbins, R.K.
Robinson, N.M.
Ronda, E.
Russell, N.J.

Sande, M.A.
Salter, A.J.
Satoh, S.
Schaffner, C.P.
Schofield, K.P.
Scholer, H.J.
Schonebeck, J.

Schubladze, A.K.
Schulman, J.L.
Schwartz, D.
Settineri, R.A.
Shadomy, S.
Shiota, H.
Sidwell, R.W.
Simon, L.N.
Smellie, J.M.
Standen, O.D.
Stainer, W.E.
Stenier, P.
Subak-Sharpe, J.L.
Swallow, A.L.
Syomens, J.

Telegdy, L.
Tolman, R.L.
Tonew, E.M.
Tyrrell, D.A.J.

Uetsuka, A.
Uretskaya, G.Y.
Utz, J.P.

Van Landuyt, H.
Vella, R.

Warner, J.F.
Warrell, D.A.
Watt, B.
Weuta, H.
Winer, B.
Winkelman, E.
Wittowski, J.T.

Yoshimura, K.